Step-Up

A High-Yield, Systems-Based Review
for the USMLE Step 1

Contributors

Reviewers

Sharon Ransom
Temple University School of Medicine, Class of 2000
Philadelphia, Pennsylvania

Wendy A. Weeks
Temple University School of Medicine, Class of 2000
Philadelphia, Pennsylvania

David B. Sykes
Department of Molecular Pathology
Medical Scientist Training Program
University of California San Diego
San Diego, California

Case Contributors

Greg Anderson
Temple University
School of Medicine, Class of 2000
Philadelphia, Pennsylvania

Zara Cooper
Mount Sinai School of Medicine, Class of 2000
New York, New York

Keith McNellis
Temple University
School of Medicine, Class of 2000
Philadelphia, Pennsylvania

Drug List Contributor

Eugene A. Milder
Temple University
School of Medicine, Class of 2002
Philadelphia, Pennsylvania

Step-Up

A High-Yield, Systems-Based Review for the USMLE Step 1

Samir Mehta
Temple University School of Medicine
Philadelphia, PA

Edmund A. Milder
Temple University School of Medicine
Philadelphia, PA

Adam J. Mirarchi
Temple University School of Medicine
Philadelphia, PA

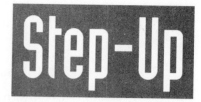

LIPPINCOTT WILLIAMS & WILKINS
A **Wolters Kluwer** Company

Philadelphia · Baltimore · New York · London
Buenos Aires · Hong Kong · Sydney · Tokyo

Editor: Elizabeth A. Nieginski
Editorial Director, Textbooks: Julie Martinez
Development Editor: Emilie Linkins
Managing Editor: Darrin Kiessling
Marketing Manager: Chris Kushner
Ilustrator: Matthew C. Chansky

530 Walnut Street
Philadelphia, Pennsylvania 19106

351 West Camden Street
Baltimore, Maryland 21201-2436 USA

Printed in the United States of America

Library of Congress Cataloging-in-Publication Data

Mehta, Samir.
   Step-up : a high yield, systems-based review for the USMLE Step 1 examination/ Samir Mehta, Edmund A. Milder, Adam J. Mirarchi.
      p. ; cm.
   Includes bibliographical references and index.
   ISBN 0–7817–3893–8
      1. Medicine—Examinations, questions, etc. I. Title: High-yield, systems-based review for the USMLE Step 1 examination. II. Milder, Edmund A. III. Mirarchi, Adam J. IV. Title.
      [DNLM: 1. Clinical Medicine—United States—Examination Questions. W 18.2 M498s 1999]
   R834.5 .M45 1999
   616'.0076—dc21

                                                                    99–052534

To purchase additional copies of this book, call our customer service department at **(800) 638-3030** or fax orders to **(301) 824-7390.** International customers should call **(301) 714-2324.**

                                                                    02 03
                                                          3 4 5 6 7 8 9 10

To my parents, Sudesh and Shobha, and to my sisters, Sonia and Sonul,

—Samir Mehta

To my parents James and Phyllis, and my siblings Eugene, Shannon and Robert

—Edmund A. Milder

To my parents Anthony and Andrea, my brother Alan, and my fiancee Sharon

—Adam J. Mirarchi

To our teachers
To our friends
And to the physicians of the future

Contents

Preface

For many first and second year medical students, the United States Medical Licensure Examination Step 1 is one of the most intimidating events of their medical school career. It often seems that there are more myths and rumors about the exam than there is information to study. The two years of medical facts, figures, and terminology that need to be organized and synthesized before taking "the boards" can leave students confused as to where to even start. STEP-UP: A High Yield, Systems Based Review for the USMLE Step 1 was conceived while three Temple University medical students were in that very same situation. The idea was made a reality after we experienced the Step 1 exam firsthand, and the result now sits in front of you.

The USMLE Step 1 has converted to CBT (Computer Based Testing). The test is a one-day, eight-hour examination, administered on Sylvan Learning Centers' computers throughout the world. While the National Board of Medical Examiners (NBME) continually updates the exam questions and makes minor adjustments to the format, the exam always consists of objective, multiple-choice questions. Scores are based on a 260-point scale, with a passing score equivalent to 179 (answering approximately 55%–65% of questions correctly). Scores for Step 1 may be available as early as ten days after administration of the exam for students taking it in the year 2000. Also, according to the 1998 statistics, nearly 93% of United States medical students passed the Step 1 examination on their first attempt.

Over the past few years, the NBME has transformed Step 1 from a subject-based examination to one that approaches the body as a whole, yet subdivided into essential systemic components. Scores that were previously broken down into subjects such as "anatomy," "biochemistry," and "pathology", are now reported in organ systems categories including "cardiovascular," "renal," and "musculoskeletal." However, while we were studying for our examinations, there were almost no systems-based review texts available.

The idea was to create a text that took a systems-based approach to the USMLE Step 1. STEP-UP was written with two major goals in mind: 1) to include only material pertinent for the Step 1 examination and 2) to present the material as efficiently as possible. Thus, while we tried to maintain a standard format, each chapter is an amalgamation of tables, figures, text,

facts, and charts presented in the format we felt best conveyed the essential material. The transitions between sections are often rapid and the text is succinct to help keep the student focused on only the relevant information. We realize that time is of the essence.

This text also has a number of additional features. The "Quick Hits" in the margins (marked by the boxing glove) are key facts that are related to the text within the body of the book and provide information that is particularly relevant to the USMLE Step 1. These "Quick Hits" can give further information on a subject, help explain a difficult topic, or provide data that bridges more than one organ system. The "At the Bedside" section is a compilation of over thirty clinical cases frequently tested on the boards. Each case is a complete history and physical with relevant figures, diagnostic and pathologic images, and a thoroughly explained differential diagnosis. Furthermore, STEP-UP provides comprehensive "Bug" and "Drug" tables in the appendix. We created these tables during our second year of medical school and have found them to be invaluable resources for Step 1 preparation and also during the pre-clinical years.

Medical schools across the country utilize a variety of curricular methods to help prepare students for the USMLE Step 1. Some use the traditional subject-based approach, others have incorporated problem-based learning, while still others have shifted to a systems-based format. Regardless of the method used at your school, this text will provide you with an avenue for preparing for the Step 1 exam, purposefully arranged in the same manner the test is now administered. We hope that students such as yourselves will also use this book as an adjunct to your daily classroom studies.

It would be hard to imagine a text that could summarize all of the important concepts students are expected to master over the first two years of medical school. We feel that STEP-UP provides an excellent foundation upon which students can build their knowledge base as high as they would like. We were once in your situation—worried about "the boards" but not knowing where to begin. We authored this book with these concerns in mind, and now offer to you a resource that we wish had been available to us. So when you sit down to begin your Step 1 exam, make sure you are ready to STEP-UP to "the boards."

Acknowledgments

We extend our thanks to the reviewers and contributors. Special thanks go to Frank Bognet, our editors at Lippincott Williams & Wilkins—Emilie Linkins, Elizabeth Nieginski, Julie Martinez, and Darrin Kiessling,—and to Matt Chansky for illustrations.

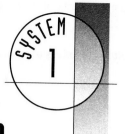

The Nervous System

DEVELOPMENT

— neural tube

I. Central Nervous System (CNS)
A. The CNS includes the **brain** and **spinal cord.**
B. It is **formed from the neural tube.**
  1. The **basal plate** of the neural tube forms **motor neurons.**
  2. The **alar plate** of the neural tube forms **sensory neurons.**
  3. The basal and alar plates are **separated** by the **sulcus limitans.**
C. **Oligodendrocytes** are responsible for **myelination,** which begins four months after conception and is finished by the second year of life.
D. The distal end of the spinal cord, the conus medullaris, is at the level of the third lumbar vertebra **(L3)** at **birth.** As the body grows, the cord "ascends" to its final resting position at the first lumbar vertebra **(L1) (Figure 1-1).**

II. Peripheral Nervous System (PNS)
— neural crest

A. The PNS includes the **peripheral nerves** and the **autonomic** and **sensory ganglia.**
B. It is **derived from neural crest cells** which give rise to:
  1. Schwann cells
  2. Pseudounipolar cells of the spinal and cranial nerve ganglia
  3. Multipolar cells of the autonomic ganglia
  4. Pia and arachnoid mater (not part of PNS)
  5. Melanocytes (not part of PNS)
  6. Epinephrine-producing chromaffin cells of the adrenal gland (not part of PNS)
C. **Schwann cells** are responsible for **myelination,** which begins four months after conception and is completed by the second year of life.

2 types of glial cells =>
- astro
- ependy
- micro

QUICK HIT For developmental and anatomic reasons, symptoms of a disk herniation are referred to the myotome and dermatome **below** the lesion. For example, a herniation of the C4-C5 disk would cause impingement of the C5 nerve root.

FIGURE 1-1 Adult derivatives of embryonic structures in the nervous system

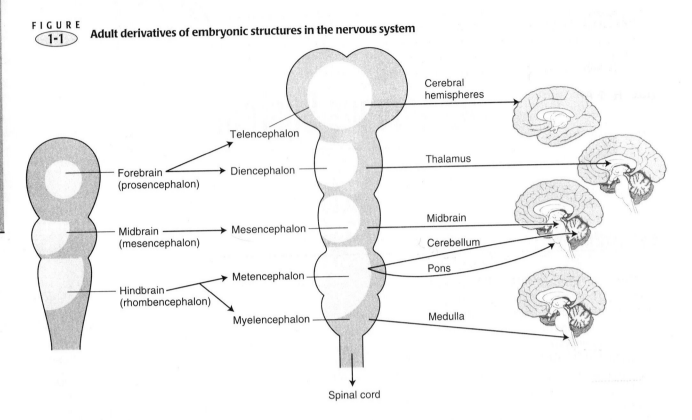

Forebrain (prosencephalon) → Telencephalon → Cerebral hemispheres

Diencephalon → Thalamus

Midbrain (mesencephalon) → Mesencephalon → Midbrain

→ Cerebellum
→ Pons

Hindbrain (rhombencephalon) → Metencephalon

Myelencephalon → Medulla

Spinal cord

CONGENITAL MALFORMATIONS OF THE NERVOUS SYSTEM

Abnormal development of the embryonal components of the nervous system can result in some of the malformations described in **Table 1-1.**

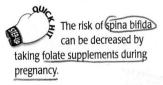

The risk of spina bifida can be decreased by taking folate supplements during pregnancy.

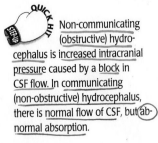

Non-communicating (obstructive) hydrocephalus is increased intracranial pressure caused by a block in CSF flow. In communicating (non-obstructive) hydrocephalus, there is normal flow of CSF, but abnormal absorption.

TABLE 1-1 Congenital Malformations of the Nervous System

Condition	Clinical Features
Fetal alcohol syndrome	• **Most common cause of mental retardation** ② Down ③ Fragile • **Cardiac septal defects** • Facial malformations including widely spaced eyes and long philtrum • Growth retardation

Spina bifida
due to ↑ AF
	• Improper closure of posterior neuropore
	• Several forms
	  - **Spina bifida occulta** (mildest form)—failure of vertebrae to close around spinal cord (tufts of hair often evident)
	  - Spinal meningocele (spina bifida cystica)—meninges extend out of defective spinal canal
	  - Meningomyelocele—meninges and spinal cord extend out of spinal canal
	  - Rachischisis (most severe form)—neural tissue is visible externally

Hydrocephaly	• Accumulation of CSF in ventricles and subarachnoid space • Due to congenital blockage of cerebral aqueducts • May be caused by **cytomegalovirus or toxoplasma infection** *TORCH'S*

(continued)

TABLE 1-1 Congenital Malformations of the Nervous System *(Continued)*	
Condition	**Clinical Features**
Anencephaly *due to ↑ AF*	• Failure of brain to develop • Due to <u>lack</u> of <u>closure</u> of <u>anterior neuropore</u> • Associated with increased alpha-fetoprotein (AFP)
Arnold-Chiari syndrome	• <u>Herniation of the</u> **cerebellar vermis** through the <u>foramen magnum</u> * Hydrocephaly * Myelomeningocele *type of* →* <u>spina bifida</u>
CSF=cerebospinal fluid	

> **QUICK HIT**
> Syringomyelia is associated with formation of Arnold-Chiari syndrome.

MAJOR RECEPTORS OF THE NERVOUS SYSTEM

Receptors of the Sympathetic and Parasympathetic Nervous System. The sympathetic and parasympathetic nervous systems exert their effects via various receptors scattered throughout the body. These effects are mediated by the substances in **Figure 1-2.**

FIGURE 1-2 Major receptors of the nervous system *(continued)*

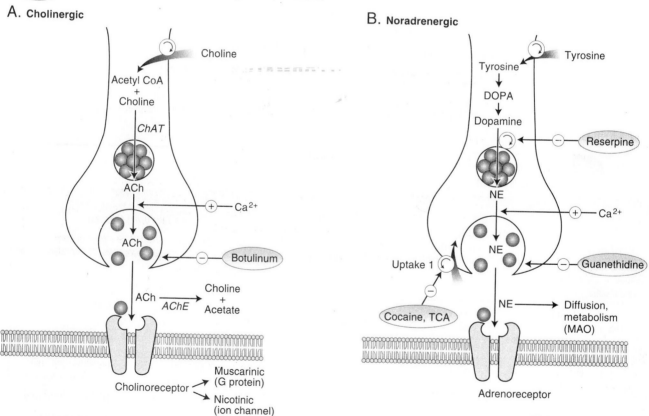

ACh=acetylcholine; AchE=acetylcholinesterase; BZ=benzodiazepines; Ca²⁺=calcium; Cl⁻=chloride; CoA=coenzyme A; DOPA=dihydroxyphenylalanine; GABA=gamma-aminobutyric acid; MAO=monoamine oxidase; NE=norepinephrine; PLP=phospholipid; TCA=tricyclic antidepressant

(text continues on page 10)

FIGURE 1-2 *(Continued)* Major receptors of the nervous system

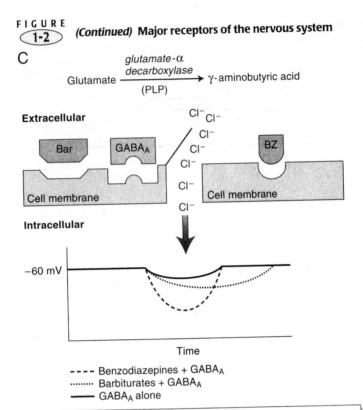

C

$$\text{Glutamate} \xrightarrow[\text{(PLP)}]{\begin{array}{c}\text{glutamate-}\alpha\\\text{decarboxylase}\end{array}} \gamma\text{-aminobutyric acid}$$

- - - - Benzodiazepines + GABA$_A$
·········· Barbiturates + GABA$_A$
——— GABA$_A$ alone

Binding of barbiturates or benzodiazepines to the GABA ionophore increases chloride ion conductance. Barbiturates increase the duration of chloride channel opening while benzodiazepines increase the amplitude of depolarization.

ACh=acetylcholine; *AchE*=acetylcholinesterase; *BZ*=benzodiazepines; *Ca²⁺*=calcium; *Cl⁻*=chloride; *CoA*=coenzyme A; *DOPA*=dihydroxyphenylalanine; *GABA*=γ-aminobutyric acid; *MAO*=monoamine oxidase; *NE*=norepinephrine; *PLP*=phospholipid; *TCA*=tricyclic antidepressant

TABLE 1-2 Receptors of the Sympathetic and Parasympathetic Nervous System

Site of Action	Sympathetic Nervous System		Parasympathetic Nervous System	
	Receptor	*Effect on site*	*Receptor*	*Effect on site*
Smooth muscle; skin and viscera	α1	Constricting	Muscarinic	Dilating
Smooth, skeletal, and cardiac muscle	α1 β2	Constricting Dilating	Muscarinic	Dilating
Smooth muscle of the lung	β2	Relax	Muscarinic	Contracting
Smooth muscle of the gastrointestinal tract	α2; β2	Relax intestinal wall; constrict sphincters	Muscarinic	Constrict intestinal wall; relax sphincter
Heart; SA node	β1	Increase heart rate	Muscarinic	Decrease heart rate
Heart; ventricles	β1	Increase contractility and conduction velocity	Muscarinic	Small decrease in contractility
Eye; radial muscle	α1	**Mydriasis** (dilation of pupil)	N/A	N/A
Eye; sphincter muscle	N/A	N/A	Muscarinic	**Miosis** (constriction of pupil)

(continued)

TABLE 1-2 Receptors of the Sympathetic and Parasympathetic Nervous System *(Continued)*

Site of action	Sympathetic nervous system		Parasympathetic nervous system	
	Receptor	*Effect on site*	*Receptor*	*Effect on site*
Eye; ciliary muscle	β2	**Relax**	Muscarinic	**Constrict** (near vision)
Bladder	β2 α1	Relax Contract sphincter	Muscarinic	Contract
Uterus	α1 β2	Contract Relax	Muscarinic	Contract
Penis	α2	Ejaculate	Muscarinic	Erection
Sweat glands	Muscarinic	Secrete	N/A	N/A
Pancreas	α2 β2	**Decrease insulin secretion** **Increase insulin secretion**	N/A N/A	N/A N/A
Liver	α1, β2	Glycolysis, gluconeogenesis	N/A	N/A
Adipose tissue	β1, β3	Lipolysis	N/A	N/A

EPI=epinephrine; *NE*=norepinephrine; *SA*=sinoatrial

● Neurotoxins and Their Effects (Figure 1-3)

FIGURE 1-3 Neurotoxins and their effects

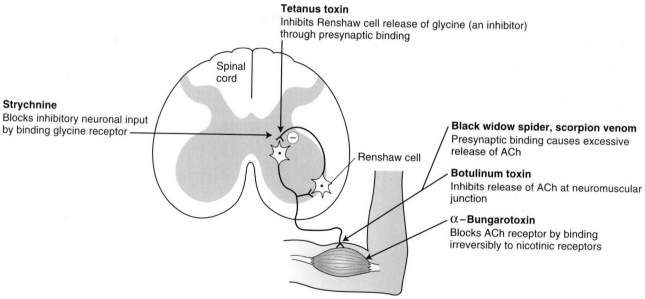

Tetanus toxin
Inhibits Renshaw cell release of glycine (an inhibitor) through presynaptic binding

Strychnine
Blocks inhibitory neuronal input by binding glycine receptor

Spinal cord

Renshaw cell

Black widow spider, scorpion venom
Presynaptic binding causes excessive release of ACh

Botulinum toxin
Inhibits release of ACh at neuromuscular junction

α–Bungarotoxin
Blocks ACh receptor by binding irreversibly to nicotinic receptors

ACh=acetylcholine

MENINGES, FLOW OF CEREBROSPINAL FLUID (CSF), AND PATHOLOGIC TRAUMA (Figure 1-4)

FIGURE 1-4 Meninges, flow of cerebrospinal fluid (CSF), and pathologic trauma

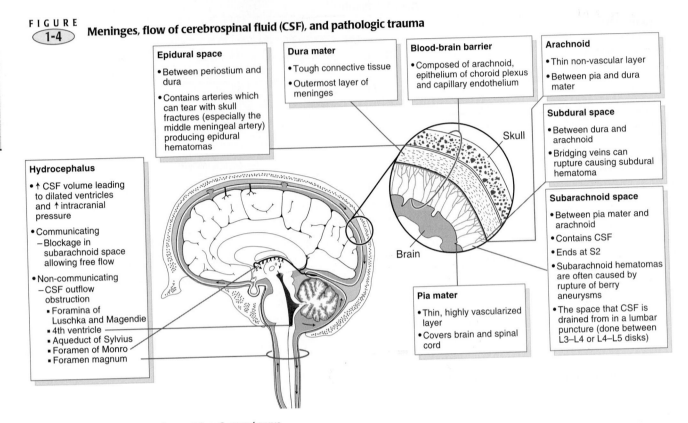

Epidural space
- Between periostium and dura
- Contains arteries which can tear with skull fractures (especially the middle meningeal artery) producing epidural hematomas

Dura mater
- Tough connective tissue
- Outermost layer of meninges

Blood-brain barrier
- Composed of arachnoid, epithelium of choroid plexus and capillary endothelium

Arachnoid
- Thin non-vascular layer
- Between pia and dura mater

Subdural space
- Between dura and arachnoid
- Bridging veins can rupture causing subdural hematoma

Subarachnoid space
- Between pia mater and arachnoid
- Contains CSF
- Ends at S2
- Subarachnoid hematomas are often caused by rupture of berry aneurysms
- The space that CSF is drained from in a lumbar puncture (done between L3–L4 or L4–L5 disks)

Pia mater
- Thin, highly vascularized layer
- Covers brain and spinal cord

Hydrocephalus
- ↑ CSF volume leading to dilated ventricles and ↑ intracranial pressure
- Communicating
  – Blockage in subarachnoid space allowing free flow
- Non-communicating
  – CSF outflow obstruction
    ▪ Foramina of Luschka and Magendie
    ▪ 4th ventricle
    ▪ Aqueduct of Sylvius
    ▪ Foramen of Monro
    ▪ Foramen magnum

Skull

Brain

CSF=cerebrospinal fluid; *L*=lumbar vertebra; *S*=sacral nerve

BLOOD SUPPLY TO THE BRAIN (Figure 1-5)

FIGURE 1-5 Blood supply to the brain *(continued)*

A. Arteries of the base of the brain and brain stem

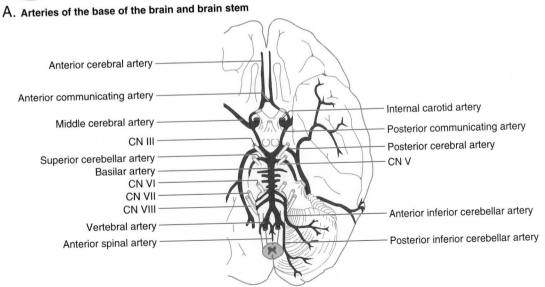

Anterior cerebral artery

Anterior communicating artery

Middle cerebral artery

CN III

Superior cerebellar artery

Basilar artery

CN VI

CN VII

CN VIII

Vertebral artery

Anterior spinal artery

Internal carotid artery

Posterior communicating artery

Posterior cerebral artery

CN V

Anterior inferior cerebellar artery

Posterior inferior cerebellar artery

CN=cranial nerve;

FIGURE
1-5 *(Continued)* **Blood supply to the brain**

B. **Arterial blood supply to the cortex**

Lateral

Medial

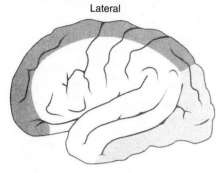
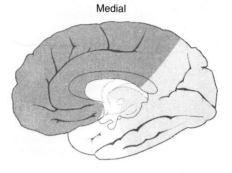

☐ Anterior cerebral artery   ☐ Middle cerebral artery   ☐ Posterior cerebral artery

C. **Venous drainage of the brain**

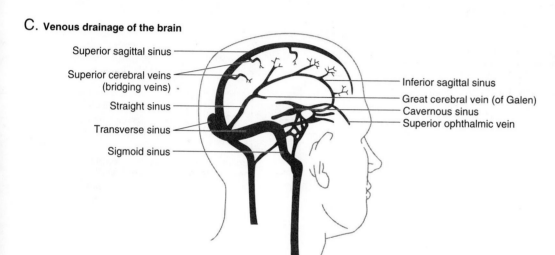

Superior sagittal sinus
Superior cerebral veins (bridging veins)
Straight sinus
Transverse sinus
Sigmoid sinus

Inferior sagittal sinus
Great cerebral vein (of Galen)
Cavernous sinus
Superior ophthalmic vein

CN=cranial nerve

LESIONS OF THE CEREBRAL CORTEX (Figure 1-6)

F I G U R E
1-6 **Lesions of the cerebral cortex**

A. Bilateral lesions

Primary somatosensory cortex (3,1,2)
- Lesion causes contralateral loss of touch, vibration and stereognosis in affected area

Primary motor cortex (4)
- Lesion causes contralateral hemiparesis in affected area

Lesion of right parietal lobe results in left-sided neglect. Patient fails to recognize that the left side of his/her body exists.

Frontal eye field (8)
- Lesion in left hemisphere causes eyes to look left. Lesion of right hemisphere causes eyes to look right

Broca's speech area of left hemisphere (44,45)
- Destruction causes Broca's (expressive) aphasia. Patient understands spoken word but cannot form fluent sentences

Primary auditory cortex (41,42)

Auditory association cortex (Wernicke's speech area of left hemisphere) (22)
- Destruction causes Wernicke's aphasia. Patient cannot understand spoken word and speech is fluid but does not make sense.

Primary visual cortex (17)
- Lesion causes visual field deficits

QUICK HIT Klüver-Bucy syndrome is a bilateral lesion of the amygdala nuclei. It results in hypersexuality, docility, and hyperorality.

B. Medial lesions

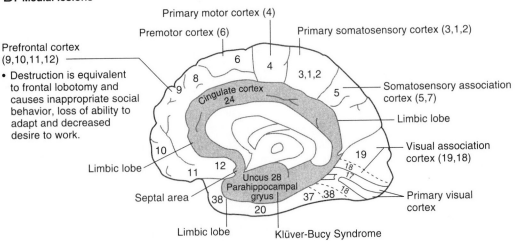

Primary motor cortex (4)
Premotor cortex (6)
Primary somatosensory cortex (3,1,2)

Prefrontal cortex (9,10,11,12)
- Destruction is equivalent to frontal lobotomy and causes inappropriate social behavior, loss of ability to adapt and decreased desire to work.

Cingulate cortex 24

Somatosensory association cortex (5,7)

Limbic lobe

Visual association cortex (19,18)

Limbic lobe

Uncus 28
Parahippocampal gryus

Septal area

Limbic lobe

Klüver-Bucy Syndrome

Primary visual cortex

(Adapted from Fix JD: *High-Yield Neuroanatomy*. Baltimore, Williams & Wilkins, 1995. p. 102)

IMPORTANT PATHWAYS OF THE SPINAL CORD (Figure 1-7)

FIGURE
1-7 **Important pathways of the spinal cord**

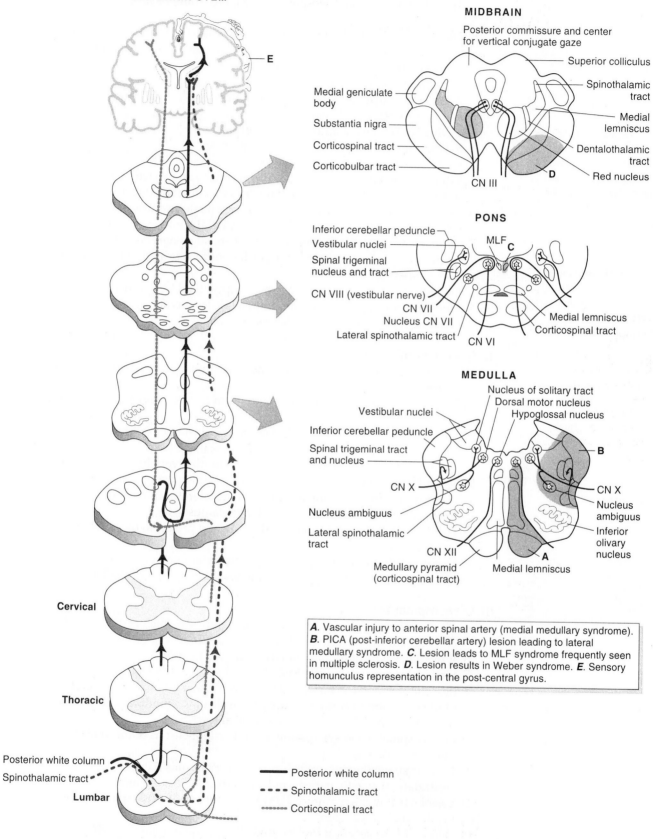

THE BRAIN STEM

MIDBRAIN

Posterior commissure and center
for vertical conjugate gaze

Superior colliculus

Spinothalamic
tract

Medial geniculate
body

Substantia nigra

Corticospinal tract

Corticobulbar tract

Medial
lemniscus

Dentalothalamic
tract

Red nucleus

CN III   D

PONS

Inferior cerebellar peduncle
Vestibular nuclei
Spinal trigeminal
nucleus and tract

MLF C

CN VIII (vestibular nerve)
CN VII
Nucleus CN VII
Lateral spinothalamic tract

CN VI

Medial lemniscus
Corticospinal tract

MEDULLA

Nucleus of solitary tract
Dorsal motor nucleus
Hypoglossal nucleus

Vestibular nuclei

Inferior cerebellar peduncle

Spinal trigeminal tract
and nucleus

CN X

Nucleus ambiguus

Lateral spinothalamic
tract

B

CN X

Nucleus
ambiguus

Inferior
olivary
nucleus

CN XII
Medullary pyramid
(corticospinal tract)

Medial lemniscus   A

Cervical

Thoracic

A. Vascular injury to anterior spinal artery (medial medullary syndrome).
B. PICA (post-inferior cerebellar artery) lesion leading to lateral
medullary syndrome. **C**. Lesion leads to MLF syndrome frequently seen
in multiple sclerosis. **D**. Lesion results in Weber syndrome. **E**. Sensory
homunculus representation in the post-central gyrus.

Posterior white column
Spinothalamic tract

Lumbar

——— Posterior white column
- - - Spinothalamic tract
········ Corticospinal tract

Dorsal column (handwritten)

I. Posterior White Column

A. The posterior white column is the ascending pathway that conveys **discriminatory touch (two-point touch), vibration, proprioception,** and **stereognosis.**

B. The posterior white column receives information at all spinal cord levels from pseudounipolar cells of dorsal root ganglia. This information is conveyed from a variety of receptors:
1. Meissner's corpuscles (rate of applied stimulus)
2. **Pacinian corpuscles (vibration stimulus)**
3. Joint receptors (joint position)
4. Muscle spindles (length of a muscle)
5. **Golgi tendon organs (tension** on a muscle)

C. First order neurons of the dorsal root ganglia enter at the dorsal horn and ascend in the **fasciculus gracilis (lower limb)** and **fasciculus cuneatus (upper limb)** and synapse in the nucleus gracilis and cuneatus, respectively.

D. Second order neurons arise from these two nuclei, decussate at the level of the inferior medulla, and ascend as the **medial lemniscus.**

E. Medial lemniscus fibers synapse in the **ventral posterolateral (VPL) nucleus** of the thalamus and third order neurons project to the **cerebral cortex (areas 3,1,2).**

F. Lesions below the decussation produce ipsilateral loss of discriminatory touch, proprioception, and vibration, while lesions above the decussation produce contralateral loss of these sensations.

> **QUICK HIT**
> Muscle spindles function as the afferent limb of the myotactic (stretch) reflex (e.g., tapping knee with reflex hammer). Ventral horn motor neurons function as the efferent limb.

> **QUICK HIT**
> **Muscle spindles** are arranged **in parallel** with the extrafusal muscle fibers; **Golgi tendon organs** are arranged in **series.**

II. Spinothalamic Tract

A. The spinothalamic tract is the ascending pathway that conveys **pain** and **temperature** from the body.

B. It receives input from free nerve endings of fast (A-type) and slow (C-type) pain fibers.

C. First order neurons originate in the dorsal root ganglion, enter the spinal cord, and synapse on second order neurons in the dorsolateral tract of Lissauer [thoracic vertebra level 2 (T2) to lumbar vertebra level 3 (L3)]

D. Second order neurons ascend while decussating through the **ventral white commissure** and continue to ascend in the lateral spinothalamic tract, terminating in the VPL nucleus of the thalamus.

E. Third order neurons originate in the VPL and project to the **cerebral cortex (areas 3,1,2).**

F. Lesions of the spinothalamic tract produce contralateral loss of pain and temperature sensation beginning **one level below that of the lesion.**

III. Corticospinal Tract

A. The corticospinal tract is the descending pathway that originates in the **cerebral cortex (area 6; area 4; and areas 3,1,2)**

B. It mediates **voluntary movement** of striated muscle.

C. First order neurons project to the posterior limb of the internal capsule, descend through the middle three fifths of the midbrain's **crus cerebri,** base of the pons and **decussate in the pyramids of the medulla** and continue down the spinal cord as the corticospinal tract.

D. Corticospinal fibers synapse on second order neurons of the ventral horn via interneurons.

E. Lesions above the pyramids [upper motor neurons (**UMN**)] produce **contralateral spastic paresis** and a positive Babinski's sign.

F. Lesions below the pyramids (**UMN**) produce **ipsilateral spastic paresis** and a positive Babinski's sign.

G. Lesions of the second order neurons [lower motor neuron (**LMN**)] produce **flaccid paralysis** and fasciculations.

Important Pathways of the Brain Stem and Cerebrum

I. Trigeminothalamic Pathway

A. The trigeminothalamic pathway is the ascending pathway that conveys **pain** and **temperature from the face** (analogous to the spinothalamic tract).

B. It receives input from free nerve endings of fast (A-type) and slow (C-type) pain fibers.

C. First order neurons originate in the trigeminal ganglion and synapse on second order neurons in the spinal trigeminal nucleus (ventral trigeminothalamic tract) or principal sensory nucleus of the trigeminal nerve (dorsal trigeminothalamic tract).

D. Second order neurons of the ventral tract decussate while ascending; however, the dorsal tract neurons remain uncrossed, with termination in the VPM nucleus of the thalamus.

E. Third order neurons originate in the VPM and project to the **cerebral cortex (areas 3,1,2)**

II. Corticobulbar Tract

A. The corticobulbar tract is the descending pathway that originates in the **cerebral cortex (area 6; area 4; and areas 3,1,2)**

B. It mediates voluntary movement of the **muscles of facial expression** (analogous to the corticospinal tract).

C. First order neurons project to the genu of the **internal capsule,** descend through the middle three fifths of the midbrain's crus cerebri and synapse in the nucleus of cranial nerve (CN) VII (facial nucleus).

D. Second order neurons innervate the muscles of facial expression (orbicularis oculi, orbicularis oris, buccinator, frontalis, platysma) via the facial nerve.

E. The **upper face** (orbicularis oculi and frontalis muscles) receives **bilateral input** from the UMN and therefore is not affected by unilateral cortical lesions.

F. The **lower face** (buccinator, orbicularis oris, platysma) receives only **contralateral input.**

 Bell's palsy is an **LMN lesion** of the **facial nerve.** This lesion results in complete facial paralysis on the affected side and is characterized by loss of the nasolabial fold, drooling, and ptosis. It is often idiopathic and usually resolves spontaneously.

III. Cerebellar Pathway

A. The cerebellar pathway controls posture and balance, maintains muscle tone, and coordinates motor activity.

B. The **dentothalamic tract** is the major cerebellar tract.
  1. It originates in the dentate nucleus of the cerebellum.
  2. It projects to the ventrolateral nucleus of the thalamus (not the VPL) via the superior cerebellar peduncle.
  3. Thalamic fibers within the tract project to area 4 (primary motor cortex).
  4. Cerebral fibers within the tract project to corticospinal neurons.
  5. The pons receives cerebral fibers and sends fibers to the cerebellum where they terminate on mossy fibers.

C. Damage to one side of the cerebellum results in ipsilateral findings. Patient will fall toward affected side **(positive Romberg sign).**

 In Friedreich's ataxia (autosomal recessive), the most common congenital ataxia, the brain shows diffuse neuronal loss involving the posterior white columns, the dentate nuclei, and the spinocerebellar tract. These patients commonly have diabetes and heart disease.

IV. Vestibulocochlear Pathways

A. **Auditory pathway**
  1. The auditory pathway originates from hair cells in the organ of Corti in the cochlea.
  2. Signals are sent down bipolar cell axons and are then relayed to the cochlear nuclei of the pons via the spiral ganglion.

THE NERVOUS SYSTEM

3. Signals are sent to higher CNS areas and relayed to the cerebral hemisphere via the **medial geniculate body of the thalamus.**
4. Fibers terminate in the transverse temporal gyri **(areas 41 and 42).**
5. Due to the bilateral projection of information in the auditory pathway, one-sided lesions of this pathway at any point beyond the cochlear nuclei do not produce hearing loss.
6. Lesions of the cochlear nerve itself will produce ipsilateral hearing loss.

B. **Vestibular pathway**
1. Hair cells of the three **semicircular canals** encode **angular acceleration** and **deceleration.**
2. Hair cells of the **utricle** encode **linear acceleration.**
3. Information is passed via the vestibular nerve to the vestibular nuclei of the low pons.
4. Fibers then project to
   a. the spinal cord
   b. the cerebellum
   c. the thalamus
   d. CN III, IV, and VI via the medial longitudinal fasciculus (MLF).
5. **Nystagmus.** Nystagmus is mediated by the vestibular and oculomotor nuclei, the medial longitudinal fasciculus (MLF), and the muscles of ocular movement controlled by cranial nerves III, IV, and VI **(Table 1-3).**

> **QUICK HIT**
> Tonotopic localization of sound in the cochlea is due in part to the increasing thickness of the basilar membrane as it ascends toward the helicotrema. The **base** of the cochlea (closest to the oval window) is sensitive to **high frequency sounds.** The **apex** of the cochlea is sensitive to **low frequency sounds.**

> **QUICK HIT**
> Linear acceleration sensed by the utricle and saccule can cause nausea and vomiting. Dimenhydrinate and scopolamine can prevent motion sickness. These drugs work best if used before the onset of symptoms.

TABLE 1-3 Direction of Movement in Types of Nystagmus

Form of Nystagmus	Direction of Movement during Fast Phase	Direction of Movement during Slow Phase
Rotary nystagmus (i.e., while spinning in a circle)	Same as direction of rotation	Opposite direction of rotation
Post-rotary nystagmus (i.e., after spinning in a circle)	Opposite direction of rotation	Same as direction of rotation
Caloric nystagmus		
• Warm water placed in one ear	Toward the ear with warm water placed in it	Away from the ear with warm water placed in it
• Cold water placed in one ear	Away from the ear with cold water placed in it	Toward the ear with cold water placed in it

V. Visual Pathways (Figure 1-8)

FIGURE
1-8

Visual pathways. (A) Legend for lesions: 1) total blindness 2) bitemporal hemianopia–common lesion caused by superiorly growing pituitary tumor, 3) right hemianopia, 4) right upper quadrantopia, 5) right lower quadrantopia, 6) right hemianopia with macular sparing. (B) Light shined in one eye causes constriction of both pupils. (C) Abduction of one eye results in adduction of the other eye in individuals with an intact medial longitudinal fasciculus (MLF), and normal lateral conjugate gaze.

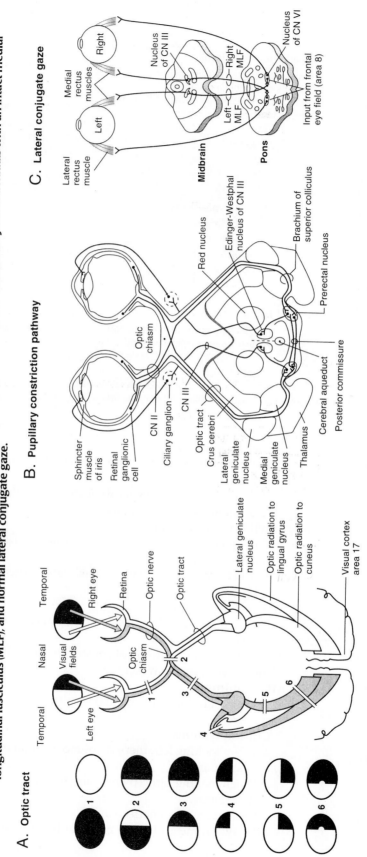

A. Optic tract

B. Pupillary constriction pathway

C. Lateral conjugate gaze

CN=cranial nerve; MSL=medial longitudinal fasciculus (Adapted from Fix JD: *High-Yield Neuroanatomy*, Baltimore, Williams & Wilkins, 1995. p. 74–75)

MUSCLES OF THE EYE (Figure 1-9)

FIGURE
1-9   Muscles of the eye

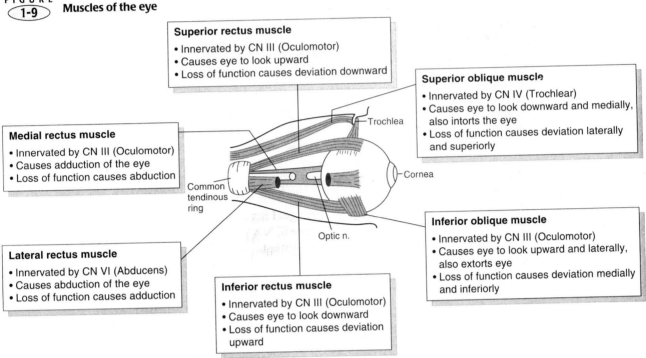

Superior rectus muscle
• Innervated by CN III (Oculomotor)
• Causes eye to look upward
• Loss of function causes deviation downward

Superior oblique muscle
• Innervated by CN IV (Trochlear)
• Causes eye to look downward and medially, also intorts the eye
• Loss of function causes deviation laterally and superiorly

Medial rectus muscle
• Innervated by CN III (Oculomotor)
• Causes adduction of the eye
• Loss of function causes abduction

Inferior oblique muscle
• Innervated by CN III (Oculomotor)
• Causes eye to look upward and laterally, also extorts eye
• Loss of function causes deviation medially and inferiorly

Lateral rectus muscle
• Innervated by CN VI (Abducens)
• Causes abduction of the eye
• Loss of function causes adduction

Inferior rectus muscle
• Innervated by CN III (Oculomotor)
• Causes eye to look downward
• Loss of function causes deviation upward

Trochlea — Cornea — Common tendinous ring — Optic n.

(Adapted from Chung, Kyong Won: *BRS Gross Anatomy, 2nd edition.* Baltimore, Williams & Wilkins, 1991, page 302.)

Horner's syndrome is often caused by **Pancoast's tumor**, a lung neoplasm that invades the cervical sympathetic chain.

A. **Horner's syndrome**
1. This syndrome is caused by a lesion of the sympathetic trunk above the 8th cervical vertebra (C8).
2. Clinical features of the syndrome include ipsilateral **ptosis, anhydrosis, flushing of skin,** and **myosis.**

B. **Argyll Robertson pupil**
1. This sign is seen in syphilis, systemic lupus erythematosus (SLE), and diabetes mellitus.
2. It presents as a pupil that **accommodates** to near objects but **does not react to light.**

C. **Marcus Gunn pupil**
1. This sign is caused by a lesion of the afferent portion of the light reflex pathway.
2. The affected pupil does not constrict to direct light input, but the consensual reflex is intact.

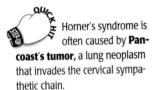

The Marcus Gunn pupil can be diagnosed using the **swinging flashlight test.** Shining a flashlight in the normal pupil causes constriction of both pupils. Swinging the flashlight quickly to the affected eye causes paradoxical dilation of the affected pupil.

D. **MLF syndrome**
1. A bilateral lesion of the medial longitudinal fasciculus causes this syndrome.
2. **Clinical features**
   a. When looking left, there is absence of right eye adduction and left eye nystagmus.
   b. When looking right, there is absence of left eye adduction and right eye nystagmus.
   c. Convergence is unaffected.
3. MLF syndrome is often seen in **multiple sclerosis.**

E. **Uncal herniation**
1. The uncus of the temporal lobe is forced through the opening of the tentorium.
2. Clinical features (See Figure 1-8).
   a. Compression of CN III occurs, leading to
      (i) Ophthalmoplegia (paralysis of one or more of the ocular muscles)
      (ii) Dilated ("blown") pupil
   b. Compression of the corticospinal tract occurs leading to ipsilateral hemiparesis.
   c. Compression of the posterior cerebral artery occurs, leading to contralateral homonymous hemianopsia.

VI. Taste

A. The **solitary** nucleus of the medulla receives taste sensation via the solitary tract from 3 sources:
1. The anterior two thirds of the tongue via the **chorda tympani** nerve of the facial nerve (CN VII)
2. The posterior third of the tongue via the **glossopharyngeal** nerve (CN IX)
3. The epiglottic region of the pharynx via the **vagal** nerve (CN X)

CN 7 taste ⅔ ant
CN 11 post ⅓

B. Neurons carrying taste sensation ascend in the ventral tegmental tract to the VPM nucleus of the thalamus.
C. The VPM nucleus of the thalamus sends fibers to the parietal lobe.

CN 12 damage Rt deviates tongue Rt.

VII. Limbic System

A. Mediates behavior and emotion, specifically:
1. Feeding
2. Feeling (emotion)
3. Fighting
4. Fleeing
5. Sexual activity

4 F's 1 sex.

B. Primarily controlled by the hypothalamus and autonomic nervous system
C. Other important areas include:
1. Anterior nucleus of thalamus
2. Cingulate gyrus
3. Mamillary bodies
4. Septal area
5. Hippocampus
6. Amygdala

QUICK HIT

Lesions of the mamillary bodies are produced from thiamine deficiency, commonly seen in chronic alcoholism. Damage results in **Korsakoff's syndrome**, characterized by confusion, severe memory impairment, and confabulation, which is **irreversible.**

CLASSIC LESIONS OF THE SPINAL CORD (Figure 1-10)

FIGURE
1-10 Classic lesions of the spinal cord

A

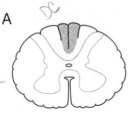

DC

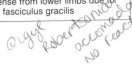

Tabes dorsalis

- Seen in tertiary syphilis
- Bilateral loss of touch, vibration and tactile sense from lower limbs due to lesion of fasciculus gracilis

Argyll Robertson accomodate no react

B

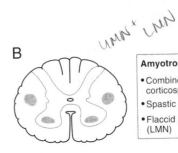

UMN + LMN   *ALS*

Amyotrophic lateral sclerosis

- Combined UMN and LMN lesion of corticospinal tract
- Spastic paresis (UMN sign)
- Flaccid paralysis with fasciculations (LMN)

Brown-Séquard Syndrome

- Ipsilateral loss of touch and vibration and tactile sense below lesion due to posterior white column lesion
- Contralateral loss of pain and touch due to loss of spinothalamic tract
- Ipsilateral spastic paresis below lesion due to lesion of corticospinal tract
- Ipsilateral flaccid paralysis at level of lesion due to loss of LMN
- If lesion occurs above T–1, Horner's syndrome on side of lesion will result

C

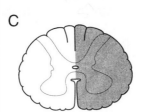

D

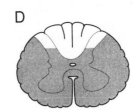

Spinal artery infarct

- Bilateral loss of pain and temperature one level below lesion due to loss of spinothalamic tract
- Bilateral spastic paresis below lesion due to lesion of corticospinal tract
- Bilateral flaccid paralysis at level of lesion due to loss of LMN
- Loss of bladder control due to lesion of corticospinal tract innervation of S2–S4 parasympathetics
- Bilateral Horner's syndrome if above T-2

Subacute combined degeneration
(Vitamin B12 deficiency)

- Bilateral loss of touch, vibration and tactile sense due to posterior white column lesion
- Bilateral spastic paresis below lesion due to lesion of corticospinal tracts

E

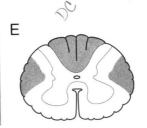

DC

F

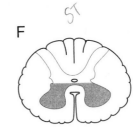

ST

Syringomyelia

- Bilateral loss of pain and temperature one level below due to lesion of ventral white commissure (spinothalamic tract)
- Bilateral flaccid paralysis of level of lesion due to loss of LMN

LMN=lower motor neuron; *UMN*=upper motor neuron

HYPOTHALAMUS (Figure 1-11)

Hypothalamus

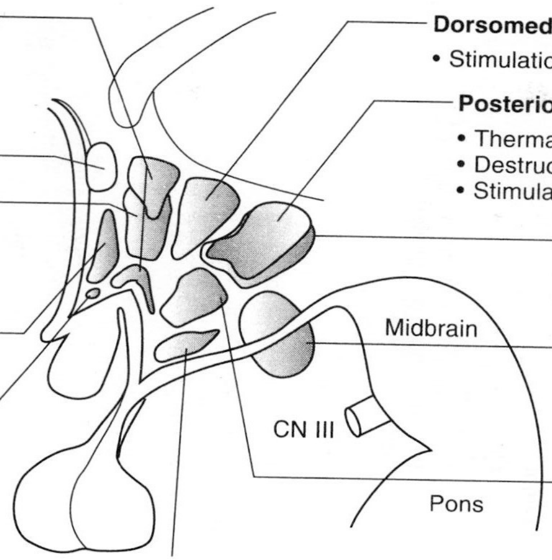

Paraventricular and supraoptic nuclei
- Regulate water balance
- Produce ADH and oxytocin
- Destruction causes diabetes insipidus

Anterior commissure

Anterior nucleus
- Thermal regulation (dissipation of heat)
- Stimulates parasympathetic NS
- Destruction results in hyperthermia

Preoptic area
- Contains sexual dimorphic nucleus
- Regulates release of gonadotropic hormones

Suprachiasmatic nucleus
- Receives input from retina
- Controls circadian rhythms

Dorsomedial nucleus
- Stimulation results in obesity and savage behavior

Posterior nucleus
- Thermal regulation (conservation of heat)
- Destruction results in inability to thermoregulate
- Stimulates the sympathetic nervous system

Lateral nucleus
- Stimulation induces eating
- Destruction results in starvation

Mamillary body
- Receives input from hippocampal formation
- Contains hemorrhagic lesions in Wernicke's encephalopathy

Ventromedial nucleus
- Satiety center
- Destruction results in obesity and savage behavior

Arcuate nucleus
- Produces hypothalamic releasing factors
- Contains DOPA-nergic neurons that inhibit prolactin release

Midbrain

CN III

Pons

ADH=antidiuretic hormone; *DOPA*=dihydroxyphenylalanine; *NS*=nervous system (Redrawn from Fix JD: *High-Yield Neuroanatomy.* Baltimore, Williams & Wilkins, 1995. p. 84)

THALAMUS (Figure 1-12)

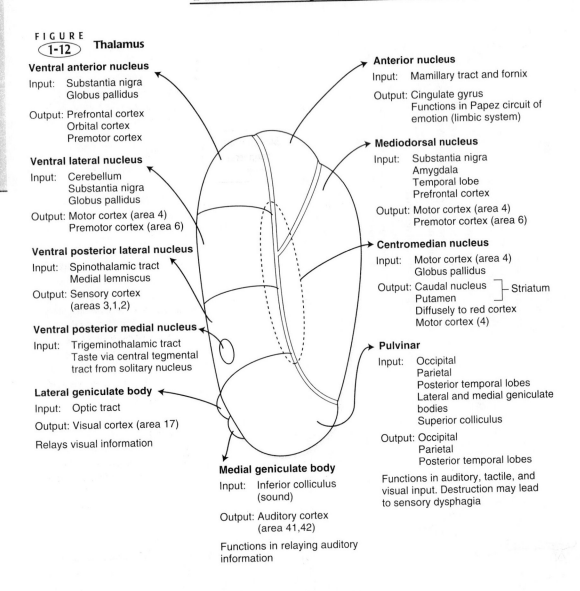

FIGURE 1-12 Thalamus

Ventral anterior nucleus

Input: Substantia nigra
Globus pallidus

Output: Prefrontal cortex
Orbital cortex
Premotor cortex

Ventral lateral nucleus

Input: Cerebellum
Substantia nigra
Globus pallidus

Output: Motor cortex (area 4)
Premotor cortex (area 6)

Ventral posterior lateral nucleus

Input: Spinothalamic tract
Medial lemniscus

Output: Sensory cortex
(areas 3,1,2)

Ventral posterior medial nucleus

Input: Trigeminothalamic tract
Taste via central tegmental
tract from solitary nucleus

Lateral geniculate body

Input: Optic tract

Output: Visual cortex (area 17)

Relays visual information

Medial geniculate body

Input: Inferior colliculus
(sound)

Output: Auditory cortex
(area 41,42)

Functions in relaying auditory
information

Anterior nucleus

Input: Mamillary tract and fornix

Output: Cingulate gyrus
Functions in Papez circuit of
emotion (limbic system)

Mediodorsal nucleus

Input: Substantia nigra
Amygdala
Temporal lobe
Prefrontal cortex

Output: Motor cortex (area 4)
Premotor cortex (area 6)

Centromedian nucleus

Input: Motor cortex (area 4)
Globus pallidus

Output: Caudal nucleus ⎤
Putamen   ⎦ Striatum
Diffusely to red cortex
Motor cortex (4)

Pulvinar

Input: Occipital
Parietal
Posterior temporal lobes
Lateral and medial geniculate
bodies
Superior colliculus

Output: Occipital
Parietal
Posterior temporal lobes

Functions in auditory, tactile, and
visual input. Destruction may lead
to sensory dysphagia

CRANIAL NERVES

The twelve cranial nerves arise from various nuclei within the brain stem and cortex and serve multiple functions in the body. Their extracranial course is important for locating lesions, which can be tested by asking the patient to perform simple tasks. **Table 1-4** outlines important information about cranial nerves I though XII.

(text continues on page 22)

TABLE 1-4 Cranial Nerves

Nerve	Site of exit from the skull	Function	Fiber types	Common lesions	Test
I-Olfactory	Cribriform plate	Smell	SVA	Cribriform plate fracture; Kallmann's syndrome	Smell
II-Optic	Optic canal	Sight	SVA	See Figure 1-8	Snellen chart; peripheral vision
III-Oculomotor	Superior orbital fissure	**Parasympathetic** to **ciliary** and **sphincter muscles;** medial rectus, superior rectus, inferior rectus, inferior oblique	GVE, GSE	Transtentorial (uncal) herniation; **diabetes;** Weber's syndrome	"H" in space; pupillary light reflexes; convergence
IV-Trochlear	Superior orbital fissure	Superior oblique muscle	GSE	Head trauma	"H" in space
V-Trigeminal			SVE, GSA	Tic douloureux (trigeminal neuralgia)	Facial sensation; open jaw **(deviates toward lesion)**
V1-Ophthalmic	-Superior orbital fissure	-Sensory from medial nose, forehead			
V2-Maxillary	-Foramen rotundum	-Sensory from lateral nose, upper lip, superior buccal area			
V3-Mandibular	-Foramen ovale	**Muscles of mastication,** tensor tympani, tensor veli palatini; sensory from lower lip, lateral face to lower border of mandible			
VI-Abducens	Superior orbital fissure	Lateral rectus muscle	GSE	**Medial inferior pontine syndrome**	"H" in space

(continued)

(Handwritten annotations: "Sensory touch"; "motor -corneal reflex in 5 out 7 - move")

QUICK HIT

Medial inferior pontine syndrome results in ipsilateral lateral rectus paralysis with contralateral spastic hemiparesis and loss of sensation of pain and temperature.

TABLE 1-4 Cranial Nerves *(Continued)*

Nerve	Site of exit from the skull	Function	Fiber types	Common lesions	Test
VII-Facial	Internal acoustic meatus	Parasympathetic to lacrimal, submandibular, and sublingual glands; **muscles of facial expression and stapedius, stylohyoid muscle, posterior belly of digastric muscle;** sensory from anterior ⅔ of tongue (including taste **via chorda tympani**)	GVE, SVE, GSA, SVA	**Bell's palsy**	Wrinkle forehead; show teeth; puff out cheeks; close eyes tightly
VIII-Vestibulocochlear	Internal acoustic meatus	Equilibrium; hearing	SSA	**Acoustic schwannoma**	Hearing; nystagmus (slow phase toward lesion)
IX-Glossopharyngeal	Jugular foramen	Parasympathetic to parotid gland; stylopharyngeus muscle; sensory from pharynx, middle ear, auditory tube, carotid body and sinus, external ear, posterior third of tongue (including taste)	GVE, SVE, GSA, GVA, SVA	Posterior inferior cerebellar artery (**PICA**) infarct	Gag reflex (no response ipsilateral to lesion)
X-Vagus	Jugular foramen	Parasympathetic to body viscera; laryngeal and pharyngeal muscles; sensory from trachea, esophagus, viscera, external ear, epiglottis (including taste)	GVE, SVE, GSA, GVA, SVA	Thyroidectomy, **PICA** infarct	Gag reflex (**uvula deviates away from lesion**)

(handwritten annotations: "motor", "Sensory ant ⅔ taste", "motor gag", "sensory post ⅓ taste")

(continued)

TABLE 1-4 Cranial Nerves (Continued)

Nerve	Site of exit from the skull	Function	Fiber types	Common lesions	Test
XI-Accessory	Jugular foramen	Sternocleido-mastoid and trapezius muscles	SVE	**PICA** infarct	Turning head (weakness turning away from lesion); raising shoulder against resistance (ipsilateral)
XII-Hypoglossal	Hypoglossal canal	Intrinsic tongue muscles	GSE	Anterior spinal artery infarct	Tongue protrusion **(deviates toward lesion)**

GSA=general somatic afferent; GSE=general somatic efferent; GVA=general visceral afferent; GVE=general visceral efferent; SSA=special somatic afferent; SVA=special visceral afferent; SVE=special visceral efferent

CONTENTS OF THE CAVERNOUS SINUS (Figure 1-13)

FIGURE
1-13   Contents of the cavernous sinus

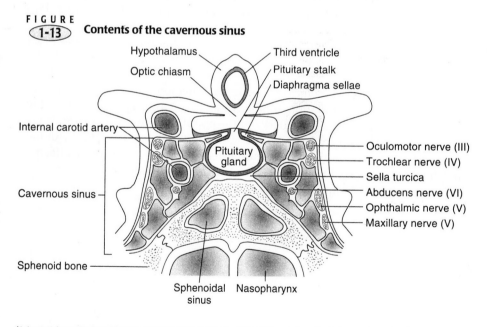

(Adapted from Bushan V, Le T, Amin C: First Aid for the USMLE Step 1. Stamford, Connecticut, Appleton & Lange, 1999. p. 110)

SLEEP (Figure 1-14)

FIGURE 1-14   The sleep cycle

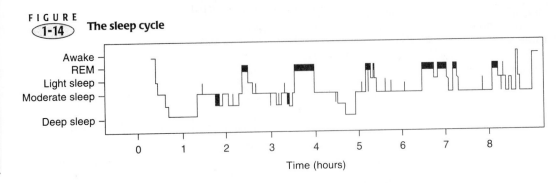

Stages of REM sleep in the young adult. As sleep progresses, slow wave sleep decreases and REM sleep episodes increase in duration and frequency. In the elderly, there is decreased slow wave sleep, increased awakenings, early sleep onset, and early morning awakenings. Solid bars indicate REM sleep.

QUICK HIT The time spent in REM sleep decreases with aging and with the use of some drugs (i.e., benzodiazepines).

QUICK HIT Slow wave sleep, which is the deepest, most relaxed sleep, is the sleep stage in which night terrors, bed-wetting, and sleepwalking occur.

Sleep-wake cycles are based on circadian rhythms controlled by the suprachiasmatic nucleus of the hypothalamus. **Serotonin** released from the raphe nuclei of the brain stem is important in initiating sleep, while the **reticular activating system** maintains alertness.

Stage 1 of sleep (when an individual is alert and relaxed) shows **alpha waves** on electroencephalograph (EEG). **Stages 3 and 4** of sleep are called delta sleep and show **slow waves** on EEG. Dreaming occurs during rapid eye movement (REM) sleep, which normally occurs at 90-minute intervals. During this period of "paradoxical sleep" the EEG registers beta waves which mirror those seen in the alert individual in the waking state.

The common sleep disorders include insomnia, narcolepsy, and sleep apnea. Insomnia affects 30% of the population. It is associated with anxiety and leads to daytime sleepiness. Narcolepsy is seen in 0.04% of the population and is characterized by sudden onset of sleep with rapid onset of REM sleep. It may be associated with hallucinations and cataplexy (sudden loss of muscle tone). Central sleep apnea, affecting less than 0.5% of the population, involves an absence of respiratory effort (for a discussion of obstructive sleep apnea, see Respiratory System.)

SEIZURE TYPES

Seizures are paroxysmal events caused by abnormal and excessive discharges from CNS neurons triggered by a variety of causes **(Table 1-5).**

TABLE 1-5	Seizure types			
Type	**Patient**	**Presentation**	**Pathology**	**Treatment**
Simple partial seizures	All ages	Malfunction of one muscle or muscle group No loss of consciousness Sensory distortions	Single focus in brain No spread, localized muscular manifestations With chronicity, may progress to generalized muscular manifestations	Phenytoin; carbamazepine
Jacksonian seizures	All ages (subtype of simple partial)	Expanding area of motor malfunction	Original focus spreads to adjacent areas of cortex	Carbamazepine
Complex partial seizures	First seizure during first two decades of life may be caused by fever in children 6 months to 5 years of age (febrile seizure)	Incontinence Jaw movements (or other automatisms) Loss of consciousness Elaborate sensory distortions	Single focus	Phenytoin; carbamazepine
Absence (petit mal) seizures	Begin at 2–3 years of age Often end with puberty	1–5 second loss of consciousness Several episodes per day Blank stare with rapid blinking	Original focus rapidly **spreads across both hemispheres**	Ethosuximide, valproic acid
Tonic clonic (grand mal) seizures	Most common type Encountered in different clinical settings, often in patients with metabolic disorders	Sudden loss of consciousness Loss of postural control and continence Tonic phase (static extension) Clonic phase (jerking movements) Recovery period with exhaustion and disorientation	Original focus rapidly spreads across both hemisphere	Phenytoin; carbamazepine

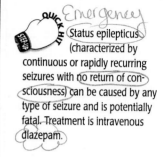

Emergency Status epilepticus (characterized by continuous or rapidly recurring seizures with no return of consciousness) can be caused by any type of seizure and is potentially fatal. Treatment is intravenous diazepam.

DEGENERATIVE DISEASES

Degeneration in specific parts of the CNS can lead to focal or systemic loss of function. Many of the degenerative diseases affecting the CNS are irreversible, and are listed in **Table 1-6**.

TABLE 1-6	Degenerative Diseases		
Disease	**Etiology**	**Clinical Manifestation**	**Notes**
Vitamin B12 deficiency	Strict vegetarian diet; **pernicious anemia;** fundal gastritis type A; *Diphyllobothrium latum*	**Megaloblastic anemia; peripheral neuropathy;** myelin **degeneration of posterior white columns** and lateral corticospinal tracts	Megaloblastic anemia, but not neuropathy, corrected with high doses of folate
Parkinson's disease	Unknown; similar symptoms may be due to depression, hydrocephaly, MPTP intoxication	**Resting tremors; masked facies; muscular rigidity;** shuffling gait; **Lewy bodies; decrease in dopamine** due to depletion of cells of substantia nigra and locus ceruleus	Usually appears after age 55; therapy with dopamine precursors or ACh inhibitors
Pick's disease	Autosomal dominant	Resembles Alzheimer's; **Pick's bodies** are seen; cerebral atrophy	Onset from 50–60 years of age; more frequent in women
Poliomyelitis	Poliovirus (RNA); fecal-oral; replicates in pharynx; spreads to CNS	Aseptic meningitis; **death of anterior horn cells** in spinal cord; paralysis	Killed (Salk) and live, attenuated (Sabin) vaccine available; Sabin vaccine given to children because of IgA response, longer action, and availability of oral form
Rabies	**Rhabdovirus** (RNA); spread via saliva	Laryngeal spasm resulting in fear of water; CNS excitability; **Negri body** inclusions; hippocampal degeneration	Treatment via passive and active immunization at distant sites
Spongiform encephalopathy Kuru **Creutzfeldt-Jakob** Subacute sclerosing panencephalitis (SSPE) Progressive multifocal leuko-encephalopathy	Slow virus infection; viral or prion Unknown agent, cannibals affected Prions, health care workers affected Persistent measles virus lacking M protein virus (papovavirus); infection of oligodendrocytes	Cerebellar degeneration; ataxia; dementia; demyelination; mental deficiency; **vacuolization of the brain**	No therapy; rapid death after onset

(continued)

TABLE 1-6 Degenerative Diseases *(Continued)*

Disease	Etiology	Clinical Manifestation	Notes
Tay-Sachs disease	Autosomal recessive; **deficiency of hexosaminidase A** with increase in GM_2 ganglioside	Mental retardation; **cherry-red spot on macula;** muscular weakness; seizures	Fatal; prenatal diagnosis possible; usually affects cells of CNS
Thiamine deficiency	Severe malnutrition (may be secondary to alcoholism)	**Degeneration of mamillary bodies** Wernicke's encephalopathy and Korsakoff's syndrome—psychosis manifested with confusion, ataxia, and confabulation Dry beri-beri—polyneuropathy with peripheral sensory/motor loss Wet beri-beri—dry beri-beri with cardiovascular symptoms	**Wernicke's** encephalopathy **(reversible)** and **Korsakoff's** syndrome **(irreversible)** are both secondary to deficiency caused by alcoholism
Wilson's disease	Autosomal recessive; **decreased ceruloplasmin**	Copper accumulation; liver cirrhosis; **Kayser-Fleischer ring** in cornea	Hepatolenticular **degeneration of the basal ganglia**

ACh=acetylcholione; *CSF*=cerebrospinal fluid; *CNS*=central nervous system; *GABA*=γ-aminobutyric acid; *HIV*=human immunodeficiency virus; *IgA*=immunoglobin A; *MPTP*=1-methyl-4-phenyl-1,2,3,6-tetrahydropyridine; *RNA*=ribonucleic acid

> **QUICK HIT** Niemann-Pick disease, a deficiency of **sphingomyelinase,** also presents with a **cherry-red spot** on the macula.

DEMYELINATING DISEASE

Loss of the neuronal sheath can lead to impaired nerve conduction, which in turn causes deficits and disease **(Table 1-7).**

TABLE 1-7 Demyelinating Diseases of the Nervous System

Disease	Etiology	Clinical Manifestation	Notes
Amyotrophic lateral sclerosis (ALS) (Lou Gehrig's disease)	No specific pattern of inheritance, though autosomal dominant in 5% of cases (similar symptoms with some heavy metal poisonings, infections, or tumors)	**Both upper and lower motor neuron signs;** loss of lateral corticospinal tracts and anterior motor neurons leading to muscle atrophy	Most common motor neuron disease; rapidly fatal course
Guillain-Barré syndrome	Post-viral autoimmune reaction involving peripheral nerves	Muscle weakness and paralysis **ascending upward** from the lower extremities	Young adults; **albuminocytologic dissociation** pathognomonic (high albumin, low cell count)

(continued)

> **QUICK HIT** Werdnig-Hoffmann disease is an infantile, autosomal recessive, lower motor neuron disease similar to ALS.

TABLE 1-7 Demyelinating Diseases of the Nervous System *(Continued)*

Disease	Etiology	Clinical Manifestation	Notes
Huntington's disease	Chromosome 4; **C-A-G triple base repeat** with anticipation	Degeneration of **caudate nucleus;** onset at 30–40 years of age; athetoid movements; muscular deterioration; dementia	Usually involves ACh and GABA neurons
Krabbe's disease	Autosomal recessive; decrease in β-galactocerebrosidase	Loss of myelin from globoid cells and peripheral nerves; mental retardation; blindness; paralysis; **globoid bodies** in white matter	Usually affects infants; **rapidly fatal**
Metachromatic leukodystrophy	Autosomal recessive defect of arylsulfatase A	Progressive paralysis and dementia; loss of myelin; accumulation of sulfatides; nerves stain **yellow-brown** in color; ataxia	Fatal in first decade
Multiple sclerosis	Unknown; more common in northern Europe; more common in women	Multiple focal areas of demyelination; variable course; **Charcot's triad:** intention tremor, scanning speech, nystagmus	Most common demyelinating disease; increased CSF immunoglobulin

ACh=acetylcholine; *CSF*=cerebrospinal fluid; *CNS*=central nervous system; *GABA*=γ-aminobutyric acid

The triad of jaundice, right upper quadrant (RUQ) pain, and fever is also known as Charcot's triad and is associated with cholangitis.

DISEASES CAUSING DEMENTIA

Dementia is a deterioration in cognitive ability where mental faculties, such as attention span, judgment, memory, mood, and behavior are affected. Dementia is a chronic condition **(Table 1-8).**

TABLE 1-8 Diseases Causing Dementia

Disease	Etiology	Clinical Manifestation	Notes
Dementia due to HIV disease	Macrophages, infected with HIV, enter CNS	Onset prior to immunodeficiency; slow thinking; ataxia; *Toxoplasma gondii* on autopsy	**Most common CNS manifestation of HIV**
Dementia of the Alzheimer type	Unknown; possibly **chromosome 21;** degeneration of nucleus basalis of Meynert; decreased choline acetyltransferase	Progressively worsening memory loss; **neurofibrillary tangles; senile plaques** (amyloid beta / **A4** protein); Hirano bodies	**Most common cause of dementia;** age of onset is usually 65 years (younger in Down syndrome patients)
Multi-infarct dementia	Cerebral atherosclerosis	Sudden onset; intermittent signs of dementia and motor deficits	**Second most common cause of dementia** (most common is Alzheimer's)

CNS=central nervous system; *HIV*=human immunodeficiency virus

Dementia is loss of cognitive function without an altered level of consciousness. Delirium is an altered level of consciousness accompanied by disordered cognition.

Toxoplasma gondii can infect the immunocompromised individual via 3 routes: undercooked meat, cat feces, or in utero. It is the most common CNS infection in AIDS patients.

ACUTE MENINGITIS

Meningitis is an infection of the meninges resulting in an inflammatory reaction characterized by severe headache, fever, photophobia, and positive **Kernig's** and **Brudzinski's signs.** Immunocompetent adults generally have *Streptococcus pneumoniae* or *Neisseria meningitidis* as the cause of their meningitis. Conditions predisposing an individual to acute bacterial meningitis due to pneumococcus include: distant foci of infection (such as otitis, sinusitis, or pneumonia), sickle cell disease (due to asplenism), alcoholism, or trauma with loss of meningeal integrity. Patients with a deficiency of complement components C5-C8 are at a greater risk of developing meningococcal meningitis. *Haemophilus influenzae* is a common cause of meningitis in children, although these numbers are decreasing due to widespread use of a capsular polyribitol phosphate vaccine conjugated to diphtheria toxoid **(Table 1-9).**

TABLE 1-9	Causes of Meningitis in Various Age Groups
Age Group	**Causes**
Newborns	Group B streptococci *Escherichia coli* Listeria
Children	*Haemophilus influenzae B* *Streptococcus pneumoniae* *Neisseria meningitidis* Enteroviruses
Adolescents and Young Adults	Enteroviruses *Neisseria meningitidis* *Streptococcus pneumoniae* Herpes simplex virus
Elderly	*Streptococcus pneumoniae* Gram-negative rods Listeria

Immunocompromised adults are at a risk for developing meningitis due to *Listeria monocytogenes*. A lumbar puncture showing organisms with a thick capsule when stained with india ink suggests *Cryptococcus neoformans* is the causal organism and the infected individual is most likely immunocompromised due to HIV infection. A lumbar puncture (LP) is often performed to confirm a suspected diagnosis of meningitis. The LP usually shows increased neutrophils, increased protein, and decreased glucose. However, if the cerebrospinal fluid (CSF) contains increased lymphocytes and a normal glucose level, viral factors such as enterovirus, human immunodeficiency virus (HIV), or herpes simplex virus type 2 (HSV-2) should be considered **(Table 1-10).**

TABLE 1-10 Evaluation of Cerebrospinal Fluid to Determine the Cause of Meningitis

Laboratory Test	Finding indicating bacterial cause	Finding indicating viral cause	Finding indicating fungal cause
CSF Pressure	↑	N	↑
Lymphocytes	N	↑	↑
Neutrophils	↑	N	N
Glucose	↓	N	↓
Protein	↑	N	↑

↑=increased; ↓=decreased; N=normal

NERVOUS SYSTEM TUMORS

Nearly 50% of the tumors occurring within the nervous system are primary tumors. **Table 1-11** lists nervous system tumors in order of clinical significance.

TABLE 1-11 Nervous System Tumors

Tumor	Presentation	Significant Features
Glioblastoma multiforme (Grade IV astrocytoma)	Cerebral hemisphere tumor; irregular mass with necrotic center surrounded by edema seen on CT; **pseudopalisading** arrangement of cells	**Most common primary intracranial neoplasm;** poor prognosis; neural tube origin
Meningioma	**Psammoma bodies;** slowly growing; originates in arachnoid cells; follows sinuses	Second most common primary CNS tumor; usually occurs in women; resectable; neural crest origin
Medulloblastoma	Ataxic gait; projectile vomiting; cerebellar mass; highly malignant; tightly packed cells in rosette pattern	**Most common intracranial tumor of childhood;** neural tube origin
Retinoblastoma (Rb)	Retinal tumor in children	**Two-hit theory** = Rb is a tumor suppressor gene; require deletion of both copies (chromosome 13); neural tube origin
Craniopharyngioma	Papilledema; endocrine abnormalities; **bitemporal hemianopsia**	Enlarged sella turcica; **most common supratentorial brain tumor in children; ectodermal origin** (Rathke's pouch)
Schwannoma	Hearing loss; ataxic gait; positive Romberg's sign; increased intracranial pressure; hydrocephalus; benign	Usually occurs in the cerebellopontine angle and involves CN VIII; seen **bilaterally in NF-2;** third most common primary intracranial tumor; neural crest origin
Neuroblastoma	Occurs in cerebral hemispheres; related to neuroblastoma of adrenal gland	Increasing **N-myc amplification** directly proportional to worsening prognosis; seen in children; neural crest origin

(continued)

QUICK HIT

Tumors of the CNS are usually intracranial, with **adult tumors** commonly **supratentorial** and **childhood** tumors usually **infratentorial.**

QUICK HIT

Psammoma bodies are also seen in papillary adenocarcinoma of the thyroid, serous papillary cystadenocarcinoma of the ovary, and malignant mesothelioma.

TABLE 1-11	Nervous System Tumors *(Continued)*	
Tumor	**Presentation**	**Significant Features**
Ependymoma	Hydrocephalus; blocked 4th ventricle; rosettes surround 4th ventricle	Seen in children; neural tube origin
Metastatic neoplasms	Headache; focal defects; formation of discrete nodules in brain	Nearly half of all intracranial neoplasm; usually blood borne; commonly from lung, breast, GI, thyroid, kidney, GU, and melanoma

CNS=central nervous system; *CT*=computed tomography; *GI*=gastrointestinal; *GU*=genitourinary; *NF-2*=neurofibromatosis-type 2

NERVOUS SYSTEM THERAPEUTICS

Autonomic Nervous System and Neuromuscular Junction Therapeutics

Acetylcholine
Albuterol
Amphetamine
Atenolol
Atropine
Clonidine
Cocaine
Dobutamine
Dopamine

d-Tubocurare
Epinephrine
Ipratropium
Isoproterenol
Muscarine
Neostigmine
Nicotine
Norepinephrine
Phenylephrine

Physostigmine
Pilocarpine
Prazosin
Propanolol
Reserpine
Scopolamine
Succinylcholine
Terbutaline

Anticancer Therapeutics

CCNU (N-(2-chlorethyl)-N-cyclo-hexyl-N-nitrosourea)

Cytosine arabinoside
Methotrexate

Thiotepa
Vincristine

Antidepressant Therapeutics

Amitriptyline
Fluoxetine
Imipramine

Nortriptyline
Paroxetine

Sertraline
Tranylcypromine

Anti-epileptic Therapeutics

Carbamazepine
Diazepam

Ethosuximide
Phenobarbital

Phenytoin
Valproic acid

Anti-manic Therapeutics

Lithium

Antimicrobial Therapeutics

Acyclovir
Ampicillin
Cephalosporin

Chloramphenicol
Gentamicin
Penicillin G

Valacyclovir
Vancomycin

Anti-psychotic Therapeutics

Chlorpromazine
Clozapine

Fluphenazine
Haloperidol

Risperidone
Thioridazine

Anxiolytic Therapeutics

Alprazolam	Flumazenil	Oxazepam
Chlordiazepoxide	(antagonist)	Buspirone
Diazepam	Lorazepam	

CNS and PNS (Endogenous) Therapeutics

Acetylcholine	Dopamine	Norepinephrine
Adenosine	GABA	Serotonin (5-HT)
Aspartate	Glutamate	
Bradykinin	Histamine	

CNS Stimulants

Amphetamine	Cocaine	Ephedrine
Caffeine		

General Anesthetics (Inhalation and Intravenous)

Alfentanil	Isoflurane	Nitrous Oxide
Enflurane	Ketamine	Propofol
Fentanyl	Midazolam	
Halothane	Morphine	

Local Anesthetics

Benzocaine	Lidocaine	Procaine

Opioids

Agonists	Morphine	Nalbuphine
Codeine		Naloxone
Diphenoxylate	*Mixed or Antagonists*	Naltrexone
Meperidine	Buprenorphine	Pentazocine
Methadone	Butorphanol	

Drugs for Treatment of Parkinson's Disease

Amantadine	Carbidopa/Levodopa	Selegiline
Benztropine	Pergolide	Trihexyphenidyl
Bromocriptine		

Sedative-Hypnotics

Flurazepam	Temazepam	Zolpidem
Phenobarbital	Triazolam	

PSYCHIATRY AND BEHAVIORAL SCIENCE

● Drugs of Abuse and Dependence (Table 1-12)

Quick Hit

Substance abuse is defined as use of psychoactive substances for at least 1 month with interference in the user's life, but without meeting the criteria for dependence. Substance dependence involves craving, withdrawal, and tolerance.

TABLE 1-12 Drugs of Abuse and Dependence

Drug	Mechanism	Intoxication Effect	Withdrawal Effects
Alcohol	Unknown; possible effect at GABA receptor directly on membranes	Sedation; hypnosis; slurred speech; ataxia; loss of motor coordination; Wernicke-Korsakoff syndrome	Malaise; tachycardia; tremors; seizures; **delirium tremens;** death

(continued)

TABLE 1-12 **Drugs of Abuse and Dependence** *(Continued)*

Drug	Mechanism	Intoxication Effect	Withdrawal Effects
Amphetamine	Release of intracellular stores of catecholamines	Insomnia; irritability; tremor; hyperactive reflexes; arrhythmias; anorexia; psychosis	Lethargy; depression; hunger; craving for drug resulting in bizarre psychological behavior; anxiety
Barbiturates	**Potentiation of GABA** action on chloride by **increase of duration** of chloride channel opening	Mental sluggishness; anesthesia; hypnosis	Restlessness; anxiety; tremor; death
Caffeine	Translocation of Ca²⁺; inhibition of phosphodiesterase (increase in cAMP, cGMP)	Insomnia; anxiety; agitation	Lethargy; irritability; headache
Cocaine	Blockade of norepinephrine, serotonin, and dopamine re-uptake	Hallucinations; anxiety; arrhythmias; nasal problems; sudden death	Craving; depression; excessive sleeping; fatigue
LSD	5-HT agonist action in the midbrain	Pupillary dilation; increased blood pressure and body temperature; piloerection; hallucinations	Flashbacks
Marijuana	Unknown; THC is active compound; possible endogenous receptors in brain	Increased appetite; visual hallucinations; increased heart rate; decreased blood pressure Impairment of short-term memory and mental activity	
Nicotine	Low doses—ganglionic stimulation; high doses—ganglionic blockade	**Increased heart rate and blood pressure;** irritability; tremors; intestinal cramps	Irritability; anxiety; restlessness; headaches; insomnia; difficulty in concentrating
Opioids (heroin)	Inhibition of adenylate cyclase by opioid receptors within the CNS	Constipation; **pinpoint pupils;** potentially lethal via **respiratory depression;** sedation	Insomnia; diarrhea; sweating; fever; piloerection
Phencyclidine (PCP)	Inhibition of dopamine, serotonin, and norepinephrine re-uptake	Hostile, bizarre behavior; hypersalivation; anesthesia	Sudden onset of violent behavior

cAMP=cyclic adenosine monophosphate; *cGMP*=cyclic guanosine monophosphate; *GABA*=γ-aminobutyric acid; *5-HT*=5-hydroxy tryptamine (serotonin); *LSD*=lysergic acid diethylamide; *THC*=tetrahydrocanniabinol

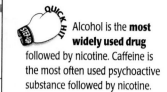 Alcohol is the **most widely used drug** followed by nicotine. Caffeine is the most often used psychoactive substance followed by nicotine.

Dependence is mediated by dopamine, the neurotransmitter linked to the pleasure and reward center.

● Defense Mechanisms (Table 1-13)

TABLE 1-13 Defense Mechanisms

Mechanism	Characteristics	Example
Acting out	Stress is dealt with through actions; immature	After the death of his brother, a priest breaks all the windows in his church
Denial	Not accepting the reality of a situation; immature	A single woman refuses to consider the possibility of pregnancy after having unprotected intercourse and missing two periods
Displacement	Feelings for causal source are transferred to another object; immature	A man kicks his dog after getting fired from his job
Dissociation	Loss of memory or change in personality due to stressor; immature	A woman who was sexually abused as a child develops another personality
Identification	Behavior patterned after another; immature	A teenager smokes pot because his favorite rock star does
Intellectualization	Reason is used to cope with anxiety; immature	A pediatrician starts reading textbooks and journal articles about his wife's cancer
Isolation of affect	Events are separated from emotion; immature	An airline passenger describes an emergency landing to his family without any emotion
Projection	One's own characteristics are applied to another; immature	A flirtatious man accuses his wife of cheating
Rationalization	Analytical reason is used to justify unacceptable feelings; immature	A man claims that his DUI arrest would never have happened if his softball team had won
Reaction formation	Feelings are denied and opposite actions are performed; immature	A woman who wants to cheat on her husband instead buys him a new car
Regression	Stress-induced behavior that involves returning to a child-like state; immature	Medical students have a food fight during their lunch break on the day of board examinations
Repression	Holding back an unacceptable feeling or idea from reaching consciousness; immature	A recent widower feels no sense of loss
Splitting	Feelings or stressors are placed in distinct, opposite compartments (i.e., either all good or all bad); immature	A woman in a doctor's office describes how much she hates the nurses, but loves the receptionist, hates her boss and co-workers, but loves the security guard
Altruism	One unselfishly assists others; mature	A woman donates her entire estate to her favorite charities upon her death
Humor	Humor is used to reduce stress; mature	While stuck in an elevator, a young man makes jokes to ease the tension
Sublimation	Unacceptable impulse is directed into a socially accepted action; mature	A boy getting into a lot of fights as a kid decides to become a professional boxer
Suppression	Conscious effort to suppress thoughts or feelings; mature	A recent widower actively refuses to think about his deceased wife while packing her things away

● Personality Disorders (Table 1-14)

TABLE 1-14	Personality Disorders	
Disorder	**Characteristics**	**Example**
CLUSTER A Paranoid	Hostile; suspicious; mistrustful; usually male	A patient being readied for surgery yells at the doctor on rounds because he feels they are gossiping about him
Schizoid	Voluntarily socially withdrawn without psychological problems; usually male	A 52-year-old computer programmer lives alone, is not married, has no friends, and is content
Schizotypal	Odd behavior, thoughts, and appearance without psychosis	A woman wears much layered clothing and inappropriately applied makeup, and only talks to people with brown-colored hair
CLUSTER B Histrionic	Dramatic; overemotional; sexually provocative; unable to maintain close friendships; usually female	A woman exaggerates her suffering over a mild cold, and behaves seductively toward physician
Narcissistic	Grandiosity, hypersensitivity to criticism, and lack of empathy	A resident refuses to put an IV line in an uninsured child because he feels it is beneath him and he only wishes to operate with the best surgeon in the hospital
Antisocial	Inability to conform to societal rules; criminal behavior; more often males	A multiple rapist has no concern for his victims or the law
Borderline	Unstable; impulsive; suicide attempts; usually female	After an argument with her boyfriend, a woman chases him out of her home with a frying pan and then calls him at home and tells him she loves him
CLUSTER C Avoidant	Shy; withdrawn; fear of rejection; usually female	A businesswoman defers speaking during presentations to her project partner and has few friends
Obsessive-compulsive	Rigid; perfectionist; stubborn; orderly. Found twice as often in males	A businessman works long hours on a project, holding up both the project deadline and his personal life, in vain attempts to make it perfect
Dependent	Defers decision-making; not comfortable with an authority position; insecure; usually female	A third-year resident often accepts on-call duty for other residents, never speaks up when talked down to by the junior residents, and has trouble writing orders
Passive-aggressive	Obstinate; inefficient; procrastinating; non-compliant	School student intentionally does poorly on homework because he does not like teacher

● Psychoses and Other Neuropsychiatric Disorders (Table 1-15)

TABLE 1-15 Psychoses and Other Neuropsychiatric Disorders

Disorder	Characteristics	Neurotransmitter(s) Involved	Treatment	Notes
Anorexia nervosa	Body weight less than 85% of predicted		Antidepressants; cyproheptadine; family therapy	Higher incidence in females and **upper middle socioeconomic classes;** amenorrhea; decreased libido
Attention-deficit hyper-activity disorder (ADHD)	Hyperactive; poor attention span; highly sensitive to stimuli		Amphetamines (methylphenidate)	More common in **male children**
Bipolar disorder	Rapid speech, decreased need for sleep, hyper-energetic state, impaired judgment followed by a state of depression	Decreased serotonin	**Lithium**	
Bulimia nervosa	Purging after binge eating; **normal weight;** abuse of laxatives		Behavioral therapy; psychotherapy fluoxetine; MAOI	Normal libido; no amenorrhea (unlike anorexics); erosion of tooth enamel
Delirium	Impaired cognitive processes; diurnal variation in mood (worse at night— **"sundowning"**); illusions and hallucinations	Autonomic dysfunction	Treat the underlying cause	**Most common** problem in hospitalized psychiatric patients
Dissociative disorders	Psychological factors resulting in memory loss and loss of function		Psychotherapy; hypnotherapy; medication for associated symptoms	Includes: amnesia, fugue, identity disorder, depersonalization
Generalized anxiety disorder	Generalized, persistent anxiety; tension; insomnia; irritability	Decreased serotonin, norepinephrine, GABA	Buspirone; benzodiazepines; **SSRI's**	Anxiety for more than **6 months**
Major depressive disorder	**Early morning waking;** anhedonia; depressed mood; suicidal thoughts	Decreased norepinephrine and serotonin	SSRI's; TCA's or MAOI's; electroconvulsive therapy; hospitalization	Decreased REM latency and slow wave sleep; more common in women

(continued)

Dissociative disorders result in retrograde amnesia, while head trauma results in anterograde amnesia.

TABLE 1-15 Psychoses and Other Neuropsychiatric Disorders *(Continued)*

Disorder	Characteristics	Neurotransmitter(s) Involved	Treatment	Notes
Obesity	120% of total predicted body weight		Dieting and exercise; strict fad dieting ineffective; surgery not useful	Lower socioeconimic groups; genetics play a role; increased risk of disease
Obsessive-compulsive disorder	Recurrent thoughts and actions; patients are distressed by repetitive actions	Decreased serotonin	Behavioral therapy; clomipramine; trazodone; SSRI's	EEG changes
Panic disorder	Discrete, episodic periods of intense anxiety or discomfort; palpitations; chest pain; sweating; fear of dying	Decreased serotonin, norepinephrine, GABA	Imipramine; behavior therapy	Associated with mitral valve prolapse; young women predominantly affected; genetic component
Phobias	Irrational, situational fear	Decreased serotonin, norepinephrine, and GABA	Systemic desensitization; propranolol useful for physiologic manifestations	
Post-traumatic stress disorder (PTSD)	Result of trauma; hypervigilance; nightmares; flashbacks	Decreased serotonin, norepinephrine, and GABA	Counseling; group therapy; benzodiaze-pines for symptoms	The first 3 months after the trauma is acute PTSD; symptoms lasting longer than 3 months after the trauma is chronic PTSD
Schizophrenia	Autism; blunted affect; loose associations; ambivalence; auditory hallucinations; **negative symptoms** (i.e., flattened affect, lack of motivation, withdrawal); **positive symptoms** (i.e., hallucinations, hyperexcitability	Increased dopamine; increased norepinephrine in paranoid schizophrenia	Antipsychotics with a trial period of 3–5 weeks; clozapine has decreased extrapyramidal side effects (as opposed to haloperidol)	Occurs in young adults; enlarged lateral and 3rd ventricles; patients oriented ×3 (person, place, and time); types include disorganized, catatonic, and paranoid

QUICK HIT

Münchausen's syndrome is a factitious disorder where the patient fakes illness in order to receive medical attention. An example would be a nurse purposely injecting him or herself with insulin to receive medical attention. **Münchausen's by proxy** is a syndrome whereby the attention seeker feigns or creates illness in another, usually his or her child, to gain medical attention.

TABLE 1-15 Psychoses and Other Neuropsychiatric Disorders *(Continued)*

Disorder	Characteristics	Neurotransmitter(s) Involved	Treatment	Notes
Somatoform disorders	Symptoms of disease occur without related pathology		Psychotherapy and therapeutics may help; variable response	Patients truly believe in having illness whereas factitious disorders are the result of faking illness
Tourette's syndrome	Involuntary motor and vocal movements	Improper dopamine regulation	Haloperidol	Onset occurs in childhood

EEG=electroencephalograph; *MAOI*=monoamine oxidase inhibitor; *GABA*=γ-aminobutyric acid; *SSRI*=selective serotonin reuptake inhibitor; *TCA*= tricyclic antidepressant

● **Non-pharmacological Therapeutic Modalities (Table 1-16)**

TABLE 1-16 Non-Pharmacologic Therapeutic Modalities

Therapy	Characteristics	Notes
Biofeedback	Gaining control over physiology via continuous information; motivation and practice required	Used for hypertension, migraine headaches, and tension headaches
Classical conditioning	A **reflexive, natural behavior** is elicited in **response to a learned stimulus;** (e.g., ringing of a bell causing salivation)	**Aversive conditioning** pairs an unwanted response to a painful stimulus; stages include acquisition, extinction, and recovery
Cognitive therapy	**Negative thinking** is reorganized into self-affirming, positive thoughts	Short-term psychotherapy used to treat depression and anxiety
Electroconvulsive therapy (ECT)	Electric current introduced into brain to alter neurotransmitter function; improvement seen faster than with pharmacological regimens	Used for **major depression;** safe; effective; retrograde amnesia is major side effect
Operant conditioning	Behavior that is not part of the natural repertoire is learned by altering the reward **(reinforcement)**	Reinforcement can be positive or negative; reward schedule includes continuous, fixed, or variable
Psychoanalysis	Intensive treatment based on recovering and integrating past experiences from the unconscious via free association; based on **Freud's theories**	**Id**—sexual drives and aggression; **ego**—controls instinct and interacts with the world; **superego**—morality and conscience
Systemic desensitization	Classical conditioning technique where relaxation procedures are combined with increasing doses of anxiety-provoking stimuli	Used to **eliminate** phobias
Token economy	Positive reinforcement where a reward is used to elicit a desired response	Seen often in mental hospitals or parents dealing with children

QUICK HIT

Behavior learned through a variable interval schedule of reinforcement is most difficult to extinguish. Behavior learned through a fixed schedule is easiest to extinguish.

ETHICS AND THE ROLE OF THE PHYSICIAN

The role of the nervous system in the manifestation of psychological problems is under debate. The occurrence of certain psychopathology has been linked to neurotransmitters and the lack of regulation in certain parts of the CNS.

Communication skills are essential to determine physical and psychological problems of patients. Establishing trust and confidence via facilitation, reflection, and an open-ended clinical interview allows the physician to gather physical, psychological, and social information. If an individual suffers from psychopathology, proper steps must be taken not to alienate, offend, or judge the patient. On the other hand, the individual's problems must be dealt with directly.

When presenting therapeutic options or advice, the physician should be forthright, direct, and honest. In making an assessment of any patient, the physician needs to be aware of the problems afflicting certain groups. For instance, it is important to remember that in elderly patients, sexual changes occur (i.e., men have slower erections and women have increased vaginal dryness and decreased vaginal length), sleep may decrease, suicide rate may increase, and depression becomes more prevalent.

Although the physician must be **nonmaleficent** (not intending to do harm) and **beneficent** (doing what's best for the patient), patient autonomy ultimately prevails in making the final decision about treatment. The physician must consider the patient's ability to make decisions based on communication skills, level of understanding about medicine, stability, consistency, and soundness of mind. Physicians have a **duty** to provide medical care to their patients and if **breach** of this duty directly leads to **damage,** the physician has been **negligent** and therefore is **liable** for malpractice. The breach of duty due to negligence and the damages caused by it represent a **tort.**

Prior to making a final decision regarding patient care, physicians should make an effort to obtain an **informed consent** which indicates that the patient understands the risks and benefits of therapy. Disheartening as it may be, terminal disease may require the physician to explain to the patient and his family that further intervention is not appropriate since maximal treatment has failed and it seems to be a reasonable conclusion that the goals of care will not be reached. **Advance directives** from the patient, either written or oral, may assist the physician in coming to a conclusion about when to terminate treatment measures.

Information about the patient must remain confidential unless the patient poses a risk to self or to others; information concerning the patient's own disease, diagnosis, or prognosis cannot be withheld from the patient, despite the wishes of the family.

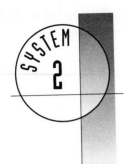

The Cardiovascular System

DEVELOPMENT

I. Heart

A. The cardiovascular system is derived from the mesoderm.

B. Paired **endocardial heart tubes** form in the cephalic region of the embryo.

C. Lateral and cephalocaudal folding causes the heart tubes to join together and lie in a ventral location, between the primitive mouth and the foregut.

D. The primitive heart dilates into five areas, shown in Figure 2-1. The five embryologic regions and their adult derivatives are as follows.

FIGURE 2-1 **Embryological development of the heart**

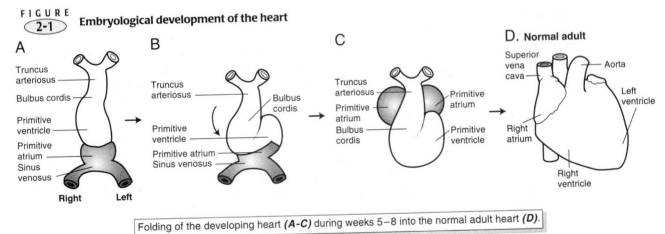

Folding of the developing heart **(A-C)** during weeks 5−8 into the normal adult heart **(D)**.

(Adapted from Dudek RW, Fix JD: *BRS Embryology*, 2nd ed. Baltimore, Williams & Wilkins, 1998.)

1. **Truncus arteriosus** → proximal aorta and proximal pulmonary artery
2. **Bulbus cordis** → smooth parts of the right ventricle (conus arteriosus) and left ventricles
3. **Primitive ventricle** → right and left ventricles
4. **Primitive atrium** → right and left atria
5. **Sinus venosus** → smooth part of right atrium, the coronary sinus, and oblique vein

E. The lumen of the truncus arteriosus and bulbus cordis is divided into the aorta and pulmonary trunk by the **aorticopulmonary septum.**

F. The septum primum, septum secundum, and atriovenous (AV) cushion form the atrial septum.

G. The **foramen ovale** is a communication between the right and left atria that is formed by the walls of the septum primum and septum secundum.

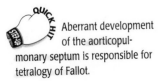

Aberrant development of the aorticopulmonary septum is responsible for tetralogy of Fallot.

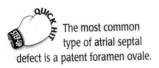

The most common type of atrial septal defect is a patent foramen ovale.

1. It allows blood to flow from the venous side of the circulation to the arterial side without passing through the lungs due to higher pressure on the venous side during gestation.
2. **After birth,** the foramen ovale **closes** due to increased arterial pressure which pushes the septum primum against the atrial septum.
H. The aorticopulmonary septum, the right and left bulbar ridges, and the atrioventricular cushion form the interventricular septum.

II. Arterial Vessels

A. **Aortic arches.** Initially, there are 6 paired aortic arches. Arches 3, 4, and 6 play a significant role in the adult.
   1. Arch 3 helps to form the adult common carotid arteries bilaterally.
   2. **Arch 4** helps to form the **aorta** on the left and the proximal subclavian artery on the right.
   3. **Arch 6** helps to form the **ductus arteriosus** and part of the **pulmonary trunk.**
B. **Paired dorsal aortae** are paired vessels that run along the length of the embryo. They coalesce to form the descending aorta.

III. Venous Vessels

A. The paired vitelline, umbilical, and cardinal veins form the definitive adult structures.
B. The **vitelline veins** help form the ductus venosus and hepatic sinusoids, the inferior vena cava, the portal vein, and the superior and inferior mesenteric veins.
C. **Umbilical veins**
   1. No adult vascular structures are formed by these veins.
   2. The left umbilical vein connects to the ductus venosus and carries oxygenated blood from the placenta to the fetus.
   3. Left umbilical vein gives rise to ligamentum teres.
D. **Cardinal veins**
   1. The anterior cardinal veins help form the internal jugular vein and the superior vena cava.
   2. The posterior cardinal veins help form the inferior vena cava, common iliac veins, azygos vein, and renal veins.

QUICK HIT

The umbilical circulation is one of the only places in the body (along with the pulmonary circulation) where an artery does not carry oxygenated blood. The paired umbilical arteries carry deoxygenated blood to the placenta while the **singular umbilical vein** brings oxygenated blood back to the fetus.

[Handwritten notes:]

R→L shunts   3T's   (PROVe)
- tetrology of Fellot
- transposition of GV   mother w/ diabetes } early cyanosis
- truncus arteriosus

pulm sten / VH / overid aorta / SD

L→R shunts   VSD > ASD > PDA. } late cyanosis
can lead to R→L Eisenmenger syndrome.

● **Fetal Circulation (Figure 2-2)**

FIGURE
2-2 **Fetal circulation**

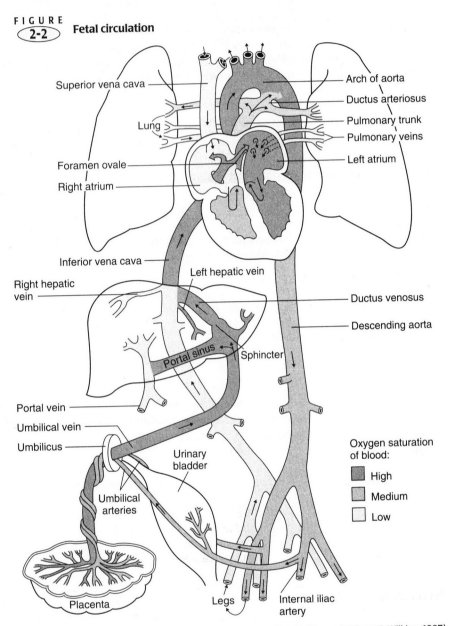

(Adapted from Lilly LS: *Pathophysiology of Heart Disease,* 2nd edition. Baltimore, Williams & Wilkins, 1997.)

● **Congenital Defects of the Heart and Great Vessels (Table 2-1)**

QUICK HIT

Down syndrome is associated with endocardial cushion defects, which may manifest as atrial septal defect (ASD) or ventral septal defect (VSD).

TABLE 2-1	Congenital Defects of the Heart and Great Vessels

Anomaly	Pathology	Clinical Presentation	Notes
Atrial septal defect (ASD)	**Secundum ASD** (defect of septum primum or septum secundum) Primum ASD (low) Sinus venosus ASD (high)	**Left to right shunt;** asymptomatic into 4th decade; murmur; right ventricular hypertrophy	Much higher incidence in females (3:1); 90% are secundum type

murmur heard @ pulm (systolic) tricuspid (diastolic)

(continued)

TABLE 2-1 Congenital Defects of the Heart and Great Vessels *(Continued)*

Anomaly	Pathology	Clinical Presentation	Notes
Coarctation of the aorta ↑ UL ↓ LL	Infantile (proximal to PDA); adult (constriction at closed ductus arteriosus, distal to origin of left subclavian artery)	Symptoms depend on extent of narrowing; infant presents with lower limb cyanosis and right heart failure at birth; adult asymptomatic with upper limb hypertension, rib notching on radiograph from collateral circulation through intercostal arteries, and **weak pulses in lower limbs**	Much higher incidence in males (3:1) and females with **Turner's syndrome** -45 XO -web neck -dwarf -amenorrhea -fibrous streak
Patent ductus arteriosus (PDA) L → R	Failure of closure of the ductus arteriosus; may be due to premature birth with **hypoxemia** or structural defects	Continuous **machinery murmur**	Second most common CHD VSD > ASD > PDA
Tetralogy of Fallot R → L (ulm stenlo VRH ver aorta ver VSD) PROVe	Defective development of the infundibular septum; Results in **overriding aorta, ventricular septal defect, pulmonary stenosis, hypertrophy of the right ventricle**	Cyanosis (may not be present at birth); right-to-left shunt; boot-shaped heart	Survival to adulthood possible; patient assumes **squatting position** to relieve symptoms
Transposition of the great vessels R → L	Aorta drains right ventricle; pulmonary artery from left ventricle; **separate pulmonary and systemic circuits**	Incompatible with life unless shunt present; cyanosis (present at birth)	caused usually by Diabetic mother
Ventricular septal defect (VSD) L → R	Membranous VSD Single muscular VSD	Left to right shunt; **loud holosystolic murmur means small defect;** large defects can present as heart failure at birth; small defects can close spontaneously	Much higher incidence in males; most common congenital heart defect (33%); 90% are membranous type

CHD=congenital heart defects; *PDA*=patent ductus arteriosus

PHYSIOLOGY AND PATHOLOGY OF HEART FUNCTION

Properly timed and integrated myocyte contraction is essential to normal heart function. Cardiac myocytes (Figure 2-3) have **gap junctions** that allow for rapid relay of electrical signals between them. Electrical impulses are transmitted via the electrical conduction system composed of the sinoatrial (SA) node, atrioventricular (AV) node, and His-Purkinje cells (Figure 2-4). Normally, the sinoatrial node is the pacemaker of the heart. The node exhibits automaticity in which spontaneous **phase 4 depolarization** generates rhythmic action potentials (APs). These electrical signals propagate from the SA node through the atrial tissue and cause it to contract. Further propagation leads to excitation of the AV node, the ventricular bundles, and lastly the

→ Na slow depolarizes in

THE CARDIOVASCULAR SYSTEM

FIGURE
2-3

Histology of cardiac myocyte. A longitudinal section of cardial muscle cells is shown.

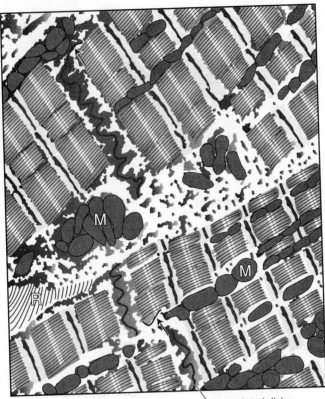

Intercalated disks

↑=arrowheads indicate location of gap junctions; *M*=mitochondria; *R*=reticular fibers.

ventricular tissue. The nodal tissues are dependent on Ca^{2+} for their phase 0 depolarization while the muscular cardiac tissue uses Na^+ for phase 0 excitation. The AV node transmits APs more slowly than the SA node. This feature provides for three important functions. It causes the atria to contract before the ventricles, while allowing time for the ventricles to repolarize and prepare to receive their next electrical signal. Furthermore, it prevents excessively rapid beats from reaching and damaging the ventricular tissue. The conduction system of the heart can best be visualized on an electrocardiogram (ECG). ECG plots can determine disturbances along the cardiac conduction path.

Chronotropic effects on the heart cause a change in heart rate by affecting the rate of depolarization of the SA node. **Inotropic** effects cause a change in contractility of the heart. Greater contractility allows the heart to squeeze harder and increase cardiac output. Increased intracellular Ca^{2+}, either drug-mediated or due to sympathetic β-receptor stimulation, allows for an increased inotropic effect. The preload and afterload also affect the function of the heart. A greater **preload** due to increased filling of the ventricles causes additional stretch of the myocytes, which induces stronger contraction and has a positive effect on contractility. **Afterload** is equivalent to aortic pressure. It is influenced by the total peripheral resistance of the body. A higher afterload means the heart must work harder or cardiac output will fall. The cardiovascular system is constantly working to maintain homeostatic equilibrium.

Hormonal systems also respond to changes in homeostasis. A major influence on cardiac work is exerted by the **renin-angiotensin-aldosterone (RAA) axis.** Whereas the baroreceptors attempt to maintain adequate pressures in the vascular system over a short-term period, the RAA system helps to regulate pressure over a longer period of time. The RAA axis responds to changes in arterial pressure by altering salt and

FIGURE 2-4 Heart anatomy and signal conduction

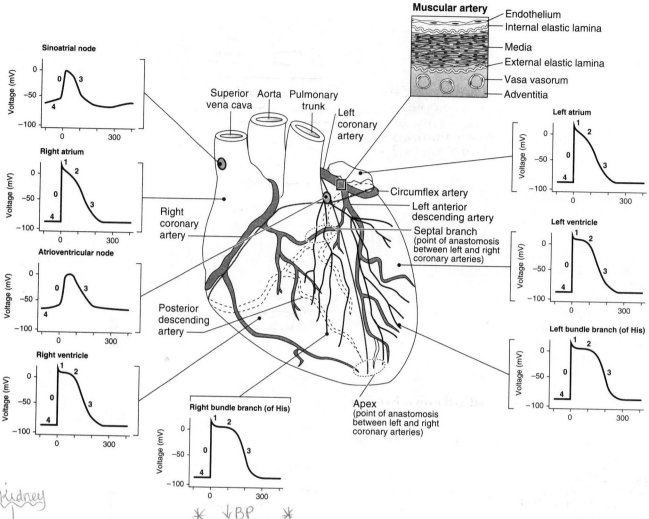

Kidney

* ↓BP *

water retention by the kidneys. Low blood pressure causes an increased release of renin, which converts angiotensinogen from the liver to angiotensin I. Angiotensin I travels to the lung where it is cleaved to angiotensin II (Ang II or vasopressin) by angiotensin-converting enzyme (ACE). Ang II stimulates constriction of arterioles and increases release of aldosterone (salt and water retention—see System 5 "Renal System"), both of which increase blood pressure. Abnormal tension, either high or low, in the vascular system must be present for several days before this system is fully engaged. **Atrial natriuretic peptide** (ANP) also responds to blood pressure changes. An increase in blood pressure causes stretch of atrial myocytes, which then release ANP. ANP lowers blood pressure by inhibiting contraction of smooth muscle, increasing salt and water excretion, and inhibiting the release of renin. **Anti-diuretic hormone** (ADH), also known as arginine-vasopressin (AVP), is involved in the response to rapid blood loss. When released from the pituitary, it works on the kidney to reduce urine output and retain water, while simultaneously constricting arterioles to increase peripheral resistance (Figure 2-6).

(↑ H₂O in principle cells)
retention.   CT.

* hypovolemia
* ↑ plasma osmolarity

QUICK HIT The baroreceptor reflex greatly affects total peripheral resistance. The carotid bodies, located at the bifurcation of the carotid vessels, sense arterial pressure. Afferent signals via cranial nerve (CN) IX induce efferent signals via CN X to influence heart rate. Increased blood pressure causes an increase in vagal output and a reduction of heart rate and blood pressure. A decrease in blood pressure causes a decrease in vagal output.

ANP trigger w/ ↑BP
⊖ Renin
↑ excretion of Na + H₂O
⊖ sm m contraction

FIGURE
2-5 ECGs of important arrhythmias.

Normal ECG

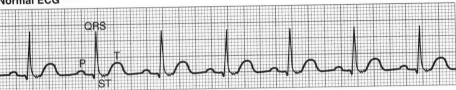

- P wave is atrial depolarization (atrial repolarization usually occurs during the QRS and remains unseen in ECG)
- PR interval (.12–.2 seconds) measures time between atrial and ventricular depolarization
- QRS interval (normally less than .1 second) reflects the duration of ventricular depolarization
- T wave is ventricular repolarization

QUICK HIT

class Ia

Torsades des Pointes
(twisting of the points):
ventricular tachycardia often
due to anti-arrhythmic drugs,
especially quinidine. It is characterized by a long QT interval and
a "short-long-short" sequence
prior to the inception of
tachycardia. The ECG shows a
series of upward pointing QRS
complexes followed by a series
of downward pointing complexes.

Sustained ventricular tachycardia

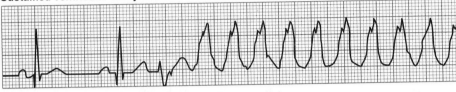

- Constant QRS morphology and fairly regular cycle length
- Initiating beat morphology may differ from ongoing VT
- AV dissociation a hallmark but not always present, nor easy to identify when present

Ventricular fibrillation

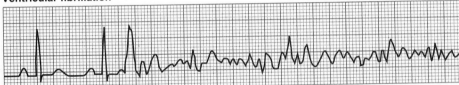

- Undulation baseline, no organized electrical activity
- Incompatible with life
- Atria may be dissociated, still in sinus rhythm

Atrial flutter

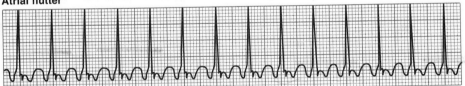

- A regular, saw-toothed pattern of atrial activity, usually very near 300/min
- Discrete, organized atrial activity on intracardiac electrograms
- Usually even-numbered AV conduction ratio (2:1, 4:1)

Atrial fibrillation

not true P waves

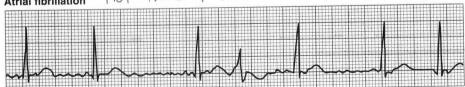

- Undulating, low amplitude atrial activity on ECG
- Intracardiac electrogram shows chaotic rapid spikes
- Variable conduction pattern as AV node is constantly bombarded with impulses; "long-short" sequences yield wide QRS complexes (aberrant, "Ashman" beats)

(continued)

FIGURE
2-5 *(Continued)* **ECGs of important arrhythmias.**

Wolff-Parkinson-White syndrome

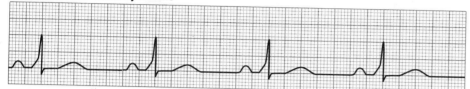

- Accessory atrioventricular conductions
- Anterograde or retrograde conduction
- Tachyarrhythmias
- Blurred QRS (referred to as δ-wave)

> **QUICK HIT**
> Myocardial infarctions can cause both second degree and third degree heart block.

TABLE 2-2 **Conduction Anomalies**

	Pathology	Notes	ECG
First degree heart block	AV nodal anomaly lengthens PR interval (greater than 0.2 sec) *asympt.*	May be due to drugs (e.g., beta blockers, digitalis and Ca++ channel blockers)	
Second degree heart block: Mobitz type 1 (Wenckebach)	Defect in AV node; progressively increasing PR interval until QRS wave is lost DROPPED BEAT	Relatively common; usually **does not require treatment** *asympt.*	
Second degree heart block: Mobitz type 2	**Defect in His-Purkinje system;** constant PR interval with random dropped QRS complexes 2:1 2P waves 1 QRS	Less common and more dangerous than Mobitz type 1; **pacemaker** *sympt*	
Third degree heart block	No electrical connection between atria and ventricles; atria and ventricles contract independently *everything on own*	His-Purkinje system sets rate of ventricular contraction; pacemaker may be necessary	

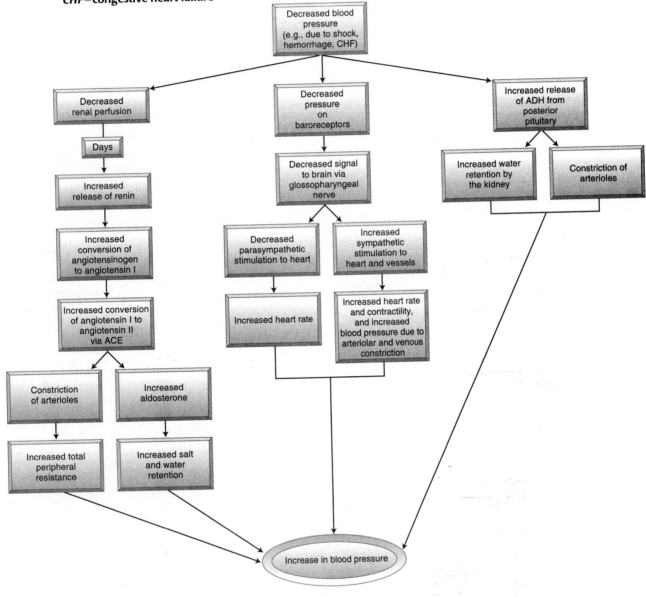

FIGURE 2-6 Blood pressure control mechanisms. *ACE*=angiotensin-converting enzyme; *ADH*=antidiuretic hormone; *CHF*=congestive heart failure

The physiologic function of the heart can be represented in several ways (e.g., pressure-volume loops and the cardiac cycle) (Figure 2-7). The effects of cardiac output, total peripheral resistance, contractility, preload, and afterload are represented on the **Frank-Starling curve.** Cardiac output is measured using the Fick principle (Figure 2-8) and normal output is approximately 5 L/min.

FIGURE 2-7 Physiologic cardiovascular relationships

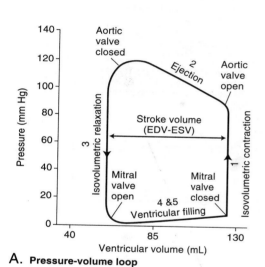

A. Pressure-volume loop

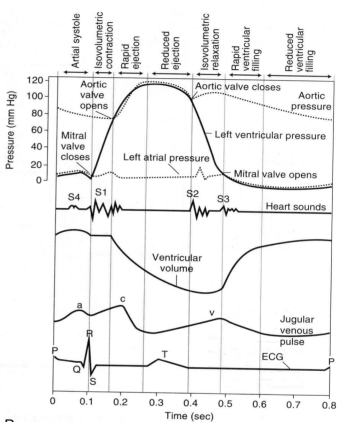

B. The Cardiac cycle

C. Progression of the action potential through cardiac muscle cells

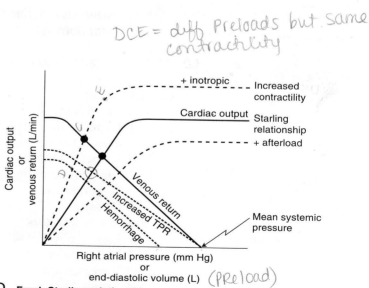

DCE = diff preloads but same contractility

(PReload)

D. Frank-Starling relationship

(Adapted from Bushan V, Le T, Amin C: *First Aid for the USMLE Step 1.* Stamford, Connecticut, Appleton & Lange, 1998. p. 284–285)

FIGURE
2-8 **Important cardiovascular equations**

$CO = \dfrac{O_2\ consumption}{([O_2]\ pulmonary\ vein -\ [O_2]\ pulmonary\ artery)}$	**The Fick equation** is used to calculate either cardiac output (CO) or oxygen (O_2) consumption
$CO = SV \times HR$	CO = cardiac output SV = stroke volume HR = heart rate
$R \propto \dfrac{1}{r^4}$	This relationship shows how arteriolar diameter can effectively control systemic resistance. For instance, if the radius (r) is increased by 2, the resistance (R) drops 16 fold.
$Q = \dfrac{\Delta P}{R}$	Q = flow ΔP = Aortic pressure - right atrial pressure or pressure difference R = resistance
$MBP = CO \times TPR$ $MAP =$	MBP = mean blood pressure (equivalent to ΔP) CO = cardiac output (equivalent to Q) TPR = total peripheral resistance (equivalent to R)
Series resistance: $R_{total} = R_1 + R_2 + R_3 + R_4 \ldots$	
Parallel resistance: $\dfrac{1}{R_{total}} = \dfrac{1}{R_1} + \dfrac{1}{R_2} + \dfrac{1}{R_3} + \dfrac{1}{R_4} \ldots$	This relationship lowers resistance when the body recruits unused parallel vessels (especially in capillary beds)

ATHEROSCLEROSIS

I. Atherosclerosis is defined as lipid deposition in the intima of arteries leading to vascular fibrosis and calcification.

II. It is the leading cause of mortality in the United States.

III. Risk factors
   A. **Major risk factors**
      1. **Hyperlipidemia:** high cholesterol, high triglycerides, decreased high-density lipoproteins (HDL) (< 35) (see Table 2-3 later in the chapter)
      2. **Diabetes mellitus**
      3. **Cigarette smoking**
      4. **Hypertension**
      5. **Obesity**
   B. **Minor risk factors**
      1. Lack of physical activity
      2. Male gender
      3. Increased age
      4. Family history
      5. Oral contraceptives, decreased estrogens, or premature menopause
      6. Type A personality
      7. Elevated homocystein level

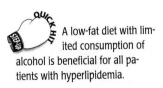
A low-fat diet with limited consumption of alcohol is beneficial for all patients with hyperlipidemia.

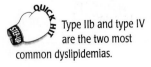
Type IIb and type IV are the two most common dyslipidemias.

IV. Pathogenesis

A. Atheroma formation

1. Monocytes adhere to vessel walls, enter tissue, and become macrophages.
2. Macrophages are transformed into **foam cells** after engulfing oxidized low-density lipoprotein (LDL).
3. Foam cells accumulate in the intima.
4. Foam cells release factors causing the aggregation of platelets, the release of fibroblast growth factor, and the accumulation of smooth muscle.
5. Upon formation of plaque, calcification occurs.
6. The central core of the plaque consists mainly of cholesterol.

B. Complications

1. Plaque rupture
2. Development of fatty streaks
3. Ischemic heart disease or myocardial infarction
4. Stroke
5. Renal arterial ischemia
6. Death

QUICK HIT Vitamin E inhibits the oxidation of LDL and its subsequent absorption by macrophages. Compounds such as superoxide, nitric oxide, and hydrogen peroxide promote oxidation of LDL and blood vessel injury.

QUICK HIT HDL works to remove cholesterol from tissues and plaques, therefore exerting a protective effect. HDL is increased by exercise.

V. Familial Dyslipidemias (Table 2-3)

TABLE 2-3 Familial Dyslipidemia

Familial Dyslipidemias	Elevated	Blood Lipid Levels	Pathology (see System 4, Gastrointestinal System)	Clinical Picture	Treatment
Hyperchylomicronemia I	Chylomicrons *[trigly → tissues, choles → liver]*	↑↑TG	Lipoprotein lipase deficiency	Increased vascular and heart disease	Low-fat diet
Hypercholesterolemia IIa	LDL	↑Cholesterol	**Decreased LDL receptors** *[on liver]*	Greatly increased vascular and heart disease; **xanthomas**	Cholestyramine/ colestipol, lovastatin (and niacin for homozygotes) *[⊖ HMG CoA reductase]*
Combined Hyperlipidemia IIb	LDL, VLDL *[choles, trig, from both liver]*	↑TG, ↑Cholesterol	Hepatic overproduction of VLDL	Increased vascular and heart disease	Cholestyramine/ colestipol, lovastatin (and niacin for homozygotes)
Dysbetalipoproteinemia III	IDL, VLDL	↑TG, ↑Cholesterol	Altered apolipoprotein E	Increased vascular and heart disease; xanthomas	Niacin and clofibrate or lovastatin
Hypertriglyceridemia IV	VLDL	↑↑↑TG, normal to ↑Cholesterol	Hepatic overproduction (with possible decreased clearance) of VLDL	Increased vascular and heart disease; obese, **diabetic, pregnant,** and **alcoholic** patients	Weight loss; low fat diet; niacin and clofibrate or lovastatin (if necessary)
Mixed Hypertriglyceridemia V	VLDL, Chylomicrons	↑↑↑TG, ↑Cholesterol	Overproduction or decreased clearance of VLDL and chylomicrons	Obese and diabetic patients	Diet modification; niacin and clofibrate or lovastat in (if necessary)

LDL=low density lipoproteins; *TG*=triglycerides; *VLDL*=very low density lipoproteins

THE CARDIOVASCULAR SYSTEM

HYPERTENSION

I. Essential

* A. **Most common** type (90% of cases)
  B. Unknown etiology
  C. Risk factors
    1. Family history
    2. Race (more common in blacks)
    3. Obesity
    4. Cigarette smoking
    5. Physical inactivity
  D. **Characteristics**
    1. Blood pressure greater than 140/90 on **three separate occasions**
    2. Hypertrophy of left ventricle
    3. Onion-skinning of vessel walls
    4. Retinal hemorrhages
  E. **Essential hypertension predisposes to ischemic heart disease** (see next section).

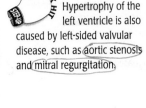 Hypertrophy of the left ventricle is also caused by left-sided valvular disease, such as aortic stenosis and mitral regurgitation.

II. Secondary hypertension refers to elevated systemic arterial pressure associated with a condition known to cause hypertension.

  A. **Renal diseases.** These are the **most common cause** of secondary hypertension.
    1. Renal parenchymal disorders
    2. Unilateral renal artery stenosis
      a. **Atherosclerosis** (more common in black males)
      b. **Fibromuscular dysplasia** (more common in white females)
    3. The renin-angiotensin axis is activated.
  B. **Endocrine causes**
    1. Primary aldosteronism
    2. Pheochromocytoma ↑ cateocholamines
    3. Hyperthyroidism

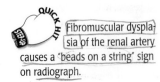 Fibromuscular dysplasia of the renal artery causes a "beads on a string" sign on radiograph.

III. Malignant (emergent) hypertension

  A. Accelerated course results in end-organ damage in days
  B. End-organ damage occurs to the following organ systems:
    1. CV—vascular damage, aortic dissection
    2. Pulmonary—pulmonary edema
    3. Renal—"flea-bitten kidneys," azotemia
    4. Ocular—fundal hemorrhages, papilledema
    5. Central nervous system (CNS)—encephalopathy, seizures, coma
  C. Early death from cerebrovascular accidents (CVA) is the result of this type of hypertension.
  D. **Young black males** are the usual victims of this type of hypertension.

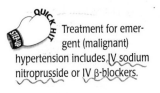 Treatment for emergent (malignant) hypertension includes IV sodium nitroprusside or IV β-blockers.

IV. Aneurysms (Table 2-4)

TABLE 2-4 Aneurysms

Type of Aneurysm	Etiology	Characteristics
Arteriovenous fistula	Abnormal communication between arteries and veins; usually secondary to **trauma**	Ischemic changes; aneurysm formation; **high output cardiac failure**
Atherosclerotic	**Atherosclerotic** disease; coronary artery disease	Usually in the **descending** aorta; located between renal arteries and iliac bifurcation
Berry	Congenital medial weakness at the bifurcations of the cerebral arteries	Saccular lesions in cerebral vessels (especially at the **circle of Willis**); hemorrhage into **subarachnoid** space
Dissecting	**Hypertension;** cystic medial necrosis; **Marfan's**	**Tearing pain;** longitudinal separation of tunica media of aortic wall
Syphilitic	Tertiary syphilis; obliteration of the vaso vasorum; necrosis of the media	Involves **ascending** aorta; aortic valve insufficiency
Mycotic (infectious)	Inflammation secondary to bacterial infection; usually salmonella	Involves abdominal aorta

ISCHEMIC HEART DISEASE

I. Defined as an **inadequate supply of oxygen** relative to demand resulting in damage to cardiac tissue.

II. Ischemic heart disease is most often caused by **atherosclerosis.**

III. **Four types** of ischemic heart disease
   A. Angina pectoris
      1. Paroxysmal attacks of retrosternal pain, heaviness, or squeezing chest pain occur and may radiate to the neck, jaw, shoulders, or arms. Angina pectoris is often associated with diaphoresis and nausea.
      2. Imbalance between cardiac perfusion and cardiac demand is characteristic. Ninety percent occlusion of coronary vessel produces symptoms.
      3. **Three types** of angina pectoris
         a. **Stable angina**
            (1) **Most common** form
            (2) Induced by exercise
            (3) Relieved by rest
            (4) Results from chronic stenosis of coronary arteries
         b. **Prinzmetal's (variant) angina**
            (1) **Episodic** pain occurs at rest.
            (2) Attacks are **unrelated to activity, blood pressure,** or **heart rate,** but are due to coronary artery **vasospasm.**
            (3) Significant artery stenosis is often present.

QUICK HIT

Berry aneurysms are commonly associated with **adult polycystic kidney** disease, an **autosomal dominant** disease located on chromosome 16.

QUICK HIT

Syphilis is a sexually transmitted disease caused by *Treponema pallidum* (a spirochete) that is characterized by a painless, hard chancre. Untreated syphilis can result in rashes, lymphadenopathy, condylomata lata) and **Argyll Robertson pupils (pupils accommodate, but do not constrict).**

QUICK HIT

Exercise tolerance testing is a good way to diagnose subacute coronary occlusion. **Thallium 201** scans reveal perfusion defects. Technetium (^{99m}Tc) scans are useful for imaging MI's.

QUICK HIT

Cocaine use can also result in coronary vasospasm resulting in myocardial ischemia. In general, cocaine works by inhibiting the reuptake of endogenous catecholamines (dopamine, norepinephrine, and epinephrine). On the other hand, amphetamines stimulate the release of endogenous catecholamines.

c. **Unstable angina**
  (1) This type occurs at rest or with **increasing frequency, severity,** or **duration.**
  (2) It is preceded by less and less activity.
  (3) It produces pain of longer and longer duration.
  (4) It is induced **by ruptured atherosclerotic plaque** with subsequent thrombosis and embolization.
  (5) Activated platelets help cause thrombosis and vasospasm.
  (6) Microinfarcts may be caused.

B. **Myocardial infarction (MI)**
  1. Lack of adequate perfusion to cardiac tissue leads to myocyte death in affected area.
  2. MI is most often caused by **atherosclerosis** with plaque rupture and thrombus.
  3. The endocardium is most vulnerable to ischemia (due to decreased blood flow during systole) and therefore most likely to infarct.
  4. In a transmural infarct (see below), the full thickness of the ventricular wall is affected within 3–5 hours.
  5. **Two types** of myocardial infarction are possible.
    a. **Non-transmural (Non-Q-wave) infarcts**
      (1) Diffuse coronary atherosclerosis is found.
      (2) This causes overall reduction of coronary flow.
      (3) Rupture or thrombosis eventually results, followed quickly by clot lysis.
      (4) Loss of perfusion to inner one third of muscular wall of ventricle occurs.
      (5) **ST segment depression** is seen on ECG.
    b. **Transmural infarct**
      (1) Atherosclerotic plaques rupture.
      (2) Platelet-mediated thrombosis occludes vessel.
      (3) Occluded vessel stops flow of blood to entire muscular wall.
      (4) **ST segment elevation** is seen on ECG.
  6. Cardiac enzymes are released when myocytes are damaged (Figure 2-9).

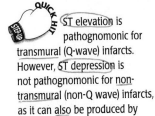

The **left anterior descending** artery is the most common artery involved in acute MI. Infarcts of this artery affect the left ventricle near its apex, or the anterior portion of the interventricular septum.

ST elevation is pathognomonic for transmural (Q-wave) infarcts. However, ST depression is not pathognomonic for non-transmural (non-Q wave) infarcts, as it can also be produced by digitalis drugs.

FIGURE
2-9 Myocardial infarction enzyme release and timeline of histologic changes.

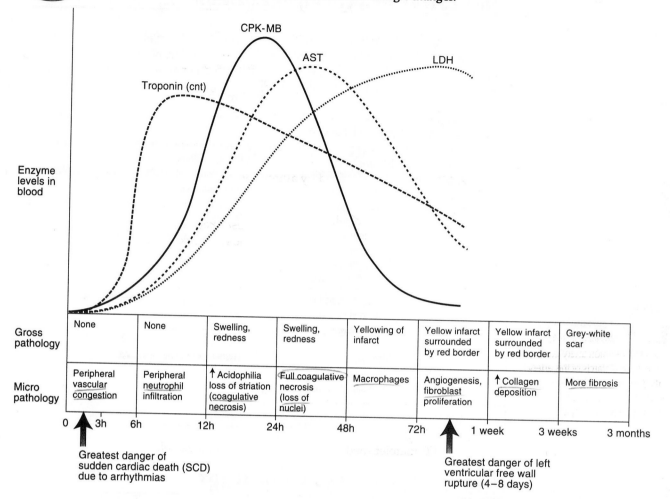

Gross pathology	None	None	Swelling, redness	Swelling, redness	Yellowing of infarct	Yellow infarct surrounded by red border	Yellow infarct surrounded by red border	Grey-white scar
Micro pathology	Peripheral vascular congestion	Peripheral neutrophil infiltration	↑ Acidophilia loss of striation (coagulative necrosis)	Full coagulative necrosis (loss of nuclei)	Macrophages	Angiogenesis, fibroblast proliferation	↑ Collagen deposition	More fibrosis

0   3h   6h   12h   24h   48h   72h   1 week   3 weeks   3 months

Greatest danger of sudden cardiac death (SCD) due to arrhythmias

Greatest danger of left ventricular free wall rupture (4–8 days)

7. Complications
   a. Heart block
   b. Arrhythmia
   c. Myocardial rupture occurs most commonly during first week post-MI.
   d. Papillary muscle rupture
   e. Mural thrombus with possible embolization
8. Remodeling and scar formation occur over a period of 3–6 months after an infarct (see Fig 2–9).

C. Chronic Ischemic Heart Disease (CIHD)
   1. Congestive heart failure (CHF) that results from ischemic cardiac damage leads to CIHD.
   2. Hypertrophy of the heart and cardiac decompensation occur due to infarction.
   3. CIHD is most often found in the elderly.

D. Sudden cardiac death
   1. This is unexpected death from cardiac failure occurring less than two hours post-MI.
   2. This is caused less commonly by a congenital anomaly.
   3. Marked atherosclerosis is usually present.
   4. The mechanism of death is almost always due to arrhythmia.

QUICK HIT Re-entry is the most common cause of arrhythmias. Re-entry requires a circuit, refractory tissue (unidirectional block), slow conduction velocity, and an initiating event (usually a premature beat).

CONGESTIVE HEART FAILURE (Table 2-5)

Congestive heart failure is a clinical diagnosis where the heart is unable to pump an adequate amount of blood to meet the metabolic needs of the body. A number of factors play a role in congestive heart failure, including hormonal changes (RAA and sympathetic activation), peripheral vasoconstriction, and myocardial dysfunction.

TABLE 2-5 Congestive Heart Failure (CHF)		
	Etiology	**Clinical Manifestations**
Left-Sided CHF	Ischemia (CAD) Hypertension Left-sided valvular disease Myocarditis Cardiomyopathy Congenital heart disease Pericardial disease	**Pulmonary edema** Dyspnea on exertion/fatigue **Orthopnea** Paroxysmal nocturnal dyspnea Hyperventilation Reduction in renal perfusion (activates RAA axis) **S3**
Right-Sided CHF	Left-sided heart failure Left-sided lesions **Cor pulmonale** Myocarditis Cardiomyopathy Right-sided valvular disease	Hepatomegaly/ascites (**nutmeg liver**) Splenomegaly **Peripheral edema** (especially pitting edema of the ankles) **Distention of neck veins** Renal hypoxia

CAD=coronary artery disease; *RAA*=renin angiotensin aldosterone (system)

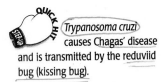

Cor pulmonale is right heart failure secondary to lung disorders which leads to pulmonary arterial hypertension.

INTRINSIC DISEASES OF THE HEART

I. Myocarditis
   A. This is defined as **inflammation of the cardiac muscle.**
   B. **Etiology**
      1. **Viral etiology** is the most common cause (usually **Coxsackie B** virus)
      2. Human immunodeficiency virus (HIV) (via toxoplasmosis and metastasis of Kaposi's sarcoma) may cause myocarditis.
      3. Bacterial causes include *Staphylococcus aureus* or *Cornybacterium diphtheriae*.
      4. Chagas' disease — cardiomyopathy + lymph enlargement.
      5. Lyme disease
      6. Hypersensitivity reactions
   C. **Physical examination**
      1. **Muffled S1**
      2. **Audible S3** heart sound
      3. Murmur of **mitral regurgitation**
      4. Cardiomegaly

II. Endocarditis
   A. Inflammation of heart lining and connective tissue.
   B. **Causes**
      1. **Rheumatic heart disease.** Endocarditis may be caused by rheumatic fever (see III).

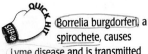

Trypanosoma cruzi causes Chagas' disease and is transmitted by the reduviid bug (kissing bug).

Borrelia burgdorferi, a spirochete, causes Lyme disease and is transmitted by the Ixodes tick. Stage 1 is marked by erythema chronicum migrans. Stage 2 is marked by cardiac and neurologic involvement. Stage 3 involves arthritis.

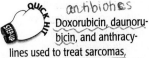

antibiotics
Doxorubicin, daunorubicin, and anthracylines used to treat sarcomas, breast cancer, lung cancer, and ALL, result in dose-dependent, irreversible cardiotoxicity.

THE CARDIOVASCULAR SYSTEM

2. **Infective endocarditis**
   a. Etiology
   (1) Bacteria, usually gram-positive cocci, or fungi (*Aspergillus* or *Candida*) are the most common causes.
   (2) Damage, surgical repair, prosthetic heart valves, or congenital abnormalities are predisposing conditions.
   (3) Vegetative growth (usually on atrial surface of valves) can throw **septic thrombi** to brain or peripheral circulation.
   (4) Endocarditis is complicated by ulcerations or rupture of chordae tendineae.
   b. Characteristics
   (1) Clinical features
   (a) Petechiae
   (b) **Janeway lesions** (peripheral hemorrhages with slight nodular character)
   (c) **Osler's nodes** (small, tender nodules on fingers and toe pads)
   (d) **Splinter hemorrhages** (subungual linear streaks)
   (e) Roth's spots (retinal hemorrhages)
   (f) Splenomegaly
   (2) The mitral and aortic valves are frequently involved.
   (3) The presence of **right-sided** valvular lesions, usually of the tricuspid, suggests **intravenous (IV) drug abuse.**

C. **Types**
   1. **Acute endocarditis**
   a. Cause is most often *Staphylococcus aureus.*
   b. Onset is rapid.
   c. Clinical features include fever, anemia, embolic events, and heart murmur.
   2. **Subacute endocarditis**
   a. Cause is most often *Streptococci viridans.*
   b. Results from poor dentition or oral surgery in patients with preexisting heart disease.
   c. Onset is over a period of 6 months.
   d. Treatment is with IV antibiotics.
   3. **Nonbacterial (marantic) endocarditis**
   a. This type is associated with metastatic cancer.
   b. Sterile fibrin deposits appear on valves.
   c. Sterile emboli cause cerebral infarct.
   4. Libman-Sacks endocarditis
   a. This is a manifestation of systemic lupus erythematosus **(SLE).**
   b. It is caused by auto-antibody damage to valves.
   c. **Vegetations form on both sides** of the valve.
   5. Carcinoid syndrome
   a. This syndrome is characterized by increased serotonin and other secretory products from a carcinoid tumor.
   b. Plaques build on **right-sided valves** of the heart.

III. Rheumatic Heart Disease
A. This is a multisystem inflammatory disorder with cardiac manifestations.
B. Pathogenesis
   1. Rheumatic heart disease usually occurs 1–4 weeks after a bout of tonsillitis caused by group A β-hemolytic streptococci.
   2. **Antigenic mimicry** occurs between streptococcal antigens and human antigens in the heart.
   3. This results in immunologic origin for rheumatic heart disease.
C. **Epidemiology**
   1. Children 5–15 years of age have the highest incidence of rheumatic fever.
   2. Incidence is decreasing since the advent of penicillin.

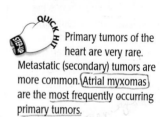

Culture-negative endocarditis can result from the **HACEK** group of organisms: Haemophilus, Actinobacillus, Cardiobacterium, Eikenella, Kingella.

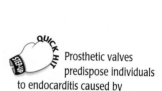

Prosthetic valves predispose individuals to endocarditis caused by Staphylococcus epidermidis.

Primary tumors of the heart are very rare. Metastatic (secondary) tumors are more common. Atrial myxomas are the most frequently occurring primary tumors.

Antiphospholipid syndrome, common in SLE, results from antibodies to phospholipids primarily producing a hypercoagulable state leading to thrombotic disorders and multiple spontaneous abortions.

D. Cardiac manifestations of rheumatic fever include the following conditions:
  1. Pancarditis—inflammation of all structures of the heart
    a. Pericarditis with effusions
    b. Myocarditis
      (1) Leads to cardiac failure
      (2) **Most common cause of early death** in rheumatic fever
    c. Endocarditis
      (1) Usually afflicts the **mitral** and **aortic** valves (areas of high stress)
      (2) Mitral—Aortic—Tricuspid—**Pulmonary** shows the order in which the valves become involved.
      (3) Early non-embolic vegetations occur.
      (4) With fibrosis and calcification, valvular damage leads to rheumatic heart disease.
E. **Other systemic manifestations** of rheumatic fever
  1. **Migratory polyarthritis**
  2. Sydenham's chorea
  3. Subcutaneous nodules
  4. Erythema marginatum
  5. Recent infection by group A streptococci (indicated by elevated anti-streptolysin O titers)
  6. **Aschoff body**
    a. Lesion characterized by focal interstitial myocardial inflammation
    b. Fragmented collagen/fibrinoid material
    c. Anitschkow myocytes: large activated histiocytes
    d. Aschoff cells: granuloma with giant cells

● **Cardiomyopathies (Table 2-6)**

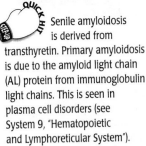

Idiopathic dilated cardiomyopathy is the most common form of cardiomyopathy. Treatment includes digitalis, ACE inhibitors, heart transplant, and sometimes chronic anticoagulation.

Senile amyloidosis is derived from transthyretin. Primary amyloidosis is due to the amyloid light chain (AL) protein from immunoglobulin light chains. This is seen in plasma cell disorders (see System 9, "Hematopoietic and Lymphoreticular System").

TABLE 2-6 Cardiomyopathies				
	Pathology	Etiology	Clinical Manifestations	Notes
Dilated	Dilated ventricles; right and left heart failure; pulmonary edema	**Idiopathic;** alcoholics; thiamine deficiency; peripartum; **coxsackie B;** *Trypanosoma cruzi;* TCA's; lithium, doxorubicin	Premature ventricular contractions; **decreased ejection fraction;** JVP; cardiomegaly; hepatomegaly	**Most common** form
Restrictive	**Stiffened heart muscle;** may result in right and left heart failure; tricuspid regurgitation	Senile or primary amyloidosis; sarcoidosis; hemochromatosis	Peripheral **edema;** ascites; JVD	Differentiate from constrictive cardiomyopathy
Hypertrophic	Ventricular and ventricular septal hypertrophy; mitral regurgitation	**Autosomal dominant;** young **athletes**	Dyspnea; syncope; S4; systolic murmur; cardiomegaly on chest radiograph	Relieved by squatting; exacerbated by physical exertion

JVD=jugular venous distention; *JVP*=jugular venous pressure; *TCA*=tricyclic antidepressant

[handwritten: Pressure ↑]
[handwritten: volume ↑]
[handwritten: also in Tetralogy of Fallot]

● Valvular Heart Diseases (Table 2-7)

TABLE 2-7	Valvular Heart Disease			
Valvular Disease	**Etiology**	**Physical Examination**	**Clinical Manifestations**	**Schematic Representation**
Mitral stenosis	Usually **rheumatic heart disease**	Cyanosis; **opening snap;** diastolic rumbling murmur	Dyspnea; orthopnea; left atrial enlargement; mid-to-late diastolic murmur	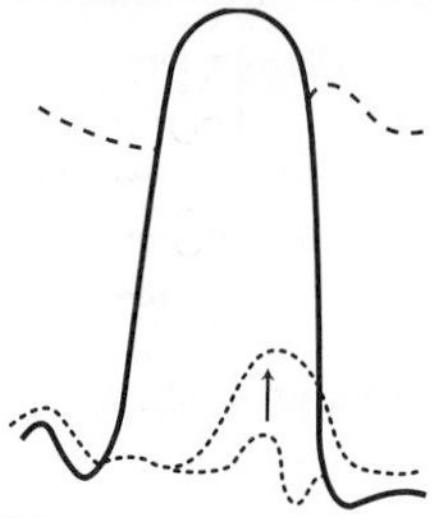
Mitral regurgitation	**Rheumatic heart disease** (50% of cases); mitral valve prolapse; hypertrophic cardiomyopathy; papillary muscle dysfunction (secondary to myocardial infarction)	Splitting of S2; **S3;** systolic murmur	Arrhythmias; infective endocarditis; dilated left atrium; holosystolic murmur	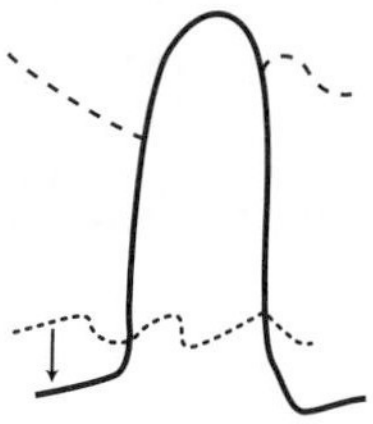
Aortic stenosis	Thickening and **calcification** of valve; bicuspid aortic valves	Delayed pulses; carotid thrill; **crescendo-decrescendo systolic ejection murmur**	Syncope; angina; death; do not administer beta-blockers; systolic ejection murmur	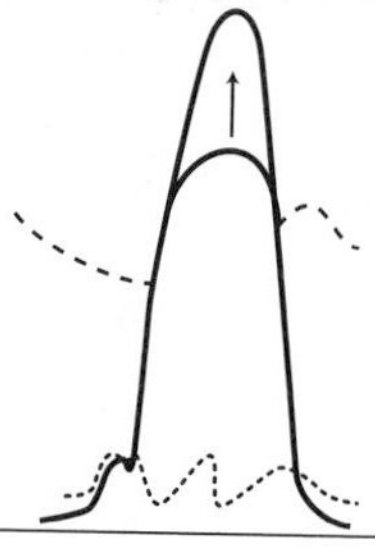
Aortic regurgitation	Rheumatic heart disease; syphilitic aortitis; nondissecting aortic aneurysm; Marfan's syndrome	Wide pulse pressure; water-hammer pulse; **S3; blowing, decrescendo diastolic murmur**	Left ventricular enlargement; dyspnea; early diastolic murmur	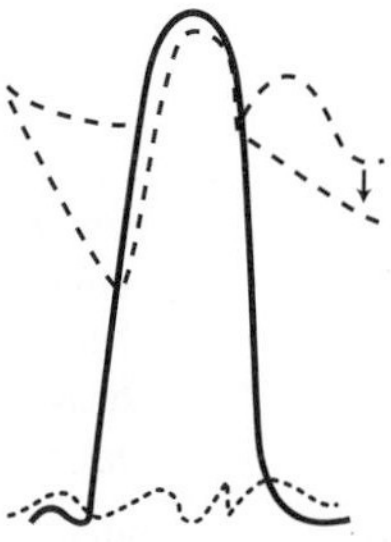

(handwritten margin notes: "diastolic", "Systolic", "Systolic", "diastolic", "Austin Flint")

QUICK HIT

Mitral valve prolapse (MVP) is the most frequently occurring valvular lesion, often found in young women or Marfan's patients, and due to tissue laxity. The murmur is exaggerated by the **Valsalva** maneuver, but reduced by **squatting**. These patients require endocarditis prophylaxis prior to surgical or dental procedures.

QUICK HIT

A midsystolic click is often indicative of mitral prolapse.

● Murmurs (Table 2-8)

TABLE 2-8 Murmurs					
Systolic			**Diastolic**		
Ejection	*Holosystolic*	*Late-systolic*	*Early*	*Mid-to-late*	*Continuous*
• Aortic valve stenosis • Hypertrophic cardiomyopathy • Pulmonic valve stenosis	• Mitral regurgitation • Tricuspid regurgitation • Ventricular septal defect	• Mitral valve prolapse	• Aortic valve regurgitation • Pulmonic valve regurgitation	• Mitral stenosis	• Patent ductus arteriosus

● Peripheral Vascular Diseases (Table 2-9)

The pathophysiology of the vasculitides is thought to be mediated by immunopathology.

Serum sickness, a generalized deposition of immune complexes, is now rare due to decreased administration of animal serum.

TABLE 2-9 Peripheral Vascular Diseases				
Disease	**Pathology**	**Vessels Affected**	**Clinical Manifestations**	**Notes**
Churg-Strauss	Eosinophilic, **granulomatous** inflammation	Small and medium vessels	**Asthma; elevated plasma eosinophils;** heart disease	May be associated with p-ANCA
Henoch-Schönlein purpura	**IgA** immune complex mediated acute inflammation; renal deposits in mesangium	Arterioles; capillaries; venules	Hemorrhagic urticaria; palpable purpura; fever; RBC casts in urine; **atopic** patient	Often associated with an **upper respiratory infection; children**
Kaposi's sarcoma	Viral origin; component of **AIDS**	Cutaneous and visceral vasculature	Malignant vascular tumor, especially in **homosexual** men	May be related to HHV-8 infection
Kawasaki's disease	Acute necrotizing inflammation	Large, medium, and small vessels	Fever; conjunctival lesions; lymphadenitis; coronary artery aneurysms	Affects **young children**
Rendu-Osler-Weber syndrome	**Autosomal dominant;** hereditary hemorrhagic telangiectasia	Dilatation of venules and capillaries	Epistaxis; GI bleeding	Increased frequency in **Mormon** population
Polyarteritis nodosa (PAN)	Anti-neutrophil antibodies (**p-ANCA**) lead to necrotizing degeneration of media; aneurysms	Small and medium arteries	Fever; weight loss; abdominal pain (GI); hypertension (renal)	Associated with **Hepatitis B infection**

(continued)

TABLE 2-9 **Peripheral Vascular Diseases** *(Continued)*

Disease	Pathology	Vessels Affected	Clinical Manifestations	Notes
Takayasu's arteritis (pulseless disease)	Inflammation leading to stenosis; **aortic arch** and the origins of great vessels	Medium and large arteries	**Loss of carotid, radial and ulnar pulses;** fever; night sweats; arthritis; visual deficits	Pathology referred to as "aortic arch syndrome"; young **Asian females**
Temporal arteritis	Nodular inflammation of branches of carotid (especially **temporal**)	Medium and large arteries	**Headache;** absence of pulse in affected vessels; **visual deficits;** polymyalgia rheumatica	Significant elevation of **erythrocyte sedimentation rate; usually elderly population** *Rx: glucocorticoids*
Thromboangiitis obliterans (Buerger's disease)	Acute, full-thickness inflammation of vessels; may extend to nerves; occlusive lesions in extremities	Small and medium arteries	Cold, pale limb; pain; **Raynaud's phenomenon;** gangrene	Typical patient is a young **Jewish** man who **smokes heavily**
Von Hippel-Lindau disease	**Autosomal dominant;** localized to chromosome ③	Visceral vasculature	**Hemangioblastomas** of the cerebellum, brain stem, and retina; hepatic, renal, and pancreatic cysts	Increased incidence of **renal cell carcinoma**
Wegener's granulomatosis	Anti-neutrophil antibodies (**c-ANCA**) causes necrotizing, **granulomatous lesions** in ⟨kidney⟩ and ⟨lung⟩	Small arteries; small veins	Cough; ulcers of sinuses and **nasal septum;** RBC casts in urine	More common in males

AIDS=acquired immune deficiency syndrome; *GI*=gastrointestinal; *HHV-8*=human herpesvirus 8; *IgA*=immunoglobulin A; *RBC*=red blood cells

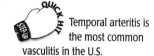

Temporal arteritis is the most common vasculitis in the U.S.

I. Diseases of the Pericardium

A. Cardiac tamponade

1. This is accumulation of fluid in the pericardial sac which causes filling defects due to compression of the heart.
   a. Blood is usually indicative of a traumatic perforation of the heart or aorta or rupture due to an MI.
   b. Serous transudate may accumulate due to edema or CHF.
2. The most common causes are neoplasms, idiopathic pericarditis, and uremia.
3. Principal features of cardiac tamponade
   a. Intracardiac pressure is elevated.
   b. **Ventricular filling** is limited.
   c. Cardiac output is reduced.

The needle for a pericardiocentesis passes through the skin, superficial fascia, pectoralis major muscle, external intercostal membrane, internal intercostal membrane, fibrous pericardium, and parietal layer of serous pericardium.

4. **Pulsus paradoxus** is a greater than normal (10 mmHg) decline in systolic arterial pressure on inspiration.
    5. **Treatment** involves pericardiocentesis (removal of fluid from the pericardial cavity).
B. **Pericarditis**
    1. Pericarditis is defined as an inflammation of the fibrous membrane covering the heart.
    2. Causes
        a. Usually idiopathic
        b. **Coxsackievirus A or B**
        c. Tuberculosis
        d. Uremia
        e. SLE
        f. Scleroderma
        g. Post-MI (Dressler's syndrome)
    3. Physical examination
        a. Jugular venous distention (JVD)
        b. Increase of jugular venous pressure (JVP) with inspiration (**Kussmaul's sign**)
        c. Pericardial **friction rub**
        d. **Distant heart sounds**
    4. Characteristics
        a. Pain exacerbated by inspiration
        b. Pain relieved by sitting
        c. Cardiomegaly
        d. Hypotension
        e. **ST elevation** on ECG
    5. Persistent, acute pericarditis leads to chronic, constrictive pericarditis.
        a. Both acute and chronic pericarditis mimic right-sided heart failure.
        b. Both acute and chronic pericarditis lead to obliteration of pericardial cavity.
        c. Fibrous tissue proliferation and calcification result.

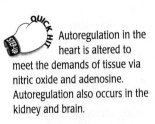

An MI also produces ST elevation. However, in an MI, ST elevation is followed by depression of the ST segment and QRS changes.

SHOCK

I. **Shock is defined as a metabolic state in which oxygen delivery is not adequate to meet oxygen demand.**

II. **Signs and symptoms**
    A. Tachycardia
    B. Hypotension
    C. Oliguria
    D. Mental status changes
    E. Weak pulses
    F. Cool extremities

Autoregulation in the heart is altered to meet the demands of tissue via nitric oxide and adenosine. Autoregulation also occurs in the kidney and brain.

III. Types of shock (Table 2-10)

TABLE 2-10 Shock		
Type of Shock	**Mechanism**	**Clinical causes**
Cardiogenic	Pump failure	Cardiac arrhythmias; heart failure; intracardiac obstruction; myocardial infarction
Hypovolemic	Volume loss	Blood, electrolyte, fluid, or plasma loss; burns, severe vomiting, or diarrhea
Obstructive	Extracardiac obstruction of blood flow	Aortic dissection; cardiac tamponade; pulmonary embolism
Septic	Increased venous capacitance	Gram-negative endotoxemia; direct toxic injury; DIC
Neurogenic	Massive peripheral vasodilation	Severe cerebral, brain stem, or spinal cord injury
Anaphylactic	Increased venous capacitance stimulated by histamine release	Type I hypersensitivity reaction to exogenous stimulus (e.g., food allergy, bee sting)

DIC=diffuse intravascular coagulation

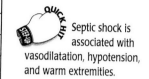

Septic shock is associated with vasodilatation, hypotension, and warm extremities.

IV. Clinical manifestations of shock
  A. Acute tubular necrosis
  B. Necrosis in the brain
  C. Fatty change in the heart and liver
  D. Patchy hemorrhages in the colon
  E. Pulmonary edema

● Cardiovascular Manifestations of Systemic Diseases (Table 2-11)

TABLE 2-11 Cardiovascular Manifestations of Systemic Diseases	
Disease	**Sequelae**
Diabetes mellitus	• Large vessel atherosclerosis • Myocardial infarctions • Coronary artery disease • Restrictive cardiomyopathy
Hyperthyroidism	• Palpitations • Systolic hypertension • Fatigue • Sinus tachycardia
Hypothyroidism	• Reduced cardiac output • Reduced heart rate • Reduced blood pressure • Reduced pulse pressure • Cardiomegaly • Bradycardia
Kwashiorkor or marasmus	• Thin, pale, flabby heart • Low cardiac output and systolic pressure
Malignant carcinoid	• Right-sided heart lesions • Coronary artery spasm

(continued)

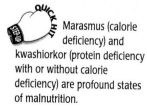

Marasmus (calorie deficiency) and kwashiorkor (protein deficiency with or without calorie deficiency) are profound states of malnutrition.

TABLE 2-11 Cardiovascular Manifestations of Systemic Diseases	
Disease	**Sequelae**
Obesity	• Increased total blood volume • Increased cardiac output • Hypertension • Coronary artery disease • Cardiac hypertrophy
Pheochromocytoma	• Hypertension • Myocardial necrosis • Left ventricular hypertrophy
Rheumatoid arthritis	• Pericarditis • Coronary arteritis
Systemic lupus erythematous (SLE)	• Pericarditis • Libman-Sacks endocarditis • Antiphospolipid syndrome
Thiamine deficiency	• High-output cardiac failure • Tachycardia • S3 • Systolic murmur

THERAPEUTICS

Antihypertensives

Captopril *ACE*
Clonidine *sympato*
Enalapril *ACE*
Furosemide *loop*
Hydralazine *vaso dil*

Hydrochlorothiazide *Thiazide*
Losartan *Ang II ⊖*
Metoprolol *B*
Nifedipine *Ca chan block*
Nitroglycerin *vasodil*

Prazosin *∝*
Propranolol *B*
Verapamil *Ca block*

Antianginal

Diltiazem *Ca chan block* Nitroglycerin *vasodil* Propranolol *B.*
Nifedipine *" "*

Antiarrhythmics (Figure 2-10)

FIGURE 2-10 Antiarrhythmic drugs

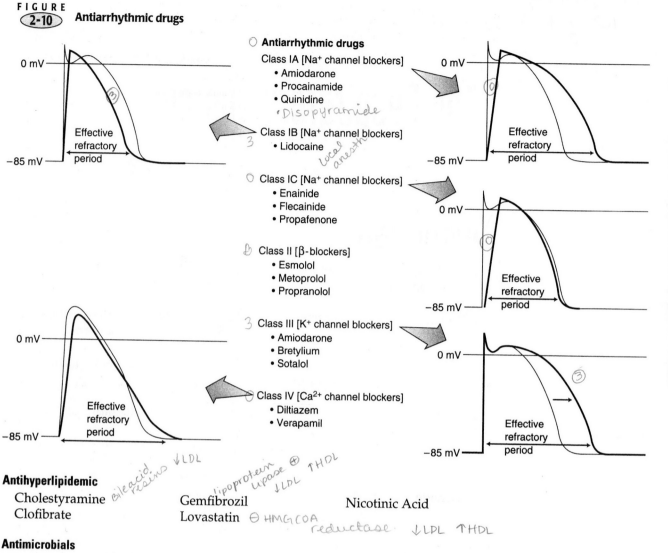

○ **Antiarrhythmic drugs**

Class IA [Na⁺ channel blockers]
- Amiodarone
- Procainamide
- Quinidine
- Disopyramide

Class IB [Na⁺ channel blockers]
- Lidocaine   *local anesth*

○ **Class IC [Na⁺ channel blockers]**
- Enainide
- Flecainide
- Propafenone

Class II [β-blockers]
- Esmolol
- Metoprolol
- Propranolol

3 **Class III [K⁺ channel blockers]**
- Amiodarone
- Bretylium
- Sotalol

○ **Class IV [Ca²⁺ channel blockers]**
- Diltiazem
- Verapamil

Antihyperlipidemic

Cholestyramine   *bile acid resins ↓LDL*

Clofibrate

Gemfibrozil   *lipoprotein lipase ⊕ ↓LDL ↑HDL*

Lovastatin   *⊖ HMG COA reductase ↓LDL ↑HDL*

Nicotinic Acid

Antimicrobials

Aminoglycoside   Methicillin   Tetracycline

Ampicillin   Penicillin   Vancomycin

Chloramphenicol

Immunosuppressive

Glucocorticoids   Cyclosporine

binds to cyclophyllin
✱ Tacrilemus very potent.

QUICK HIT

Cyclosporine is used to prevent acute rejection of heart and renal transplants by inhibiting T-helper cell activation (via inhibition of IL-2).

Inotropic

Digoxin   Dobutamine   Dopamine

Digitalis

Myocardial Infarction

Aspirin   Ticlopidine

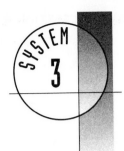

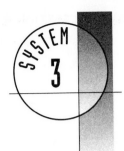

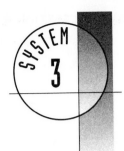

The Respiratory System

DEVELOPMENT

I. The **lung bud** forms from the foregut during week 4 of embryological development.

II. The lining of the lower respiratory tract is derived from **endoderm**, while the connective tissue cartilage and muscle are derived from **mesoderm.**

III. Normal development causes the lung bud to completely separate from the esophagus at the level of the larynx.

IV. Incomplete separation causes a **tracheoesophageal (TE) fistula** (Figure 3-1).

FIGURE
3-1 **Tracheoesophageal fistula**

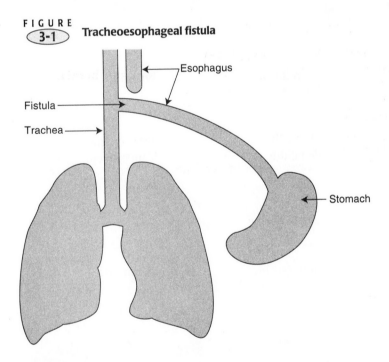

A. In the most common form of TE fistula, the esophagus ends in blind pouch and air enters the stomach.
B. Signs and symptoms of the most common form of TE fistula:
   1. Copious secretions
   2. Possible aspiration with respiratory distress
   3. Inability to pass nasogastric tube

V. Stages of bronchial development

A. **Pseudoglandular period** (5–17 weeks)
1. During this period, the primary bronchi are formed, followed by secondary, tertiary, and segmental bronchi.
2. Bronchi appear as glandlike structures organized in tubules.
3. Respiration is not yet possible in this stage.

B. **Canalicular period** (15–25 weeks)
1. Respiratory bronchioles and terminal sacs begin to develop.
2. Vascular structures begin to form around sacs.
3. Respiration is possible only in the very latest weeks.

C. **Terminal sac period** (24 weeks to birth)
1. Vascular structures and terminal sacs continue to proliferate.
2. Cells differentiate into Type I (blood–air barrier) and Type II (surfactant-producing) pneumocytes.
3. Respiration is possible **after week 25.**
4. The amount of surfactant is the primary determinant of survival.

D. **Alveolar period** (29 weeks—8 years of age)
1. The majority of alveoli develop after birth.
2. As the child grows, the lung increases in size due to proliferation of respiratory bronchioles and terminal sacs.

VI. Diaphragm muscle

A. This is the primary muscle used for breathing.
B. The diaphragm muscle separates the pleural and peritoneal cavities.
C. It is formed from fusion of the following structures:
1. **Septum transversum**
2. Paired **pleuroperitoneal membranes**
3. **Dorsal mesentery** of the **esophagus**
4. **Body wall**
D. It is innervated by the phrenic nerve (C 3,4,5).
E. Improper formation of this muscle can lead to a **diaphragmatic hernia,** a condition with serious complications.
1. Abdominal contents are forced into the pleural cavity.
2. Lung hypoplasia results.
3. Hernias appear most often on the **left side** (posterolateral).
4. Diaphragmatic hernia is associated with polyhydramnios.
5. Diaphragmatic hernia presents at birth as a flattened abdomen, cyanosis, and inability to breathe.

QUICK HIT
The primary molecule of surfactant is dipalmitoyl-diphosphatidyl choline (lecithin). A lecithin: sphingomyelin ratio of 2:1 is the normal ratio of surfactant molecules in a newborn. A ratio below 2:1 can result in neonatal respiratory distress, especially in cesarean section delivery.

QUICK HIT
The sternocleidomastoid and the internal and external intercostals are accessory muscles of respiration. They are used when there is an increased demand for oxygen (such as in exercise) or in disease states.

PHYSICS AND FUNCTION OF THE LUNG

I. Lung Volumes
● Capacities and Volumes in the Normal Lung (Figure 3-2)

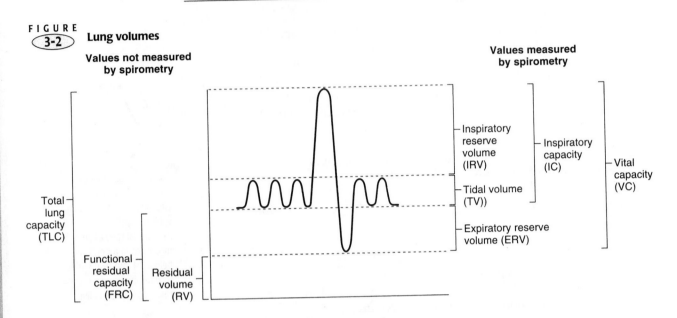

FIGURE 3-2 Lung volumes

Values not measured by spirometry

Values measured by spirometry

● Volumes and Pressure During the Breathing Cycle (Figure 3-3)

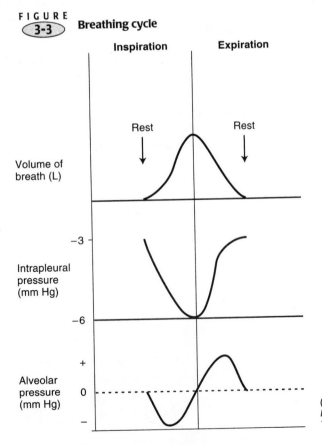

FIGURE 3-3 Breathing cycle

(Redrawn from Costanzo LS, *BRS Physiology*. Baltimore, Williams & Wilkins, 1995, p 113)

● Spirometry Tracing—Normal versus Diseased (Figure 3-4)

FIGURE
3-4 Spirometry tracings: normal versus diseased

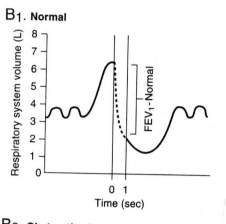

B₁. **Normal**

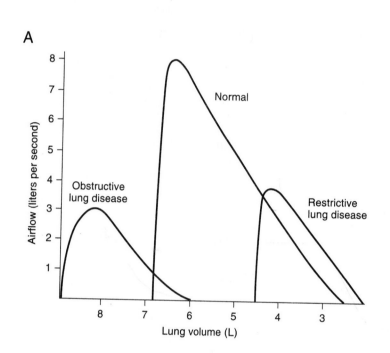

A

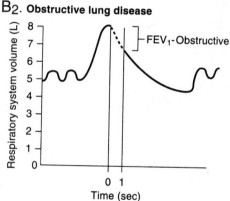

B₂. **Obstructive lung disease**

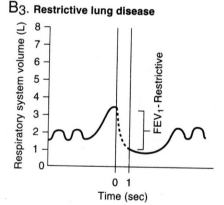

B₃. **Restrictive lung disease**

II. Compliance

A. Defined as $\Delta V/\Delta P$, where V is volume and P is pressure, compliance decribes the ability of the chest wall and lung to expand when stretched.
   1. At functional residual capacity (FRC), the lungs have a tendency to collapse.
   2. This force is balanced by the chest wall, which has a tendency to expand.
   3. Low compliance implies a stiff chest wall or lung (seen in **pulmonary fibrosis**).
   4. High compliance implies a flaccid lung (seen in **emphysema**) (See Figure 3-4).

B. **Surfactant** plays an important role in lung compliance.
1. Alveoli have a tendency to collapse.
2. An alveolus with a small radius has more collapsing pressure than an alveolus with a large radius, according to **Laplace's law:**

$P \propto T/r$, where P is pressure required to prevent alveolar collapse, T is surface tension, and r is alveolar radius.

3. Surfactant reduces the pressure and prevents collapse by reducing the intermolecular forces between liquid molecules lining the alveoli.
4. Surfactant helps increase compliance and allows the alveoli to expand.
5. **Neonatal respiratory distress** occurs in premature infants (< 37 weeks) because **Type II** (surfactant-producing) **pneumocytes** are not yet fully developed and fail to produce sufficient surfactant.
6. Atelectasis (collapsed bronchi) results from neonatal respiratory distress syndrome.

III. Airway resistance

A. Airway resistance is inversely proportional to the fourth power of the radius (formula $R = 1/r^4$); thus, any mechanism that decreases the radius of the bronchi will greatly affect the airway resistance.
B. **The airway radius** is under the control of the parasympathetic and sympathetic nervous systems.
1. **Parasympathetic nervous system**
   a. Causes **constriction** of the airways
   b. Mediated by direct stimulation, airway irritation, and slow-reacting substance of anaphylaxis (SRS-A) (see IV A).
   c. Stimulates mucus secretion
2. **Sympathetic nervous system**
   a. Causes **dilation** of airways
   b. Used as treatment for allergy and asthma (β_2-agonists)
   c. Functions in fight-or-flight autonomic reflexes; dilates airways to help provide oxygen in times of stress

IV. Ventilation and perfusion

A. **Ventilation/Perfusion (V/Q) ratio:** The ratio of the rate of alveolar ventilation to the rate of pulmonary blood flow.
B. Varies over the entire lung (higher in the apices, lower in the bases in an upright patient), but is 0.8 on average.
C. Airway obstruction
1. Causes a reduction in ventilation
2. V/Q is reduced (to zero in complete airway occlusion)
3. A V/Q of zero is considered a shunt and no gas exchange will occur (areas that are perfused, but not ventilated).
D. Blood flow obstruction
1. Blockage of a pulmonary artery or smaller vessel causes a reduction in perfusion.
2. A perfusion value of zero yields an infinite V/Q ratio.
3. A V/Q of infinity is considered **physiologic dead space.**
E. Pulmonary embolism results in increased V/Q ratio.
F. Blood flow and ventilation vary over the regions of the lung (Figure 3-5).

QUICK HIT

Allergies and allergic asthma release histamine, which is a powerful constrictor of airway smooth muscle and causes increased airway resistance.

QUICK HIT

SRS-A is a combination of the leukotrienes C_4 and D_4 (LTC_4 and LTD_4). In the treatment of asthma, zileuton blocks production of leukotrienes by inhibiting the lipoxygenase enzyme, while Zafirlukast blocks leukotriene receptors. Leukotriene A_4 (LTA_4) is a precursor to leukotriene B (LTB_4, LTC_4, and LTD_4). LTB_4 is responsible for chemotaxis of neutrophils and adhesion of white blood cells.

QUICK HIT

Anatomic shunts are passageways of blood flow that go from the venous circulation to the arterial circulation without passing through the lungs. Normally about 2% of the cardiac output is shunted. However, it can be as much as 50% in certain congenital malformations (e.g., Tetralogy of Fallot produces a right to left shunt).

QUICK HIT

There are two types of dead space:
(1) **Anatomic dead space,** measured by the **Fowler method,** is usually about 150 ml.
(2) **Physiologic dead space,** measured by the **Bohr method,** is generally considered to be the volume of the lung that does not eliminate CO_2.

THE RESPIRATORY SYSTEM

FIGURE

3-5   **Pulmonary circulation**

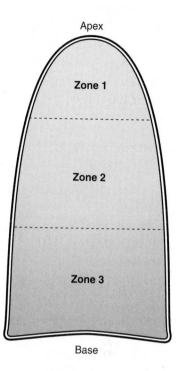

Apex

Zone 1

Zone 2

Zone 3

Base

Zone 1

- Lowest blood flow
- Alveolar pressure > Arterial pressure > Venous pressure
- Capillaries collapse due to high alveolar pressure
- Ventilation (V) is decreased less than blood flow [also called perfusion (Q)]

so: $\dfrac{V}{Q} = \dfrac{\downarrow}{\downarrow\downarrow} = \uparrow$ (Ventilation in excess of profusion)

Zone 2

- Blood flow is higher than Zone 1, but lower than Zone 3
- Arterial pressure > Alveolar pressure > Venous pressure
- Capillaries remain open because arterial pressure is greater than alveolar pressure
- Ventilation (V) is approximately equivalent to perfusion (Q)

so: $\dfrac{V}{Q} \approx 1$

Zone 3

- Highest blood flow
- Arterial pressure > Venous pressure > Alveolar pressure
- Capillaries remain open because arterial pressure is higher than both alveolar and venous pressure
- Ventilation (V) is increased less than perfusion (Q)

so: $\dfrac{V}{Q} = \dfrac{\uparrow}{\uparrow\uparrow} = \downarrow$ (Perfusion in excess of ventilation)

 QUICK HIT During exercise, pulmonary vascular resistance decreases due to dilation of the lung arterioles by metabolic products. The V/Q ratio becomes uniform over the entire lung. Conversely, during hypoxia, lack of oxygen constricts local lung vasculature, thus increasing pulmonary vascular resistance; this is opposite of what takes place in the systemic circulation, where lack of oxygen results in vasodilatation.

CONTROL OF BREATHING

I. Medulla

A. Mediates inspiration and expiration

B. Generates the basic breathing rhythm

C. Receives input via the vagus and glossopharyngeal nerves

D. Sends output via the **phrenic** nerve to the diaphragm and via the spinal nerve to the intercostals and abdominal wall.

E. The cerebral cortex can override the medulla and provide voluntary control of breathing if desired.

II. The central nervous system seeks to keep PaO_2 (partial pressure of arterial oxygen) and $PaCO_2$ (partial pressure of arterial CO_2) within a narrow range.

III. Depth and rate of respiration control these variables.

A. **Central control**

1. Chemoreceptors in the **medulla** sense the pH of the cerebrospinal fluid.

2. CO_2 crosses the blood–brain barrier and increases the **H^+ concentration** (which decreases the pH).

3. Increases in $[H^+]$ directly stimulate the central chemoreceptors which stimulate breathing.

4. Decreases in $[H^+]$ reduce stimulation of the receptors and slow respiration.

B. **Peripheral control**

1. Chemoreceptors in the **carotid bodies** and at the aortic arch bifurcation sense changes in PaO_2, $PaCO_2$, and $[H^+]$.

2. Decreases in **PaO_2** below 60 mmHg stimulate the peripheral chemoreceptors to increase rate and depth of breathing (rarely a stimulus of breathing in the absence of lung disease).

3. Increases in **PaCO₂** potentiate peripheral chemoreceptor response to PaO₂ (major direct effect of changes in PaCO₂ is on the central chemoreceptors).
4. Increases in arterial [H⁺] directly stimulate the chemoreceptors, independent of the PaCO₂ concentration (causes increased respiration in metabolic acidosis).
5. Stimulation of irritant receptors in large airways and stretch receptors in small airways inhibit inspiration.

C. **Abnormal breathing**
   1. **Cheyne-Stokes breathing**
      a. Tidal volumes variably increase and decrease and are separated by a period of apnea.
      b. This breathing abnormality is associated with drug overdose, hypoxia, and CNS depression.
   2. **Kussmaul's breathing**
      a. Rate and depth of respiration are **increased.**
      b. This abnormality is associated with diabetic ketoacidosis (DKA) and other forms of metabolic acidosis.
   3. **Sleep apnea**
      a. **Obstructive sleep apnea**
         (1) Risk factors
            (a) Middle-age
            (b) Male
            (c) Obese
            (d) Smoker
            (e) History of hypertension
            (f) History of pharyngeal malformations
            (g) Use of alcohol and other drugs
         (2) **Characteristics**
            (a) Ventilatory effort exists.
            (b) Airway is obstructed.
            (c) Apnea is terminated by self-arousal.
            (d) Apnea usually occurs in the nasopharynx or oropharynx when muscles relax during rapid eye movement (REM) sleep.
      b. **Central sleep apnea**
         (1) Ventilatory effort does not exist.
         (2) Airway is not obstructed.
         (3) Patient does not arouse self.
         (4) Central sleep apnea, like obstructive sleep apnea, occurs in the REM stage of sleep.
         (5) It is carbon dioxide threshold dependent—there is decreased chemoreceptor sensitivity to O₂ and CO₂ concentrations.
      c. **Therapy** includes weight loss (for obstructive sleep apnea) and continuous positive airway pressure (CPAP).

IV. Gas exchange

A. Diffusion of gas depends on the **partial pressure difference** between the gas in the alveolus and the gas in the blood (i.e., the difference in pressure across the blood–air barrier).

B. Partial pressure
   1. The alveolar partial pressure of oxygen (PAO₂) can be calculated as follows:

   $$PAO_2 = (760 \text{ mmHg} - 47 \text{ mmHg}) \text{ FiO}_2 - (PCO_2 / 0.8)$$

   where:
   a. 760 mmHg = total atmospheric pressure
   b. 47 mmHg = partial pressure of completely humidified air as found in the alveoli

Patients with unexplained daytime sleepiness, arrhythmias, and mood changes should be evaluated for sleep apnea.

The blood–air barrier is made up of:
1) Membrane and cytoplasm of type I pneumocytes
2) Fused basement membrane of type I pneumocytes and endothelial cells
3) Membrane and cytoplasm of endothelial cells.

c. FiO_2 = percent of air that is oxygen (normally 0.21 at sea level)

d. **$PACO_2$** = partial pressure of CO_2 in the alveoli (normally 40)

e. 0.8 = ratio of volume of CO_2 produced to the volume of O_2 consumed

2. Higher pressures will force more air into the blood and allow it to equilibrate more readily.

3. For CO_2, higher partial pressures in the blood (or lower in the alveoli) will force more CO_2 out of the blood and into the lungs, where it can be expired.

4. The amount of CO_2 delivered to the lungs and the amount of O_2 delivered to the tissues are also determined by hemoglobin concentration and red blood cell number (hematocrit) (see System 8, "Hematopoietic and Lymphoreticular System")

C. Disease affects diffusion capacity of the lung.

1. Fibrosis causes a thickening of the interstitium, which hinders perfusion across the blood–air barrier.

2. Emphysema destroys the alveolar walls and decreases the area available for gas exchange.

LUNG DEFENSES

I. Anatomical barriers

A. Impaction

1. Large particles **greater than 10 microns** fail to turn the corners of respiratory tract.

2. Common site: **nasopharynx**

B. Sedimentation

1. Medium particles between **2 and 10 microns** settle due to weight.

2. Common site: **small airways**

C. Diffusion

1. Small particles between **0.5 to 2 microns** are engulfed by alveolar macrophages (dust cells).

2. Common site: **alveoli**

D. Suspension. Particles **less than 0.5 micron** remain suspended in air.

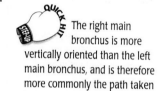

The right main bronchus is more vertically oriented than the left main bronchus, and is therefore more commonly the path taken by aspirated particles.

II. Non-specific

A. **Mucociliary escalator**

1. Particles are trapped in gel layer of upper airway.

2. Ciliary motion removes particles.

B. **Cough**

1. Cough is a bronchoconstriction that occurs to prevent penetration of particles.

2. It is also defined as deep inspiration followed by forced expiration.

Slow, deep breaths increase the deposition of dust by sedimentation and diffusion, while exercise results in higher rates of airflow and increased deposition by impaction.

III. Specific mechanisms include **secretory IgA and complement.**

ADULT RESPIRATORY DISTRESS SYNDROME AND NEONATAL RESPIRATORY DISTRESS SYNDROME

This group of diseases often leads to respiratory failure and death (Table 3-1).

TABLE 3-1	Adult Respiratory Distress Syndrome (ARDS) and Neonatal Respiratory Distress Syndrome (NRDS)	
	ARDS (Diffuse alveolar damage)	**NRDS** (Hyaline membrane disease)
Age group	*Adults*	*Premature infants*
Causes	**Shock, infection, trauma,** oxygen toxicity (free radical damage), or aspiration	**Lack of surfactant** production
Pathophysiology	Impaired gas exchange due to pulmonary hemorrhage, pulmonary edema, or atelectasis	Increased work to expand lungs; infant can clear lungs of fluids, but cannot fill lungs with air; atelectasis
Features	Respiratory insufficiency; cyanosis; hypoxemia; heavy, wet lungs; diffuse pulmonary infiltrates on radiograph; hyaline membranes in alveoli; pneumothorax may result—may be rapid and fatal	Respiratory insufficiency; cyanosis; hypoxemia; heavy, wet lungs; diffuse pulmonary infiltrates on radiograph; hyaline membranes in alveoli

QUICK HIT
Hyaline membrane disease is associated with diabetes of the mother.

QUICK HIT
Hyaline membranes are characteristic of both ARDS and NRDS but are due to distinctly different pathologic mechanisms.

PNEUMOTHORAX

I. Simple pneumothorax
A. May be caused by **spontaneous** rupture of a bleb (congenital or secondary to paraseptal emphysema) or penetrating trauma.
B. Is most commonly seen in **men 20–40 years of age.**
C. Presents as sudden chest pain, shortness of breath, **cough** and no breath sounds over the affected lung.
D. Has a 50% recurrence rate.
E. Treatment includes monitoring small defects and chest tube with vacuum for larger defects.

II. Tension pneumothorax
A. A flap of tissue allows air to enter pleural space but not to escape.
B. Pressure builds, the mediastinum is displaced, the **trachea deviates away from the lesion,** jugular venous distention (JVD) occurs, and breath sounds are uneven.
C. Cardiovascular and respiratory compromise may be rapidly **fatal.**

III. Open sucking chest wound
A. Penetrating trauma to the chest wall and pleura can cause this condition.
B. If the diameter of the lesion approaches the diameter of the trachea, air will preferentially enter through the defect.

QUICK HIT
Flail chest is caused by multiple fractures of 4 or more consecutive ribs and leads to paradoxical respirations.

PULMONARY VASCULAR DISEASES (PVD)

There are a variety of diseases which primarily affect the vasculature of the lungs (Table 3-2).

TABLE 3-2 Pulmonary Vascular Diseases			
Disease	**Etiology**	**Features**	**Complications**
Pulmonary hypertension	Primary—unknown etiology Secondary—due to COPD or increased pulmonary blood flow (as seen with a left to right shunt)	Loud **S2** **Right ventricular hypertrophy** Heart-failure cells	Leads to **cor pulmonale**
Pulmonary embolism	Commonly from proximal **deep vein thrombosis** (usually lower limb) as a result of **Virchow's triad:** blood stasis, endothelial damage (fat, infection, trauma), and hypercoagulable states	**Hemorrhagic,** red, wedge-shaped infarct Acute-onset dyspnea, chest pain, tachycardia, hypotension V/Q ratio approaches infinity Saddle embolus—an embolus lodged at the pulmonary artery bifurcation, often fatal	Can lead to cardiovascular collapse and sudden death
Pulmonary edema	Obliteration of alveoli due to intra-alveolar accumulation of fluid	Heart failure or overload leads to **increased hydrostatic pressure** Inflammatory alveolar reactions (due to drugs, pneumonia, sepsis, and uremia) leads to **increased capillary permeability**	Hypoxia
Wegener's granulomatosis	The etiology is unknown but thought to be autoimmune in nature	Focal necrotizing **vasculitis** affecting small- to medium-sized vessels. Acute necrotizing **granulomas of upper and lower respiratory tract.** Bilateral nodular and cavitary infiltrates seen on chest radiograph. Mucosal ulceration of nasopharynx seen on examination. Associated with c-ANCA.	Untreated disease is fatal within several years

c-ANCA = cytoplasmic antineutrophil cytoplasmic antibody

THE RESPIRATORY SYSTEM

QUICK HIT The clinical settings in which a pulmonary embolus can occur include cancer, multiple fractures, oral contraceptive use, prolonged bed rest, or congestive heart failure (CHF).

QUICK HIT Fat emboli are often caused by crush injury with fracture of the long bones and orthopedic surgery.

CHRONIC OBSTRUCTIVE PULMONARY DISEASE (COPD) [Table 3-3]

COPD is characterized by **airflow obstruction.** This is in contrast to restrictive pulmonary diseases which demonstrate **defective lung expansion.** Obstructive disorders have increased TLC and decreased FEV_1, while restrictive disorders show reduced lung volumes and an increased FEV_1/FVC.

Status asthmaticus is a prolonged asthmatic attack which does not respond to therapy and can be fatal.

There are many types of asthma: extrinsic (children), intrinsic (adults), exercise-induced, or cold-air-induced.

Emphysema and bronchitis often coexist in the same patient.

TABLE 3-3 Types of Chronic Obstructive Pulmonary Disease (COPD)

Disease	Pathophysiology	Clinical Features and Management
Asthma	**Increased sensitivity** of bronchioles; muscle hypertrophy; airway mucus plugs and **Charcot-Leyden crystals;** infection; emphysema; bronchitis	**Wheezing;** shortness of breath; treatment involved with inhaled β-agonists and corticosteroids
Bronchitis	Caused by persistent irritants and infections; hyperplasia of goblet cells and submucosal glands (**increased Reid index**); **excess mucus;** possible cor pulmonale	"Blue bloater"; defined as a **productive cough** for three consecutive months over two consecutive years; patients must quit **smoking**
Emphysema	Dilated alveoli; damaged alveolar walls; **decreased elastic recoil;** centrilobular, panacinar (α_1-antitrypsin deficiency), paraseptal, and irregular forms	"Pink puffer"; paraseptal type may lead to pneumothorax; patients must quit **smoking**
Bronchiectasis	**Irreversible,** pathologic bronchial dilation; chronic infection; destruction of bronchial wall; commonly due to bronchial **obstruction** (e.g., tumor)	Purulent sputum; hemoptysis; possible lung abscess; associated with cystic fibrosis and Kartagener's syndrome

INTERSTITIAL LUNG DISEASE (ILD) [Table 3-4]

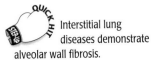

Interstitial lung disease can be a side effect of bleomycin, methotrexate, and amiodarone.

Interstitial lung diseases demonstrate alveolar wall fibrosis.

Eosinophilic granuloma, Letterer-Siwe, and Hand-Schüller-Christian are all subsets of histiocytosis X.

Sarcoidosis patients often demonstrate **anergy** when challenged with the tuberculin skin test, despite a polyclonal hyperglobulinemia.

TABLE 3-4 Interstitial Lung Disease

Disease	Pathophysiology	Population Most at Risk	Clinical Features
Eosinophilic granuloma	Presence of Langerhans-like cells and **Birbeck granules;** subset of histiocytosis X	Former **smokers**	Lesions in lung or ribs; pneumothorax
Goodpasture's syndrome	Pulmonary hemorrhage; anemia; glomerulonephritis; **anti-basement membrane antibodies**	Males; middle-aged people	**Hemoptysis;** hematuria
Idiopathic pulmonary fibrosis	Chronic **inflammation of alveolar wall;** fibrosis; cystic spaces	Sixth generation of life	**Honeycomb lung;** fatal within years
Sarcoidosis	Interstitial fibrosis; diagnosis based on biopsy showing **non-caseating granulomatous lesions;** uveitis; polyarthritis	**Young black females**	Dyspnea on exertion, dry cough, fever, fatigue and bilateral hilar lymphadenopathy
Hypersensitivity pneumonitis (Farmer's lung)	Prolonged exposure to organic antigens in atopic individuals; interstitial inflammation; alveolar damage leads to chronic, fibrotic lung	People with an occupational history of farming or bird-keeping	**Dry cough, Chest tightness** general malaise and fever

ILD is a non-infectious, non-malignant condition characterized by inflammation and pathologic changes of the alveolar wall. Differentiation and diagnosis often require histologic evaluation of the lung.

ENVIRONMENTAL LUNG DISEASES (PNEUMOCONIOSIS) [Table 3-5]

This group of diseases is often caused by workplace exposure to various organic and chemical irritants. A careful history and pulmonary function testing are often important for diagnosis.

TABLE 3-5 Environmental Lung Diseases (Pneumoconiosis)		
Disease	**Pathophysiology**	**Clinical Features**
Anthracosis	Carbon dust ingested by alveolar macrophages; visible **black deposits**	Usually asymptomatic
Asbestosis	Asbestos fibers ingested by alveolar macrophages; fibroblast proliferation; interstitial fibrosis (lower lobes); **asbestos bodies and ferruginous bodies;** pleural plaques and effusions	Increased risk of bronchogenic carcinoma and **malignant mesothelioma;** synergistic effect of asbestos and tobacco.
Coal worker's pneumoconiosis	Carbon dust ingested by alveolar macrophages forms bronchiolar **macules;** may progress to fibrosis	Plaques are asymptomatic; often benign, may progress to fibrosis; may be fatal due to pulmonary hypertension and **cor pulmonale**
Silicosis	Silica dust ingested by alveolar macrophages causing release of harmful enzymes; **silicotic nodules**	Nodules may obstruct air or blood flow; concurrent tuberculosis common **(silicotuberculosis)**
Berylliosis	Induction of cell-mediated immunity leads to non-caseating granulomas; several organ systems affected; histologically identical to sarcoidosis	Increases lung cancer

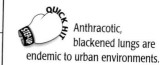

QUICK HIT Anthracotic, blackened lungs are endemic to urban environments.

QUICK HIT Silicosis is an **occupational** disease seen in individuals involved in mining, stone-cutting, and glass production.

RESPIRATORY INFECTIONS

I. Pneumonia

A. Pathogenesis

1. Most commonly, pneumonia is caused by **aspiration** from the oropharynx.
2. Alcoholism, nasogastric tubes, and obtunded states increase risk of contracting pneumonia.
3. Normal flora consists of gram-positive cocci.
4. Hospitalized patients are colonized by gram-negative rods (nosocomial infections).
5. Other portals of entry include respiratory droplets, contiguous spread, or traumatic inoculation.

B. **Clinical Manifestations**

1. **Typical pneumonia** presents with acute fever, purulent sputum, pleuritic pain, and lobar "whited out" infiltrate on chest radiograph (e.g., *Streptococcus pneumoniae*).

   2. **Atypical pneumonia** is characterized by slow onset of nonproductive cough, headache, gastrointestinal (GI) symptoms, and patchy infiltrate on chest radiograph (e.g., *Mycoplasma pneumoniae*).
C. Location of pathology and typical organisms
   1. **Lobar** (intra-alveolar infiltrate): *S. pneumoniae*
   2. **Bronchopneumonia** (bronchiolar infiltrate): *Staphylococcus aureus, Haemophilus influenza*
   3. **Interstitial** (diffuse infiltrate in alveolar wall): *Mycoplasma pneumoniae*
D. Etiology
   1. Bacterial and mycoplasma pneumonia (Table 3-6)
   2. Viral pneumonia (Table 3-7)
   3. Fungal pneumonia (Table 3-8)
E. Clinical diagnosis of pneumonia (Table 3-9 and Table 3-10)

TABLE 3-6 **Bacterial and Mycoplasma Pneumonia**

Bacteria	Presentation	Population Most at Risk	Clinical Features
Streptococcus pneumoniae	Typical	**Adults**	Most common cause of pneumonia
Haemophilus influenzae	Typical	Elderly	Complicates viral infection; chronic respiratory disease
Staphylococcus aureus	Typical	Can cause typical community-acquired pneumonia but also infects immunocompromised and hospitalized patients	Abscesses; complicates viral infection
Streptococcus agalactiae	Typical	**Neonates** (along with *E. coli*)	Similar to *S. pneumoniae*
Mycoplasma pneumoniae	Atypical	**Young adults**	Most common cause of atypical pneumonia; positive cold-agglutinin test
Legionella pneumophila	Atypical	Immunocompromised patients	Found in drinking water and air conditioners
Klebsiella *pneumoniae*	Atypical	Patients with alcoholism	Aspiration of gastric contents
Chlamydia psittaci	Atypical	**Pet bird** owners	Bradycardia; splenomegaly
Chlamydia trachomatis	Atypical	Neonates	Most common cause of preventable blindness (trachoma)
Chlamydia pneumoniae	Atypical	Young adults	Upper and lower pulmonary tract infection
Coxiella burnetii	Atypical	Dairy workers (via inhalation)	Fever
Francisella tularensis	Atypical	Patients exposed to rabbits or squirrels	Granulomatous nodules

TABLE 3-7 Viral Pneumonia

Virus	Pathophysiology	Clinical Features
Respiratory syncytial virus (Types 1 and 2)	Atypical	Also causes bronchiolitis; more common in winter months
Influenza	Atypical	**Often complicated by bacterial infection**

TABLE 3-8 Fungal Pneumonia

Etiology	Pathophysiology	Clinical Features
Histoplasma capsulatum	Atypical	Most infections are subclinical; organisms in macrophages
Coccidioides immitis	Atypical	Most infections are subclinical; "valley fever"
Pneumocystis carinii	Atypical	Often fatal

TABLE 3-9 Clinical Diagnosis of Pneumonia

	Bacterial	Viral	Mycoplasma
Age	Any; often under 2 years	Any	Young adults
Fever	>39°C	<39°C	<39°C
Onset	Abrupt	Gradual	Abrupt fever; gradual cough
Relatives	Healthy	Sick (concurrent)	Sick (2–3 weeks previous)
Cough	Productive	Dry	Paroxysmal
Pleuritic chest pain	Yes (splinting)	No	No
Physical examination	Tubular breath sounds; dull to percussion	Bilateral, diffuse rales	Rales in one or two segments
Radiographic findings	Consolidated "whited out" lobe	Diffuse; patchy; bilateral	Patchy; one or two lobes; no consolidation

QUICK HIT

Aspirin therapy for the fever of influenza and varicella zoster infections in children is contraindicated as it may cause Reye's syndrome. Clinical manifestations of Reye's syndrome include encephalopathy and potentially fatal liver damage.

QUICK HIT

Other less common sources of fungal lung infection include *Cryptococcus neoformans* and Aspergillus (resulting in a **fungus ball**) in immunocompromised individuals.

QUICK HIT

Pneumocystis carinii is sometimes classified as a parasite.

THE RESPIRATORY SYSTEM

TABLE 3-10	Most Common Causative Agents of Pneumonia By Age			
	Children (birth–20 years of age)	**Young Adults (20–40 years of age)**	**Adults (40–60 years of age)**	**Elderly (60 years of age and older)**
Causative agents in each age group	RSV *Mycoplasma pneumoniae* *Chlamydia pneumoniae* *S. pneumoniae*	*Mycoplasma pneumoniae* *S. pneumoniae*	*S. pneumoniae* *Mycoplasma pneumonia* *H. influenzae*	*S. pneumoniae* Anaerobes *H. influenzae* RSV
RSV=respiratory syncytial virus				

II. Tuberculosis (Figure 3-6)

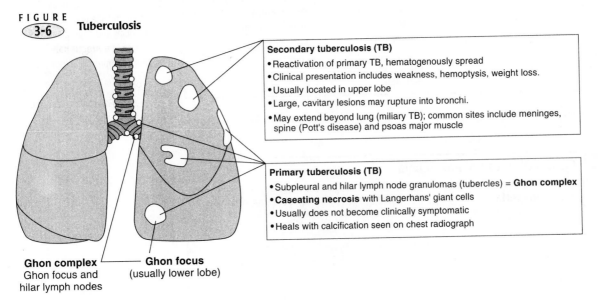

FIGURE 3-6 Tuberculosis

Secondary tuberculosis (TB)
- Reactivation of primary TB, hematogenously spread
- Clinical presentation includes weakness, hemoptysis, weight loss.
- Usually located in upper lobe
- Large, cavitary lesions may rupture into bronchi.
- May extend beyond lung (miliary TB); common sites include meninges, spine (Pott's disease) and psoas major muscle

Primary tuberculosis (TB)
- Subpleural and hilar lymph node granulomas (tubercles) = **Ghon complex**
- **Caseating necrosis** with Langerhans' giant cells
- Usually does not become clinically symptomatic
- Heals with calcification seen on chest radiograph

Ghon complex
Ghon focus and hilar lymph nodes

Ghon focus
(usually lower lobe)

> **QUICK HIT** Sudden infant death syndrome (SIDS) is the death of a child under one year of age from unexplained causes (even after autopsy). The infant is usually asleep in the prone position and has a history of an **upper respiratory infection.**

III. Upper Respiratory Infections
1. Sinusitis
   a. Results from obstructed drainage outlets of the sinuses
   b. Caused by *S. pneumoniae, H. influenzae,* Moraxella
2. Rhinitis
   a. Viral rhinitis
      (1) Commonly caused by adenovirus
      (2) Common cold
   b. Bacterial rhinitis
      (1) Often secondary to viral infection
      (2) Commonly caused by streptococcus, staphylococcus, *H. influenzae*
   c. Allergic rhinitis
      (1) Type 1 hypersensitivity reactions
      (2) Characterized by eosinophilia
3. Laryngitis
   a. Characterized by edema and inflammation of the vocal cords
   b. Caused by infection (*M. pneumonia,* parainfluenza virus) or overuse
4. Croup versus Epiglottitis (Table 3-11)

TABLE 3-11 Croup versus Epiglottitis		
	Croup	**Epiglottitis**
Organism	Parainfluenza type 2 virus	*H. influenzae*
Pathology	Inflammation of subglottic trachea	Inflamed epiglottis
Age	6 months to 2 years	1 to 5 years
Fever	< 39°C	> 39°C
Onset	Gradual (barking cough to **stridor**)	Abrupt; **stridor**
Associated symptoms	Rhinorrhea; hoarseness; conjunctivitis	None
Degree of illness	Not toxic; degree of symptoms greater than degree of illness	Toxic
Physical examination	Writhing; anxious; subglottic edema on radiograph	Quiet; "**sniffing position**"; drooling; "thumb-print" epiglottis on radiograph
Outcome	Self-limiting	Medical emergency; 90% of patients require surgery to re-establish airway

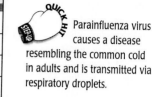

QUICK HIT Parainfluenza virus causes a disease resembling the common cold in adults and is transmitted via respiratory droplets.

CYSTIC FIBROSIS (CF)

I. CF is the **most common lethal genetic disease in whites.**

II. **Autosomal recessive** mutation occurs on chromosome 7, the cystic fibrosis transmembrane conductance regulator (CFTR) gene. This leads to
   A. Altered **chloride** and water transport in cells.
   B. Deletion of phenylalanine at position 508 (**delta F508**).
   C. High sodium and chloride concentrations on sweat test.
   D. Malfunction of exocrine glands increases mucus viscosity and leads to organ malfunction.

III. **Chronic Pulmonary Disease**
   A. Most serious complication and **leading cause of death** in patients with CF.
   B. *Pseudomonas aeruginosa* infections are common.
   C. Increased residual volume (RV) and increased total lung capacity (TLC) are characteristic of chronic pulmonary disease.
   D. Atelectasis
   E. Bronchiectasis

IV. **Pancreatic insufficiency**
   A. Nutrition deficiencies (especially of fat-soluble vitamins A, D, E, and K)
   B. **Steatorrhea**

V. **Meconium Ileus**

VI. **Treatment** of cystic fibrosis includes symptomatic treatment and gene therapy.

THE RESPIRATORY SYSTEM

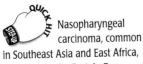

Superior sulcus tumors (**Pancoast's**) involve the apex of the lung and result in **Horner's syndrome** (ptosis, miosis, anhydrosis). **Superior vena cava syndrome** occurs when the superior vena cava is obstructed, resulting in facial cyanosis and swelling.

Nasopharyngeal carcinoma, common in Southeast Asia and East Africa, is caused by the Epstein-Barr virus.

Paraneoplastic syndrome is a clinical and biochemical disturbance caused by a neoplasm that is not directly related to the primary tumor or metastases. Secretion of parathyroid hormone (PTH)-like hormone results in hypercalcemia. Ectopic antidiuretic hormone (ADH) production leads to syndrome of inappropriate antidiuretic hormone (SIADH) with urinary retention and high urine osmolality. Adrenocorticotropic hormone (ACTH)-producing tumors lead to Cushing's syndrome.

LUNG NEOPLASMS (Table 3-12)

I. Lung neoplasms are the **leading cause of cancer death for both men and women in the United States.**

II. Lung is the **second most common type** of cancer (with the first being prostate cancer in men and breast cancer in women).

III. Lung cancer deaths among women are rising rapidly due to increased smoking in this population.

IV. Symptoms include cough, hemoptysis, airway obstruction, weight loss, and paraneoplastic syndromes.

TABLE 3-12 Lung Neoplasms

Tumor	Location and Histology	Clinical Features
Adenocarcinoma	**Peripheral;** subpleural; usually on pre-existing **scars;** glandular	**Most common type;** may be related to smoking; CEA positive; K-ras oncogenes
Bronchioalveolar	**Peripheral;** subtype of adenocarcinoma; tumor cells line alveolar walls	**Less strongly associated with smoking;** auto-antibodies to surfactant may exist
Carcinoid	Major bronchi; spread by direct extension	Increased secretion of **5-HT;** flushing; wheezing; heart disease; low malignancy
Large cell	**Peripheral;** undifferentiated; giant cells with pleomorphism	Poor prognosis; metastasis to the brain; smoking
Metastasis	**Cannonball** lesions	**Higher incidence than primary lung cancer**
Small cell (oat cell)	**Central;** undifferentiated; **most aggressive;** small, dark blue cells	Poor prognosis; increased in smokers; ectopic ACTH and ADH secretion
Squamous cell	**Central;** mass from bronchus; keratin pearls; cavitation	Increased in smokers; secretion of **PTH-like peptide**

ACTH=adrenocorticotropic hormone; *ADH*=antidiuretic hormone; *CEA*=carcinoembryonic antigen; *5-HT*=serotonin; *PTH*=parathyroid hormone

THERAPEUTICS

Antitussives, Expectorants, and Mucolytics

Acetylcysteine
Codeine

Dextromethorphan
Guaifenesin

Hydrocodone

Asthma therapeutics

Adenosine
Albuterol
Cromolyn sodium
Epinephrine

Ipratropium bromide
Prednisone
Terbutaline

Theophylline
Zafirlukast
Zileuton

Antimicrobials

Amoxicillin
Cephalosporin
Clindamycin

Erythromycin
Nafcillin
Penicillin

Trimethoprim-
   sulfamethoxazole
Vancomycin

Antineoplastic

Cisplatin

Paclitaxel

Sleep Apnea Therapeutics

Tricyclic
   anti-depressants

Antituberculosis Therapeutics

Ethambutol
Isoniazid

Pyrazinamide

Rifampin

The Gastrointestinal System

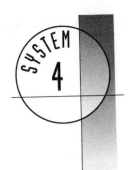
The boundaries of the epiploic foramen of Winslow (opening of the lesser sac) are the hepatoduodenal ligament (containing the common bile duct, the common hepatic artery, and the portal vein) located anteriorly, the caudate lobe of the liver located superiorly, the duodenum located inferiorly, and the inferior vena cava located posteriorly.

INNERVATION AND BLOOD SUPPLY OF THE GASTROINTESTINAL TRACT (Figure 4-1)

FIGURE
4-1

Innervation and blood supply of the gastrointestinal tract

☐ Foregut   ☐ Midgut   ☐ Hindgut

Liver

Stomach

Gallbladder   Pancreas   Splenic flexure

Gastrocolic flexure   Colon

Small intestine

Appendix

Rectum

1) Foregut
 • Derivatives
  – Esophagus
  – Stomach
  – First part of duodenum
  – Liver
  – Gallbladder
  – Pancreas
   (formed from fusion of dorsal and ventral buds)
 • Supplied by celiac trunk
 • Vagal parasympathetic nerve, thoracic nerve, and splanchnic sympathetic nerve

2) Midgut
 • Derivatives
  – Second, third, and fourth parts of duodenum
  – Jejunum
  – Ileum
  – Appendix
  – Proximal two thirds of colon (up to splenic flexure)
 • Supplied by superior mesenteric artery
 • Vagal parasympathetic nerve, thoracic splanchnic sympathetic nerve

3) Hindgut
 • Derivatives
  – Distal one third of colon including sigmoid colon and rectum to pectinate line
 • Supplied by inferior mesenteric artery
 • Pelvic splanchnic (S2-S4) parasympathetic nerve, and lumbar spanchnic sympathetic nerve

4) Ectoderm
 • Derivatives
  – Oropharynx (anterior two thirds of tongue, lips, parotid glands, tooth enamel)
  – Anus, distal rectum (from pectinate line outward)

HORMONES OF THE GASTROINTESTINAL SYSTEM (Figure 4-2)

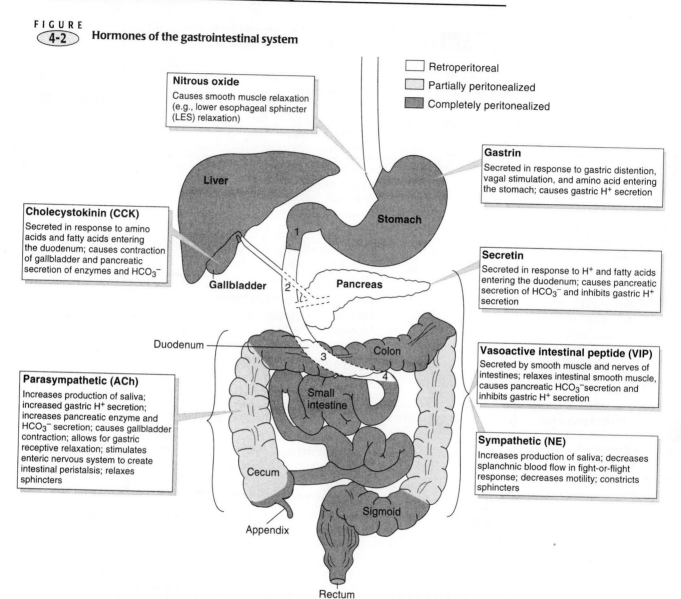

FIGURE 4-2 Hormones of the gastrointestinal system

☐ Retroperitoreal
▨ Partially peritonealized
▨ Completely peritonealized

Nitrous oxide
Causes smooth muscle relaxation (e.g., lower esophageal sphincter (LES) relaxation)

Gastrin
Secreted in response to gastric distention, vagal stimulation, and amino acid entering the stomach; causes gastric H⁺ secretion

Cholecystokinin (CCK)
Secreted in response to amino acids and fatty acids entering the duodenum; causes contraction of gallbladder and pancreatic secretion of enzymes and HCO_3^-

Secretin
Secreted in response to H⁺ and fatty acids entering the duodenum; causes pancreatic secretion of HCO_3^- and inhibits gastric H⁺ secretion

Vasoactive intestinal peptide (VIP)
Secreted by smooth muscle and nerves of intestines; relaxes intestinal smooth muscle, causes pancreatic HCO_3^- secretion and inhibits gastric H⁺ secretion

Parasympathetic (ACh)
Increases production of saliva; increased gastric H⁺ secretion; increases pancreatic enzyme and HCO_3^- secretion; causes gallbladder contraction; allows for gastric receptive relaxation; stimulates enteric nervous system to create intestinal peristalsis; relaxes sphincters

Sympathetic (NE)
Increases production of saliva; decreases splanchnic blood flow in fight-or-flight response; decreases motility; constricts sphincters

Liver, Stomach, Gallbladder, Pancreas, Duodenum, Colon, Small intestine, Cecum, Sigmoid, Appendix, Rectum

ACh=acetylcholine; H⁺=hydrogen; HCO_3^-=bicarbonate; NE=norepinephrine.

With the exception of a Meckel's diverticulum, which can remain asymptomatic throughout life, congenital malformations of the gastrointestinal (GI) tract will manifest themselves during the neonatal period.

IMPORTANT CONGENITAL MALFORMATIONS OF THE GASTROINTESTINAL SYSTEM (Table 4-1)

TABLE 4-1 Important Congenital Malformations of the Gastrointestinal System	
Malformation	**Clinical Features**
Hypertrophic pyloric stenosis	Thickening of the pylorus musculature **Projectile vomiting** Palpable knot in the pyloric region
Extrahepatic biliary atresia	Incomplete recanalization of bile duct during development Presents shortly after birth Dark urine Clay-colored stool Jaundice
Annular pancreas	Abnormal fusion of ventral and dorsal pancreatic buds forming a constricting ring around the duodenum Duodenal obstruction presents shortly after birth
Meckel's diverticulum	Persistent remnant of the vitelline duct Forms an outpouching (true diverticulum) in the ileum Ulceration and bleeding 50% contain either gastric or pancreatic tissue
Malrotation of the midgut	Normal 270° rotation is not completed Cecum and appendix lie in upper abdomen Associated with **volvulus** (twisting of intestine) causing an obstruction
Intestinal stenosis or atresia	Results from failure of the normal recanalization of the lumen May produce failure to thrive
Hirschsprung's diseases (congenital or toxic megacolon)	Failure of **neural crest cells** to migrate to colon No peristalsis Constipation and abdominal distention in newborn **Bowel movement precipitated by digital rectal examination**
Anal agenesis	Lack of anal opening due to improper formation of the urorectal septum May cause rectovesicular (anus to bladder), rectovaginal, or rectourethral fistula

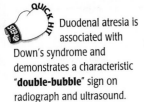

Rule of 2's for Meckel's diverticulum: 2 feet from ileocecal junction; 2 inches long; 2% of the population affected; 2 types of ectopic tissue involved (gastric or pancreatic).

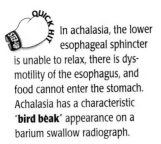

Duodenal atresia is associated with Down's syndrome and demonstrates a characteristic **"double-bubble"** sign on radiograph and ultrasound.

THE OROPHARYNX, ESOPHAGUS, AND STOMACH

I. The digestion of food begins in the oral cavity with salivary enzymes.

II. The esophagus transports food to the stomach.
   A. **The upper third** of the esophagus is **skeletal muscle.**
   B. **The middle third** is **both** skeletal and smooth muscle.
   C. **The lower third** is **smooth muscle.**
   D. The lower esophageal sphincter relaxes in preparation for the passage of food into the stomach.

III. The stomach receives and stores food.
   A. **Receptive relaxation**—the stomach relaxes to accommodate entering food (a vagovagal reflex).

In achalasia, the lower esophageal sphincter is unable to relax, there is dysmotility of the esophagus, and food cannot enter the stomach. Achalasia has a characteristic **'bird beak'** appearance on a barium swallow radiograph.

B. Three phases of gastric secretion
  1. **Cephalic phase**—the sight, smell, taste, or thought of food stimulates secretion
  2. **Gastric phase**—secretion is caused by the entry of food into the stomach
  3. **Intestinal phase**—food entering the intestine causes a feedback stimulation of gastric secretion
C. Important gastric secretions
  1. **Hydrochloric acid** is secreted by parietal cells of the fundus.
    a. Stimulated by gastrin, histamine, and vagal stimulation.
    b. Inhibited by **omeprazole** (proton pump inhibitor), **cimetidine** (H_2 blocker), chyme in small intestine via gastric inhibitory peptide (GIP) and secretin.
  2. **Intrinsic factor** is secreted by parietal cells of the fundus.
    a. Binds to vitamin B_{12} (extrinsic factor)
    b. **B_{12}-intrinsic factor** complex absorbed in **terminal ileum**.
  3. **Pepsinogen** is secreted by chief cells.
    a. Pepsinogen is converted to pepsin by the low pH of the stomach.
    b. Pepsin begins digestion of protein.
  4. **Gastrin** is secreted by the G cells of the antrum and pylorus stimulates the release of hydrochloric acid (HCl) from parietal cells.
  5. Somatostatin is secreted by a variety of cells throughout the GI tract and has a global inhibitory effect.
D. The stomach grinds food into small particles and forces it into the duodenum.
  1. Grinding (trituration) takes place in peristaltic waves occurring at a rate of 3 to 5 waves per minute.
  2. **Migrating motor complexes** (MMC), stimulated by motilin, occur in the inter-digestive period and serve to flush undigested food through the GI system.

Non-neoplastic and neoplastic disorders originating proximal to the pyloric sphincter often present with hematemesis and dysphagia as a result of alcohol and tobacco abuse.

● **Non-neoplastic Disorders of the Oropharynx, Esophagus, and Stomach (Table 4-2)**

TABLE 4-2	**Non-neoplastic Disorders of the Oropharynx, Esophagus, and Stomach**		
Disorder	**Etiology and Pathology**	**Clinical Features**	**Notes**
Sialolithiasis	Blockage of salivary gland duct preventing release of saliva; follows chronic sialadenitis (inflammation of the salivary glands)	Acute pain; usually in submandibular gland or Stensen's duct of the parotid gland	Passage of stone can be induced by stimulating secretion of saliva (e.g., by sucking on a lemon)
Pleomorphic adenoma	Increased risk with radiation exposure	Benign, recurring, mixed cell tumor of the parotid; may lead to facial nerve injury	Most frequent salivary gland tumor; more common in women 20–40 years of age

(continued)

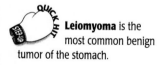

Leiomyoma is the most common benign tumor of the stomach.

TABLE 4-2 Non-neoplastic Disorders of the Oropharynx, Esophagus, and Stomach *(Continued)*

Disorder	Etiology and Pathology	Clinical Features	Notes
Esophageal variceal bleeding	Bleeding from esophageal varices due to portal hypertension	Hematemesis; signs of portal hypertension (i.e., caput medusae, ascites)	Usually treated with vasoconstrictors (vasopressin); endoscopy required for diagnosis (to rule out bleeding ulcers)
Boerhaave's syndrome	Complete rupture of the esophagus (all layers); caused by severe retching	Often presents as left pneumothorax; surgical correction necessary	Esophageal reflux disease predisposes to this condition
Mallory-Weiss syndrome	Laceration of the gastroesophageal junction; usually caused by severe retching	Post-retching hematemesis	Alcoholics at increased risk
Acute gastritis	NSAIDs; smoking; alcohol; aspirin; steroids; burn injury (Curling's ulcer); brain injury (Cushing's ulcer)	Erosive; acute inflammation; necrosis; hemorrhage; **"coffee-ground" vomitus**	Blood in the nasogastric tube
Chronic Gastritis	Type A (fundal): autoimmune pernicious anemia, aging; Type B (antral): Helicobacter pylori	Non-erosive; mucosal inflammation and atrophy of mucosa	Risk factor for gastric carcinoma
Gastric Ulcers	**H. pylori** (70% of cases); bile-induced gastritis; increased permeability of gastric mucosa; associated with use of aspirin and NSAIDs	Post-prandial pain; bleeding; perforation; obstruction	Usually near lesser curvature; not dependent on increased gastric acid secretion; not precancerous
Dumping syndrome	Post vagotomy; unimpeded passage of hypertonic food to the small intestine causing distention due to osmotic flow of water into the lumen	Nausea; diarrhea; palpitations; sweating; lightheadedness; reactive hypoglycemia	Can be prevented by eating only small meals and ingesting solids and liquids separately

NSAIDs=nonsteroidal anti-inflammatory drugs

● **Neoplastic Disorders of the Oropharynx, Esophagus, and Stomach (Table 4-3)**

TABLE 4-3 Neoplastic Disorders of the Oropharynx, Esophagus, and Stomach

Disorder	Etiology and Pathology	Clinical Features	Notes
Oral cancer	**Smoking;** chewing tobacco; alcohol	Squamous cell carcinoma; usually involves tongue	Leukoplakia (white patch on the mucus membrane that cannot be wiped off) is a common precursor lesion *(continued)*

TABLE 4-3	Neoplastic Disorders of the Oropharynx, Esophagus, and Stomach (Continued)		
Disorder	**Etiology and Pathology**	**Clinical Features**	**Notes**
Esophageal adenocarcinoma	**Barrett's esophagus;** complication of gastroesophageal reflux disease	**Columnar metaplasia of esophageal squamous epithelium;** distal third of the esophagus	More common in whites
Esophageal squamous cell carcinoma	Alcohol and tobacco use; esophagitis	Dysphagia; anorexia; pain	More common in blacks
Gastric carcinoma	**H. pylori;** gastritis; low fiber diet; nitrosamines; blood group A; high salt diet; increased incidence in Japan	Aggressive spread from antrum to nodes and liver; **Virchow's node** (enlarged supra-clavicular lymph node); **Krukenberg tumor** (metastatic disease to the ovaries from the stomach charac-terized by mucinous, signet ring cells)	More common in men over 50 years of age; infiltration of stomach walls with tumor cells and subsequent fibrosis leads to linitis plastica (leather-bottle stomach)

THE SMALL INTESTINE, LARGE INTESTINE, AND RECTUM

● Muscular Layers of the GI Tract (Figure 4-3)

FIGURE 4-3 Picture of muscular layer of the GI tract

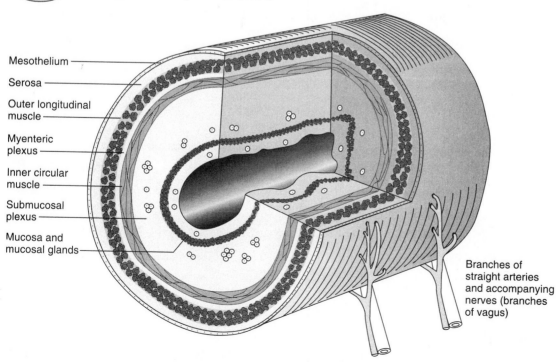

Mesothelium
Serosa
Outer longitudinal muscle
Myenteric plexus
Inner circular muscle
Submucosal plexus
Mucosa and mucosal glands

Branches of straight arteries and accompanying nerves (branches of vagus)

I. The small intestine digests and absorbs food.

A. Digestion is mediated by a variety of GI hormones including cholecystokinin (CCK), secretin, somatostatin, and others (see Figure 4-2).

B. Carbohydrates

1. Pancreatic amylase hydrolyzes glycogen, starch, and most other complex carbohydrates to disaccharides.
2. Disaccharides are broken down to monosaccharides by intestinal brush border enzymes and absorbed.
3. Monosaccharides are absorbed by a variety of mechanisms.
   a. Glucose and galactose are absorbed by sodium (Na^+) dependent transport.
   b. Fructose is absorbed by facilitated diffusion.

C. **Protein**

1. Degraded to amino acids, di- and tri-peptides by proteases produced by the pancreas.
   a. Activation of **trypsinogen to trypsin**
      (i) Auto-activated
      (ii) Activated by intestinal brush border enterokinases
   b. Trypsin degrades the peptide bonds of arginine or lysine.
   c. Trypsin also activates the other proteolytic pancreatic enzymes.
2. Proteins absorbed by an Na^+ dependent transport.
   a. Separate carriers for acidic, basic, and neutral amino acids.
   b. Di- and tri-peptides are absorbed faster than single amino acids.

D. **Fats**

1. Lipids are broken into droplets by the mixing action of the stomach.
2. **Pancreatic lipase** (and to a lesser extent salivary lipase) **hydrolyzes triacylglycerol to fatty acids and 2-monoacylglycerol.**
3. Bile salts (amphipathic molecules) emulsify the hydrolyzed products and form micelles.
4. **Micelles** allow for fat absorption (Figure 4-4).

QUICK HIT

Lactose intolerance is caused by a genetic absence or decrease in lactase. Lactose cannot be broken down; it remains in the lumen of the gut and causes osmotic diarrhea.

QUICK HIT

Often the amino acid transporter found in the intestines is identical to the amino acid transporter found in the renal tubules. As such, diseases which affect these transporters have multi-organ system effects. One of these diseases is Hartnup's, which is a defect in the intestinal and renal tubular absorption of neutral amino acids leading to excretion of tryptophan derivatives and causing pellagra-like symptoms.

The Gastrointestinal System

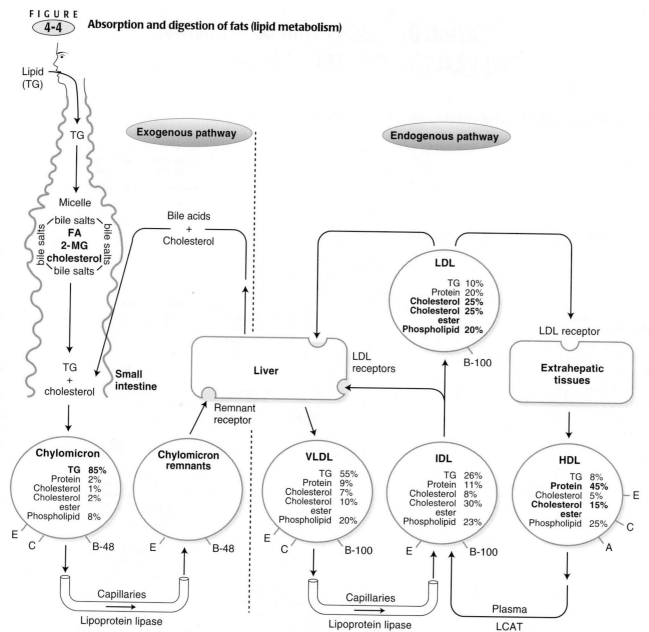

FIGURE 4-4 Absorption and digestion of fats (lipid metabolism)

FA=fatty acid; HDL=high density lipoprotein; IDL=intermediate density lipoprotein; LDL=low density lipoprotein; TG=triglyceride; MG=monoglyceride; VLDL=very low density lipoprotein; A, B, C, and E are lipoproteins involved with lipid metabolism.
(Adapted from Goldstein J, Kita T, and Brown M: Defective lipoprotein receptors and atherosclerosis. NEJM 309:288, 1983).

II. The **large intestine** stores and excretes non-digestible material.

A. Absorbs 2–3 L/day of water

B. **Secretes potassium (K+)**

C. Mediates defecation of undigested material through both voluntary and involuntary (rectosphincteric reflex) mechanisms.

LOCATION OF ABSORPTION OF VITAMINS, MINERALS, AND NUTRIENTS (Figure 4-5)

FIGURE 4-5 Location of absorption of vitamins, minerals, and nutrients

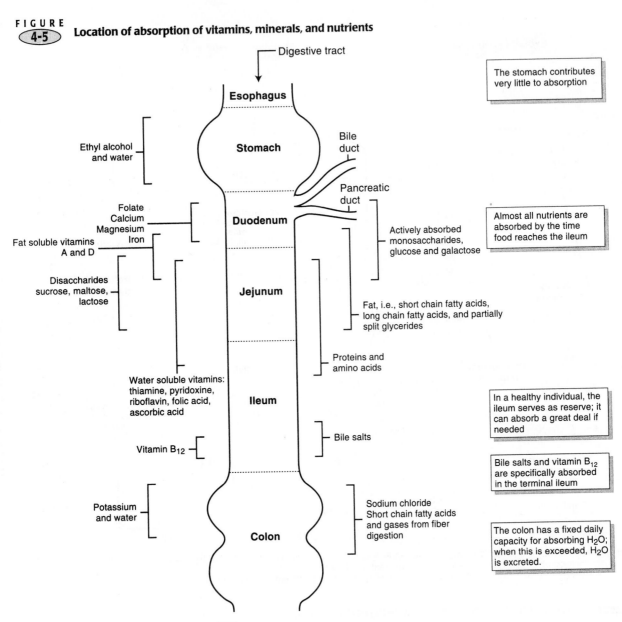

The stomach contributes very little to absorption

Almost all nutrients are absorbed by the time food reaches the ileum

In a healthy individual, the ileum serves as reserve; it can absorb a great deal if needed

Bile salts and vitamin B_{12} are specifically absorbed in the terminal ileum

The colon has a fixed daily capacity for absorbing H_2O; when this is exceeded, H_2O is excreted.

(Adapted from James P. Ryan, PhD, Physiology, 1997)

Common clinical disorders of the gastrointestinal tract, distal to the pyloric sphincter, will usually present as vague abdominal pain due to stimulation of the visceral afferent nerves. If the parietal peritoneum, innervated by the somatic afferent nerves, is irritated due to the lesion, the pain will become more localized (as is seen in acute appendicitis).

COMMON CLINICAL DISORDERS OF THE SMALL INTESTINE, LARGE INTESTINE, AND RECTUM (Table 4-4)

TABLE 4-4	Common Clinical Disorders of the Small Intestine, Large Intestine, and Rectum		
Disorder	**Etiology and Pathology**	**Clinical Features**	**Notes**
Hiatal hernia	Sac-like herniation of stomach through diaphragm; smoking; obesity	Retrosternal pain (worse in supine position); can lead to **gastroesophageal reflux disease**	Usually occurs in the sliding (vs. rolling) form
Duodenal ulcers	**Helicobacter pylori** (in 90% of cases); hypersecretion of acid; smokers; Zollinger-Ellison syndrome; blood group O; associated with NSAID use	Coffee ground vomitus; **smooth border;** clean base; black stools; pain at night or 2 hours post-prandial; perforation may result in acute pancreatitis	Not pre-cancerous
Ischemic bowel disease	Atherosclerosis of celiac artery or mesenteric artery	Abdominal pain; nausea; vomiting; stool positive for blood test	Usually affects watershed areas (splenic flexure or rectosigmoid junction)
Diverticulitis	Outpouchings of the colon obstructed with fecalith leading to inflammation or infection; low fiber diet	Usually involves the **sigmoid colon;** fever; leukocytosis; colicky pain; usually multiple in number and cause increased risk of perforation	False diverticula: pockets of mucosa and submucosa herniated through muscular layer
Appendicitis	Obstruction (usually fecalith or lymphoid hyperplasia); bacterial proliferation and mucosal invasion	Nausea; vomiting; abdominal pain that migrates from epigastrium to right lower quadrant (RLQ); pain at **McBurney's point;** psoas sign or obturator sign; increased WBC's in blood	Differential diagnosis in females includes ectopic pregnancy, ovarian torsion, ruptured ovarian cyst, and PID
Adenocarcinoma of colon and rectum	Chronic inflammatory bowel disease; low fiber diet; older age; hereditary polyposis or adenomatous disorders	**Increased CEA** (not diagnostic, used to assess treatment); rectosigmoid tumors present in an **annular manner** producing early obstruction and constipation. **Left-sided tumors present with blood in the stool, while right-sided tumors typically present with anemia, as a result of occult blood loss.**	Screen for occult blood in stool; third most common cause of cancer death (after lung and prostate/breast)
Carcinoid tumor	Arise from **neuroendocrine cells** (Kulchitsky's cells); release vasoactive peptides such as histamine, serotonin, and prostaglandins	**Increased 5-HIAA in urine;** diarrhea; **flushing;** right sided heart valve lesions; hypotension; bronchospasm	Most common tumor of the appendix, but also found in the ileum, rectum, and bronchus

CEA=carcinoembryonic antigen; 5-HIAA=5-hydroxyindoleacetic acid; NSAID=nonsteroidal anti-inflammatory drug; PID=pelvic inflammatory disease; WBC=white blood cell

QUICK HIT Posterior duodenal ulcers are associated with erosion of the gastroduodenal artery and subsequent hemorrhage.

QUICK HIT *H. pylori* infection is pharmacologically treated with "**triple therapy**". The therapeutic regimen typically includes a proton-pump inhibitor (omeprazole) and two of the following antibiotics: clarithromycin, amoxicillin, and metronidazole.

QUICK HIT Small bowel obstructions are usually due to adhesions, while large bowel obstructions are most commonly a result of neoplasms. Ileus, a common cause of temporary small bowel paralysis, commonly occurs post-operatively.

QUICK HIT Diverticulosis, the most common cause of bleeding from the lower GI tract, can be differentiated from diverticulitis because, typically, diverticulitis does not cause bleeding.

THE GASTROINTESTINAL SYSTEM

Diarrhea, the passage of abnormal amounts of fluid or semisolid fecal matter, can be mediated by a number of mechanisms. Osmotic diarrhea results when non-absorbed solutes increase intraluminal oncotic pressure, causing an outpouring of water. Surgical resection can lead to an inadequate surface for absorption of nutrients, resulting in a form of osmotic diarrhea. Active ion secretion causing obligatory water loss is termed secretory diarrhea. Altered intestinal motility, where there is an alteration of the normally coordinated control of intestinal propulsion, may also result in diarrhea (often alternating with constipation). Finally, sloughing of colonic mucosa, due to inflammation and necrosis, as often a result of infection, causes an exudative form of diarrhea.

● **Bacterial Causes of Diarrhea (Table 4-5)**

TABLE 4-5 Bacterial Causes of Diarrhea

Infectious Agent	Clinical Features	Treatment	Notes
Shigella	**Shiga-toxin** causes **bloody** diarrhea, mild to severe, 1–2 weeks in duration; fever for 3–4 days	Bismuth, ampicillin	Fecal leukocytes and stool culture necessary for diagnosis
Salmonella	**Bloody** diarrhea; fever; cramps; nausea	Supportive therapy only; no opiates	Commonly acquired from **eggs** or **poultry;** diagnosis based on stool culture; increased susceptibility in immunocompromised patients
Campylobacter jejuni	**Bloody** diarrhea; fever; crampy abdominal pain; self-limited, but may persist for 3–4 weeks	Supportive therapy or possibly erythromycin	**Leading cause of food-borne diarrhea** in United States
Vibrio cholerae	**Watery** diarrhea (**rice-water stools**), vomiting, and dehydration occur after 12–48 hours of incubation	Supportive therapy only; no opiates	Caused by **toxin;** most often occurs in underdeveloped nations
Clostridium difficile	**Watery** diarrhea caused by antiobiotic-induced suppression of normal colonic flora; **pseudomembranes** on the colonic mucosa	Metronidazole, oral vancomycin	Exotoxin mediated
Enterotoxigenic *E. coli* (Traveler's diarrhea)	**Watery** diarrhea; 3–6 days duration; occasional fever and vomiting	Bismuth, trimethoprim-sulfa, doxycycline, ciprofloxacin	Antibiotics reduce duration of infection to 1–2 days
Enterohemorrhagic *E. coli* (O157:H7)	**Shiga-like toxin** causes **bloody** diarrhea	Supportive therapy	Typically, foodborne transmission (e.g., **uncooked hamburger**); diagnosis made by stool culture
Yersinia enterocolitica	**Bloody** diarrhea; fever; cramps; nausea	Supportive therapy only; no opiates	Transmitted by food or contaminated domestic animal feces; clinically indistinguishable from Salmonella or Shigella

QUICK HIT

Salmonella requires at least 100,000 organisms to be infectious. Shigella, however, requires only 100.

QUICK HIT

Vibrio cholerae produces an exotoxin that activates adenylate cyclase in the crypt cells. The increase in cAMP activates Cl- secretory channels. Consequently, sodium and water accompany Cl- into the lumen which result in an osmotic diarrhea.

THE GASTROINTESTINAL SYSTEM

● Viral Causes of Diarrhea (Table 4-6)

TABLE 4-6 Viral Causes of Diarrhea			
Infectious Agent	**Clinical Features**	**Treatment**	**Notes**
Rotavirus	Severe, dehydrating diarrhea; vomiting; low-grade fever	Supportive therapy only	**Most common cause of diarrhea in infants;** usually occurs during **winter** months
Norwalk virus	Mild diarrhea	Supportive therapy only	Epidemics in underdeveloped countries; **affects older children and adults**

● Protozoal Causes of Diarrhea (Table 4-7)

TABLE 4-7 Protozoal Causes of Diarrhea			
Infectious Agent	**Clinical Features**	**Treatment**	**Notes**
Entamoeba histolytica	**Bloody** diarrhea; lower abdominal pain; may lead to dysentery with 10–12 bloody and mucous stools per day	Metronidazole	Caused by ingestion of viable cysts via fecal-oral route
Giardia lamblia	**Watery,** foul-smelling diarrhea; nausea; anorexia; cramps lasting weeks to months	Metronidazole	Fecal-oral transmission; often contracted while **camping**
Cryptosporidium	**Watery** diarrhea with large fluid loss; symptoms persist in immunocompromised patients; is self-limited in healthy individuals	Supportive therapy	Immunocompromised patients (especially **AIDS patients);** fecal-oral transmission of oocysts

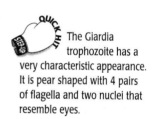

Norwalk virus, in contrast to most viruses transmitted via the fecal-oral route, is uncommon in children.

The Giardia trophozoite has a very characteristic appearance. It is pear shaped with 4 pairs of flagella and two nuclei that resemble eyes.

THE GASTROINTESTINAL SYSTEM

● Inflammatory Bowel Conditions Compared (Table 4-8)

It has been speculated that the pathogenesis of inflammatory bowel disease (IBD) is due to activation of the immune system and consequent release of cytokines and inflammatory mediators. The cause of IBD has yet to be discovered; however, there is some suggestion of a genetic component.

TABLE 4-8 Comparison of Inflammatory Bowel Conditions

	Crohn's Disease	Ulcerative Colitis
Typical patient	• Young person of Jewish descent • Bimodal age distribution: 25–40 years of age and 50–65 years of age • Female > male	• Person of Jewish descent • Recently quit smoking • Bimodal age distribution: 20–35 years of age and 65+ years of age • Male > female
Clinical findings	• Diarrhea • Abdominal pain • Fever • Malabsorption • Obstruction	• Bloody, mucous diarrhea • Abdominal pain • Fever • Weight loss • Toxic megacolon
Location	• Small Intestine • Colon • "Mouth to anus"	• Colon • Rectum
Histologic findings	• Full-thickness inflammation • **Granulomas**	• Mucosal inflammation • **Crypt abscesses**
Gross findings	• **Cobblestone appearance** • Wall thickening with narrowed lumen • **Skipped areas** • **Fistulas**	• Pseudopolyps • Widened lumen • Toxic megacolon
Diagnostic evaluation	• Colonoscopy • Barium enema • Upper GI series with small-bowel follow through	• Colonoscopy • Barium enema • Upper GI series with small-bowel follow through
Risk of malignancy	• Small increase	• Large increase
Associated systemic manifestations	• Arthritis • Eye lesions • Erythema nodosum • Pyoderma gangrenosum	• Arthritis • Eye lesions • Erythema nodosum • Pyoderma gangrenosum • Sclerosing cholangitis
Medical treatment	• Sulfasalazine • Steroids • Metronidazole	• Sulfasalazine • Steroids • Metronidazole
Indications for surgery	• Obstruction • Massive bleeding • Perforation • Refractory to medical treatment • Cancer • Toxic megacolon	• Toxic megacolon • Cancer • Massive bleeding • Failure to mature • Refractory to medical treatment

GI=gastrointestinal

MALABSORPTION SYNDROMES OF THE SMALL INTESTINE (Table 4-9)

Malabsorption may produce a variety of symptoms ranging from diarrhea to steatorrhea to specific nutrient deficiencies. For example, iron, vitamin B_{12}, fat-soluble vitamins (A, D, E, and K), or protein may be poorly absorbed and lead to systemic manifestations.

TABLE 4-9 Malabsorption Syndromes of the Small Intestine

Syndrome	Pathology	Clinical Features	Notes
Abetalipoproteinemia	Lack of apoprotein B; defective chylomicron assembly; enterocytes congested with lipid	Acanthocytes ("burr" cells) in blood; **no chylomicrons, VLDL, or LDL in blood**	Autosomal recessive
Celiac disease (non-tropical sprue)	Gluten sensitivity	Foul-smelling, pale stool; **villi of small intestine blunted;** stunted growth; symptoms disappear when gluten is removed from diet	Associated with HLA-B8 and DQW2; predisposes to T-cell lymphoma, and GI and breast cancer
Disaccharidase deficiency	Enzyme deficiency; bacterial digestion of unabsorbed disaccharide	Diarrhea; bloating	Most commonly lactase deficiency
Tropical sprue	Etiology unclear	Affects small intestine; may cause vitamin deficiencies and megaloblastic anemia	Possible infectious cause
Whipple's disease	Systemic disease caused by *Tropheryma whippelii*	Diarrhea; weight loss; lymphadenopathy; hyperpigmentation; **macrophages laden with *T. whippelii***	Older white males
Bacterial overgrowth	Bacterial overpopulation of small intestine due to stasis, raised pH, impaired immunity, or **clindamycin** therapy	Inflammatory infiltrate in bowel wall	Treat with antibiotics

GI=gastrointestinal; *HLA-B8*=human leukocyte antigen-B8; LDL=low density lipoprotein; VLDL=very low density lipoprotein

NEOPLASTIC POLYPS (Table 4-10)

Gastrointestinal polyps can be very diverse in their presentation. Individuals can be asymptomatic, as is usually the case with tubular adenomas, or can present with serious systemic manifestations such as anemia secondary to invasive cancer.

TABLE 4-10 Neoplastic Polyps		
Tubular Adenoma	**Tubulovillous Adenoma**	**Villous Adenoma**
• Usually **benign**	• Greater potential of malignancy than tubular adenoma	• Highly **malignant**
• Multiple	• Morphologically, shares features of both tubular and villous adenomas	• **Sessile** tumors • Finger-like projections
• **Pedunculated** tumors		
• Greater chance of malignancy if genetically predisposed		
• Most common polyp		

● Comparison of Polyposis Conditions (Table 4-11)

TABLE 4-11 Comparison of Polyposis Conditions		
Disease	**Inheritance**	**Clinical Features**
Familial adenomatous polyposis	Autosomal dominant	Colon lined with hundreds of polyps; potential for malignancy approaches 100%
Turcot's syndrome	Autosomal dominant	Colonic polyps and **CNS tumors;** potential for malignancy approaches 100%
Gardner's syndrome	Autosomal dominant	Colonic polyps; soft tissue and **bone tumors;** potential for malignancy approaches 100%
Peutz-Jeghers syndrome	Autosomal dominant	Benign hamartomatous polyps of the GI tract (especially the small intestine); **hyperpigmented mouth, hands and genitalia;** increased incidence of tumors of the uterus, breast, ovaries, lung, stomach, and pancreas; no malignant potential
Familial nonpolyposis syndrome	Autosomal dominant	**Defect in DNA repair** causing large number of colonic lesions (especially proximal); potential for malignancy approaches 50%

CNS=central nervous system; *DNA*=deoxyribonucleic acid; *GI*=gastrointestinal

THE HEPATOBILIARY SYSTEM

● Microscopic Organization of the Liver (Figure 4-6)

FIGURE
4-6
Microscopic organization of the liver

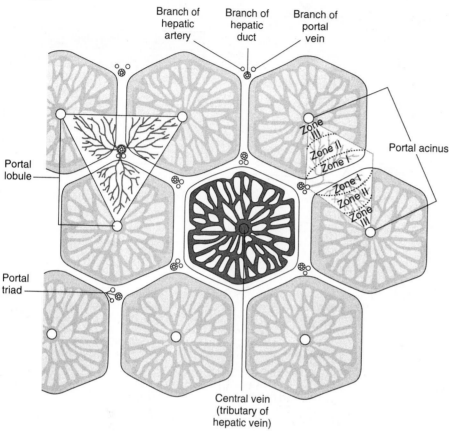

Branch of hepatic artery

Branch of hepatic duct

Branch of portal vein

Zone III
Zone II
Zone I

Portal acinus

Zone I
Zone II
Zone III

Portal lobule

Portal triad

Central vein (tributary of hepatic vein)

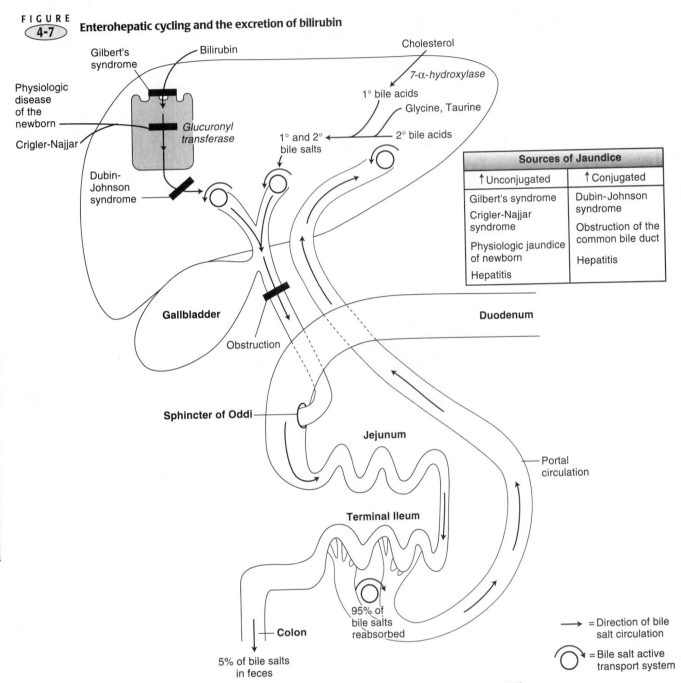

FIGURE 4-7 Enterohepatic cycling and the excretion of bilirubin

Sources of Jaundice	
↑Unconjugated	↑Conjugated
Gilbert's syndrome	Dubin-Johnson syndrome
Crigler-Najjar syndrome	Obstruction of the common bile duct
Physiologic jaundice of newborn	Hepatitis
Hepatitis	

(Adapted from Bullock J, Boyle III J, Wang MB: NMS Physiology, 3rd edition. Baltimore, Williams & Wilkins, 1995, p. 437).

Figure 4–8 (opposite). Glycolysis: 1) Hexokinase (and glucokinase in liver). **2)** Phosphofructokinase-1 (PFK-1): rate limiting step in glycolysis; induced by insulin; (+) adenosine monophosphate (AMP), fructose 2,6-bisphosphate; (−) adenosine triphosphate (ATP), citrate. **3)** Pyruvate kinase: irreversible; (+) fructose 1,6-bisphosphate in liver; (−) phosphorylation in response to increase glucagon, alanine. **4)** Pyruvate dehydrogenase: requires thiamine pyrophosphate (TPP), lipoic acid, fadin adenine dinucleotide (FAD), nicotinamide adenine dinucleotide (NAD), coenzyme A (CoA); irreversible; occurs in mitochondria; (+) pyruvate, insulin; (−) reduced nicotinamine adenine dinucleotide (NADH), acetyl CoA, phosphorylation. **Gluconeogenesis: 5)** Pyruvate carboxylase: requires biotin; (+) citrate; (−) malonyl CoA, phosphorylation. **6)** Phosphoenolpyruvate carboxykinase (PEPCK): induced by cortisol and glucagon (NOTE: substrate oxaloacetate is transported out of mitochondria as malate and converted back to oxaloacetate before reaction can occur). **7)** Fructose 1,6-bisphosphatase: induced by glucagon; (−) AMP, fructose 2,6-bisphosphate. **8)** Glucose 6-phosphatase: induced by glucagon. **9)** Phosphofructokinase-2: (+) insulin, (−) glucagon; **9a)** Works in opposite direction when phosphorylated. **Glycogenolysis: 10)** Glycogen phosphorylase and α 1,6 glucosidase: (+) AMP, phosphorylation. **Hexose monophosphate shunt: 11)** Glucose 6-phosphate dehydrogenase. **Tricarboxylic acid (TCA) cycle: 12)** Isocitrate dehydrogenase: rate limiting step; irreversible; (+) ADP, NADH. **13)** α-ketoglutarate dehydrogenase: requires TPP, lipoic acid, FAD, CoA; (−) ATP, guanosine triphosphate (GTP), NADH, Succinyl CoA. **Urea cycle: 14)** Carbamoyl phosphate synthetase 1. **15)** Ornithine transcarbamoylase. **16)** Argininosuccinate synthetase. **17)** Argininosuccinate lyase. **18)** Arginase. **Fatty acid synthesis: 19)** Acetyl CoA carboxylase: requires biotin; (+) citrate; (−) malonyl CoA, phosphorylation. *ADP*=adenosine diphosphate; *Arg*=arginine; *Asn*=asparagine; *ATP*=adenosine triphoshate; *CoA*=coenzyme A; *CO₂*=carbon dioxide; *GTP*=guanosine triphosphate; *His*=histidine; *Ile*=isoleucine; *Leu*=leucine; *Lys*=lysine; *Met*=methionine; *NAD*=nicotinamide adenine dinucleotide; *NADH*=reduced nicotinamide adenine dinucleotide; *P*=phosphate group; *Phe*=phenylalanine; *Pro*=proline; *Thr*=threonine; *Trp*=transfer ribonucleic acid proline; *Tyr*=tyrosine; *UDP*=uridine diphosphate; *Val*=valine.
(Adapted from Champe PC, Harvey RA: Lippincott's Illustrated Reviews: Biochemistry, 2nd edition. Philadelphia, J. B. Lippincott Company, 1994. p. 76)

● Important Biochemical Pathways of the Liver and Digestion (Figure 4-8)

FIGURE
4-8   Important biochemical pathways of the liver and digestion

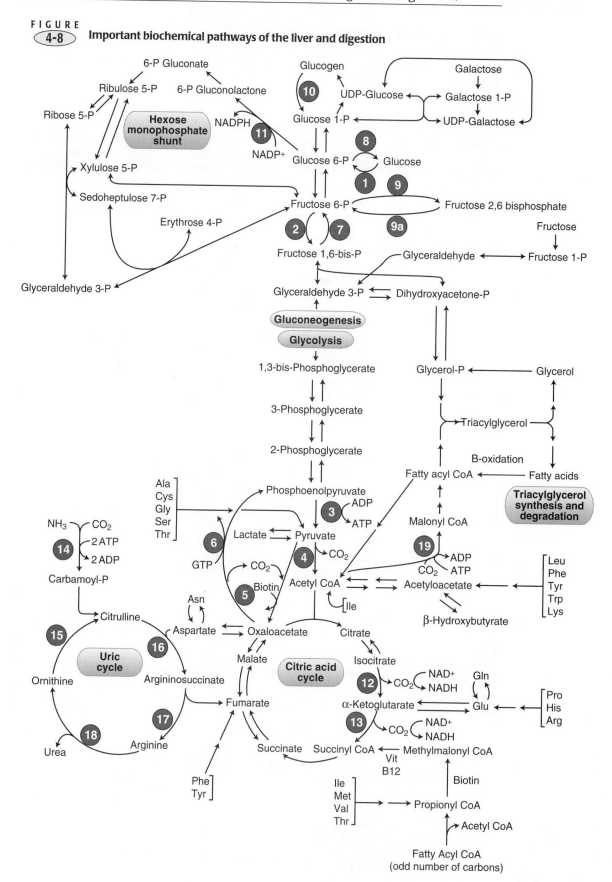

● **Glycolysis versus Gluconeogenesis versus Glycogenolysis (Table 4-12)**

As food is absorbed, the glycolysis pathway is activated and energy is stored as glycogen in the liver. Glycogenolysis provides food for the periods between regular meals. After 30 hours of fasting, all glycogen is depleted and gluconeogenesis becomes the only source of blood glucose.

(TABLE) 4-12	Glycolysis versus Gluconeogenesis versus Glycogenolysis		
	Glycolysis	**Gluconeogenesis**	**Glycogenolysis**
Description of Process	Glucose is broken down to form pyruvate and energy is released	Glucose is formed after 4–6 hours of fasting	**Glucose** is produced from glycogen stores after **2–3 hours of fasting**
Key enzymes and their regulation	Glucokinase (in liver), hexokinase (all tissues); requires ATP; (−) glucose-6-p; see enzyme 1, Figure 4-8	Pyruvate carboxylase; requires **biotin, CO$_2$,** and **ATP**; (+) acetyl CoA; see enzyme 5, Figure 4-8	Glycogen phosphorylase; (+) AMP, phosphorylation; see enzyme 10, Figure 4-8
	Phosphofructokinase-1 (PFK-1); requires ATP; **rate limiting step in glycolysis;** (+)AMP, fructose-2-6-BP; (−) ATP, citrate; see enzyme 2, Figure 4-8	Phosphenolpyruvate carboxykinase (PEPCK); requires GTP; (+) cortisol, glucagon; see enzyme 6, Figure 4-8	Phosphoglucomutase converts glucose-1-P to glucose-6-P
	Pyruvate kinase; produces ATP; (+) fructose-1-6-BP; (−) alanine, phosphorylation, ATP; see enzyme 3, Figure 4-8	Fructose-1-6-bisphosphatase;(+) glucagon; (−) AMP, fructose-2-6-BP; see enzyme 7, Figure 4-8	
	Pyruvate dehydrogenase; (+) pyruvate, insulin, ADP; (−) NADH, acetyl CoA, phosphorylation; see enzyme 4, Figure 4-8	Glucose-6-phosphatase; (+) glucagon; see enzyme 8, Figure 4-8	

ADP=adenosine triphosphate; *AMP*=adenosine monophosphate; *ATP*=adenosine triphosphate; *BP*=bisphosphate; *CoA*=coenzyme A; *CO$_2$*=carbon dioxide; *GTP*=guanosine triphosphate; *NADH*=reduced nicotinamide adenine dinucleotide

● Defective Enzyme Diseases (Table 4-13)

With a few exceptions, most defective enzyme diseases are autosomal recessive. Since the liver contains a high proportion of metabolic enzymes, it is often affected by these diseases.

TABLE 4-13	Defective Enzyme Diseases	
Disease	**Defective enzyme**	**Clinical Features**
Gaucher's disease	Glucocerebrosidase	• Accumulation of **glucocerebroside** • Hepatosplenomegaly • Erosion head of long bones (e.g., femur) • Gaucher's cells (distinctive, **wrinkled paper** appearance) found in liver, spleen, bone marrow
Niemann-Pick disease	Sphingomyelinase	• **"Foamy histiocytes"** in liver, spleen, lymph nodes, and skin • Hepatosplenomegaly • Anemia • Neurologic deterioration
von Gierke's disease	Glucose-6-phosphatase	• Accumulation of glycogen in liver and kidney • Hepatomegaly • Hypoglycemia
Cori's disease	Debranching enzyme	• Accumulation of glycogen in liver and striated muscle • Hepatomegaly • Hypoglycemia • Failure to grow
Pompe's disease	α-1,4-glucosidase (lysosomal enzyme)	• Accumulation of glycogen in liver and striated muscle • Cardiomegaly • Death due to cardiac failure before 3 years of age
Galactosemia	Galactose-1-phosphate uridyl transferase	• Accumulation of galactose-1-phosphate in many tissues • **Cataracts** • Cirrhosis • Mental retardation • Failure to thrive
Phenylketonuria	Phenylalanine hydroxylase	• Accumulation of phenylalanine • Cerebral myelin degeneration • **Mental retardation**
Maple syrup urine disease	Branched chain α-ketoacid dehydrogenase	• Inability to metabolize leucine, isoleucine, and valine • Neurologic symptoms • High mortality

QUICK HIT

McArdle's disease is a glycogen storage disease similar to von Gierke's, Pompe's, and Cori's but has no GI manifestations. It is a deficiency of muscle glycogen phosphorylase with consequent accumulation of glycogen in skeletal muscle.

THE GASTROINTESTINAL SYSTEM

● Viral Hepatitis (Table 4-14)

Viral hepatitis can lead to **direct hyperbilirubinemia,** elevated serum transaminases, icterus, hepatomegaly, but not ascites. Morphologically, changes range from multifocal hepatocellular necrosis with Councilman bodies (hepatitis A and hepatitis B) to ballooning degeneration (hepatitis B and hepatitis C) to piecemeal necrosis (hepatitis C).

TABLE 4-14 **Viral Hepatitis**

	Hepatitis A	Hepatitis B	Hepatitis C	Hepatitis D	Hepatitis E
Virus Family	Picornavirus	Hepadnavirus	Flavivirus	Delta agent	Calcivirus
Viral morphology	Single-stranded RNA	Circular, double-stranded DNA	Single-stranded RNA	Incomplete RNA	Single-stranded RNA
Mode of transmission	Fecal-oral	Sexual and parenteral, transplacental	Parenteral; limited sexual; transplacental	Sexual and parenteral; transplacental	Fecal-oral
Diagnostic test	IgM anti-HAV	HBsAg; anti-HbsAg; IgM anti-HBcAg	Anti-HCV	Anti-delta Ag	None
Severity	Mild	Moderate	Mild	Severe	Mild
Chronic infection	No	1%–2%	80%–90%	No increase over hepatitis B alone	No
Carrier state	No	Yes	Yes	Yes	No
Hepatocellular carcinoma	No	Yes	Yes	No	No
Prophylaxis and treatment	Immune globulin; vaccine	Hepatitis B immune globulin; vaccine	Interferon and Ribavirin	Hepatitis B immune globulin; vaccine	None
Notes	Incubation period of 14–15 days	**Dane particle:** viral DNA genome, DNA polymerase, HBcAg, HBeAg, HBsAg; has **reverse transcriptase;** incubation period 60–90 days	**Most frequent cause of transfusion-mediated hepatitis**	Defective in replication; **requires co-infection with hepatitis B**	Hepatitis infection in Third World nations

Ag=antigen; *DNA*=dioxyribonucleic acid; *HAV*=hepatitis A virus; *HBsAg*=hepatitis B surface antigen; *HCV*=hepatitis C virus; *IgM*=immunoglobulin M; *RNA*=ribonucleic acid

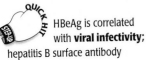

QUICK HIT

HBeAg is correlated with **viral infectivity;** hepatitis B surface antibody (HBsAb) is indicative of recovery and immunity; HBcAb acts as a marker for of hepatitis infection during the window period.

● **Cirrhosis (Table 4-15)**

Cirrhosis is a disease of the liver characterized by fibrosis and disorganization of the lobular and vascular structure due to the destruction and regeneration of hepatocytes.

TABLE 4-15 Cirrhosis

Etiology	Pathology	Clinical Manifestation	Notes
Chronic alcohol abuse	**Micronodular** fatty liver; decreased metabolism of estrogen; decreased synthesis of coagulation factors	**Jaundice;** bleeding; gynecomastia; testicular atrophy; edema; **asterixis;** portal hypertension **(esophageal varices,** spider angiomata, splenomegaly); encephalopathy	**Most common cause of cirrhosis in the United States**
Wilson's disease	**Decreased ceruloplasmin**	Copper deposits in liver, basal ganglia (causing extrapyramidal signs), and Descemet's membrane of cornea **(Kayser-Fleischer ring)**	Autosomal recessive
Hemochromatosis	Familial; increased total iron; decreased TIBC; increased ferritin; increased transferrin saturation	Iron deposits in liver; diabetes mellitus; increased skin pigmentation; cardiomyopathy	**"Bronze diabetes";** increased risk of hepatocellular carcinoma
Primary biliary cirrhosis	Autoimmune; **anti-mitochondrial antibodies**	Jaundice; pruritis; hypercholesterolemia	More common in women and middle-aged people
Posthepatitic	Chronic active hepatits due to HBV and HCV infection	Jaundice; pruritis	**Most likely cause of cirrhosis to lead to hepatocellular carcinoma** (HCC)
α-1 antitrypsin deficiency	Autosomal recessive; decreased inactivation of elastase	Jaundice; **panacinar emphysema;** pancreatic manifestations	**More severe in homozygous form** (piZZ alleles)
Congestive heart failure	Passive congestion	**Nutmeg liver**	Most often due to right heart failure

HBV=hepatitis B virus; *HCV*=hepatitis C virus

QUICK HIT
Cirrhosis often leads to portal hypertension. There are three major collateral circulation pathways that allow blood to return to the heart: (1) Left gastric to esophageal plexus to azygous to the superior vena cava (SVC) **(esophageal varices);** (2) inferior mesenteric to superior rectal to inferior rectal to inferior vena cava (IVC) **(hemorrhoids);** and (3) ligamentum teres to superficial abdominals to SVC or IVC **(caput medusae).**

THE GASTROINTESTINAL SYSTEM

● Common Clinical Disorders of the Hepatobiliary System (Table 4-16)

Hepatobiliary diseases vary in their presentation and etiology. Cholelithiasis is very common and curable with surgery, whereas hepatocellular carcinoma is much less common but usually fatal.

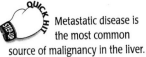

Pigment gallstones occurring in children or young adults with no history of pregnancy may be a result of a congenital hemoglobinopathy (e.g., sickle cell disease or thalassemia).

Metastatic disease is the most common source of malignancy in the liver.

Renal cell carcinoma also typically spreads via the **hematogenous route**.

TABLE 4-16	Common Clinical Disorders of the Hepatobiliary System		
Disorder	**Etiology and Pathology**	**Clinical Features**	**Notes**
Cholelithiasis (gallstones)	Very common disease; women over 40; obesity; multiparity	Steatorrhea; nausea; vomiting; bile duct obstruction; jaundice; may lead to cholangitis or cholecystitis; malignancy; positive Murphy's sign	Cholesterol stones (large); pigment stones (seen in hemolytic anemia or excess bilirubin production); mixed stones (majority)
Hepatocellular adenoma (hepatoma)	Benign tumor; women 20–30 years of age taking **oral contraceptives**	Usually found incidentally; may cause pain or hemorrhage	10% may become malignant; oral contraceptive use should be stopped
Adenocarcinoma of the gallbladder	Gallstones	Obstructive jaundice; enlarged gallbladder	**Courvoisier's law:** obstruction of common bile duct enlarges gallbladder while obstructing stones do not; due to scarring of gallbladder
Hepatocellular carcinoma	Cirrhosis; **hepatitis B; hepatitis C;** aflatoxin B (carcinogen in contaminated peanuts)	Increased α-fetoprotein; jaundice; abdominal distention; ascites	**Hematogenous spread**

THE PANCREAS

In the United States alcohol is the most common cause of pancreatic pathology.

● Common Clinical Disorders of the Pancreas (Table 4-17)

TABLE 4-17	Common Clinical Disorders of the Pancreas		
Disorder	**Etiology and Pathology**	**Clinical Features**	**Notes**
Acute pancreatitis	Gallstones (obstructing the ampulla of Vater); alcohol abuse	**Midepigastric pain radiating to back; increased serum amylase** and lipase; hemorrhage may lead to Cullen's or Grey Turner's sign; hypocalcemia	Activation of pancreatic enzymes leads to autodigestion
Chronic pancreatitis	**Alcoholism** in adults; cystic fibrosis in children	**Increased serum amylase** and lipase; **pancreatic calcifications;** epigastric pain; steatorrhea	Irreversible; leads to organ atrophy; may lead to formation of pancreatic pseudocyst

(continued)

TABLE 4-17	Common Clinical Disorders of the Pancreas		
Disorder	**Etiology and Pathology**	**Clinical Features**	**Notes**
Adenocarcinoma of the exocrine pancreas	More common in smokers	Invasive; **Trousseau's syndrome** (migratory thrombophlebitis); radiating abdominal pain; obstructive jaundice; **increased carcinoembryonic antigen** (CEA)	Poor prognosis; over 50% in head of pancreas; more common in blacks, males, patients with diabetes, and people over 60 years of age
Insulinoma (endocrine pancreas)	Originates in β cells	**Whipple's triad:** hypoglycemia, CNS dysfunction, reversal of CNS abnormalities with glucose	Most common islet cell tumor
Gastrinoma (Zollinger-Ellison syndrome)	Gastrin-secreting tumor (most commonly islet cell origin)	Recurrent peptic ulcers	Part of **MEN I**

CNS=central nervous system; *MEN*=multiple endocrine neoplasia

QUICK HIT The presence of **C-peptide** in the blood helps distinguish endogenous insulin secretions (as in an insulinoma) from exogenous insulin administration (as seen in Münchausen's syndrome).

QUICK HIT MEN I, also known as Wermer's syndrome, involves neoplasia or hyperplasia of the pancreas, the parathyroid, and the pituitary.

BUGS OF THE GASTROINTESTINAL TRACT

Bacterial

Enterobacteriaceae
Salmonella
Shigella
Escherichia coli

Vibrio cholerae
Staphylococcus aureus
Campylobacter jejuni
Helicobacter pylori

Clostridium botulinum
Clostridium difficile
Bacteroides fragilis

Parasitic
Entamoeba histolytica
Giardia lamblia

Cryptosporidium
Trichuris trichiura

Ascaris lumbricoides
Strongyloides stercoralis

Viral
Adenovirus
Coronavirus

Echovirus
Rotavirus

Norwalk agent
Reovirus

THERAPEUTICS

Drugs for treating alcohol abuse
Disulfiram

Antibiotics

Ampicillin
Ciprofloxacin
Doxycycline

Erythromycin
Metronidazole

Trimethoprim-sulfa
Vancomycin

Anti-inflammatories

Prednisone   Sulfasalazine

Anti-nausea drugs

Ondasetron   Prochlorperazine

Drugs for treating colon cancer

5-Fluorouracil   Levamisol

Drugs for treating *Helicobacter pylori* infection

Bismuth   Amoxicillin   Metronidazole
Clarithromycin   Tetracycline   Omeprazole

Laxatives and Antidiarrheals

Docusate   Loperamide   Magnesium hydroxide
Lactulose

Inhibitors of gastric secretion

Aluminum hydroxide   Lansoprazole   Omeprazole
Atropine   Metoclopramide   Ranitidine
Cimetidine   Octreotide   Sucralfate
Magnesium hydroxide   Misoprostol

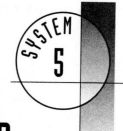

The Renal System

DEVELOPMENT

I. Intermediate Mesoderm
A. This forms the **urogenital ridges** on each side of the aorta.
B. The **nephrogenic cord** arises from this urogenital ridge and gives rise wholly or in part to the pronephros, the mesonephros, and the metanephros.

II. Pronephros
A. Forms in the fourth week
B. Quickly regresses by the fifth week
C. Non-functional

III. Mesonephros
A. Forms late in the fourth week and is functional until the permanent kidney is able to develop.
B. The **mesonephric duct** forms from the mesonephros.
   1. Forms the **ductus deferens, epididymis, ejaculatory duct,** and **seminal vesicle in the male.**
   2. Forms the **ureteric bud** from which are derived the **ureter, renal pelvis, calyces,** and **collecting tubules** in both the male and female.
   3. No important genital or reproductive derivatives of the mesonephric duct specific to females are formed.

IV. Metanephros
A. Develops into the **adult kidney.**
B. Formed during the fifth week from the **ureteric bud** and the metanephric mass (which is induced to form by contact with the ureteric bud) and begins to function in the ninth week.
C. Metanephric mesoderm forms the nephrons.
D. "Ascends" from sacral levels to low thoracic levels during its development due to longitudinal growth of the fetus.
E. Urogenital sinus forms the **bladder,** which is continuous with allantois. Allantois is equivalent to the median umbilical ligament in the adult.
F. Urethra
   1. Formed from endoderm and urogenital sinus
   2. Distal portion formed from ectoderm

V. Congenital anomalies of the renal system are described in Table 5-1.

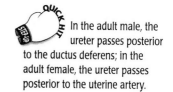

In the adult male, the ureter passes posterior to the ductus deferens; in the adult female, the ureter passes posterior to the uterine artery.

THE RENAL SYSTEM

The entire collecting system arises from **the ureteric bud.** The remainder of the renal system arises from the metanephric mesoderm.

Fanconi's syndrome is a **hereditary** or **acquired** dysfunction of the proximal renal tubules. As a result of impaired glucose, amino acid, phosphate, and bicarbonate reabsorption, it manifests clinically as glycosuria, hyperphosphaturia, aminoaciduria, and acidosis.

TABLE 5-1 Congenital Anomalies	
Anomaly	**Characteristics**
Bilateral renal agenesis (Potter's syndrome)	• Occurs when the ureteric bud does not form • **Oligohydramnios** • Limb deformities • Facial deformities • **Pulmonary hypoplasia** • Bilateral agenesis is not compatible with life
Accessory renal arteries	• Arise from the aorta • Feed a particular section of the kidney • Are end-arteries • **Cutting will produce ischemic** infarct in the area they supply
Congenital polycystic kidney disease	• Multiple small and large cysts causing renal insufficiency • Cysts are "closed"—not continuous with collecting system • Evident at birth • Death within days to weeks
Horseshoe kidney	• Inferior poles of the kidneys are fused • Ascent is arrested at the level of the inferior mesenteric artery • Increases probability of Wilms' tumor

GROSS DESCRIPTION OF THE KIDNEY

I. **Paired adult kidneys weigh approximately 150 g each.**

II. **They are located posterior to the peritoneum and at approximately the level of the first lumbar vertebra.**

III. **The right kidney is slightly lower than the left due to downward displacement by the liver.**

IV. **The left renal vein lies posterior to the superior mesenteric artery and anterior to the abdominal aorta.**

V. **The kidney is highly vascularized; it filters over 1700 liters of blood per day to produce about 1 liter of urine.**

● **The Kidney and Urinary Tract are shown in Figure 5-1.**

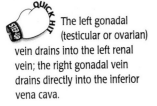
The left gonadal (testicular or ovarian) vein drains into the left renal vein; the right gonadal vein drains directly into the inferior vena cava.

THE RENAL SYSTEM

FIGURE
5-1 **The kidney and urinary tract**

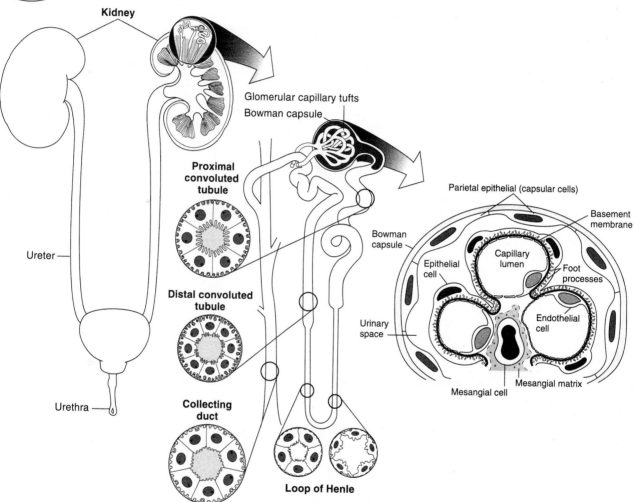

(Adapted from Damjanov I: *A Color Atlas and Textbook of Histopathology*. Baltimore, Williams & Wilkins 1996. pp. 258–259)

● **Distribution of Body Water** is shown in Figure 5-2.

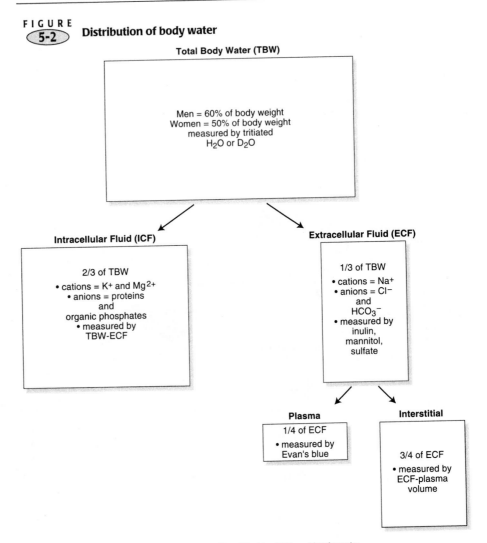

FIGURE 5-2 Distribution of body water

H_2O=water; D_2O=heavy water; Na^+=sodium; Cl^-=chloride; HCO_3^-=bicarbonate

NORMAL KIDNEY FUNCTION

I. Renal Blood Flow (RBF)
  A. 25% of cardiac output
  B. **RBF = renal plasma flow (RPF) /[1-hematocrit (Hct)]**
  C. Renal vasculature **autoregulates** RBF, keeping it constant even when arterial pressure varies from 100–200 mmHg.

II. Renal Plasma Flow (RPF)
  A. Effective RPF is measured by clearance of para-aminohippuric acid (**PAH**), which is filtered and secreted.
  B. This measurement underestimates by 10%.

III. Glomerular Filtration Rate (GFR)
  A. Normal GFR is 120 ml/min.
  B. It is measured by **inulin** clearance (filtered; not absorbed or secreted).
    1. Decreases in GFR cause a rise in BUN and creatinine levels.
    2. GFR decreases with age.

C. GFR is driven by Starling forces (filtration is always favored)(Figure 5-3).

FIGURE
5-3 **Starling forces on the glomerular capillary**

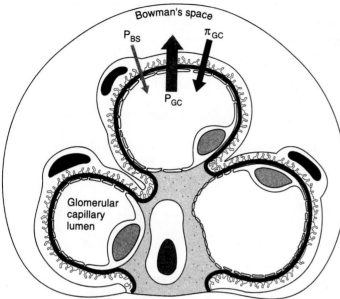

The Starling forces influence the Glomerular Filtration Rate (GFR)

$$GFR = K_F \, [(P_{GC}-P_{BS}) - (\pi_{GC}-\pi_{BS})]$$

Where K_F: the filtration coefficient of the glomerular capillaries

P_{GC}: The hydrostatic pressure exerted by the fluid in the glomerular capillary. A dilated afferent arteriole increases P_{GC}, as does a constricted efferent arteriole.

P_{BS}: The hydrostatic pressure exerted by the fluid in Bowman's space. Blockage or constriction of the ureters increases P_{BS}.

π_{GC}: The oncotic pressure of the glomerular capillary. The value of π_{GC} increases along the length of the capillary because the protein concentration in the capillary increases as water is forced into Bowman's space.

π_{BS}: The oncotic pressure in Bowman's space. This value is usually zero because the small amount of protein that enters Bowman's space is quickly reabsorbed back into the capillaries.

K_f=kidney function; P_{BS}=Bowman's space hydrostatic pressure; P_{GC}=glomerular capillary hydrostatic pressure; π_{BS}=Bowman's space oncotic pressure; π_{GC}=glomerular capillary oncotic pressure;

D. Clearance
 1. Removal of a substance from the blood by renal excretion.
 2. Determined by the amount of blood flow that contains a given amount of substance:

$$\text{Clearance} = U \times V \, / \, P = ml/min$$

  U = concentration of substance in urine in mg/ml
  V = urine volume (urine flow rate) in ml/min
  P = concentration of substance in mg/ml

 3. Factors that determine clearance
   a. Highly cleared substances (e.g., PAH) are those that are filtered and secreted.
   b. Poorly cleared substances are those that are either not filtered (e.g., protein) or reabsorbed (e.g., glucose).
   c. Reabsorption
    (i) Limited by the number of transporters for certain compounds (e.g., glucose)
    (ii) Transport maximum (T_m) is the concentration of the resorbed substance at which all transporters are saturated.
    (iii) Concentrations above T_m result in excretion of the excess.

IV. Filtration Fraction
 A. **Filtration fraction (FF) = glomerular filtration rate (GFR)/RPF**
 B. The normal filtration fraction is 20%.

V. Innervation and Hormones
 A. Juxtaglomerular apparatus (JGA) produces renin.
   1. JGA are stimulated by macula densa, which serve as baroreceptors.
   2. JGA are stimulated by the β sympathetic adrenergics in the kidney.

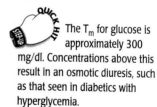

The T_m for glucose is approximately 300 mg/dl. Concentrations above this result in an osmotic diuresis, such as that seen in diabetics with hyperglycemia.

B. **Renin** cleaves angiotensinogen to **angiotensin I.**

C. Angiotensin I is cleaved to **angiotensin II** by angiotensin-converting enzyme (**ACE**) in the lung.

    1. Functions of angiotensin II

        a. Stimulates aldosterone release from the zona glomerulosa

        b. Stimulates secretion of antidiuretic hormone (ADH) and adrenocorticotropic hormone (ACTH)

        c. Acts as a potent local vasoconstrictor of the renal arterioles at low plasma levels

        d. Acts as a general systemic vasoconstrictor at high plasma levels

        e. Stimulates thirst

        f. Stimulates epinephrine and norepinephrine release from adrenal medulla

    2. Angiotensin II is inactivated to angiotensin III, a potent stimulator of aldosterone secretion but not an effective vasoconstrictor.

> **QUICK HIT**
>
> ACE inhibitors **captopril** and **enalapril** reduce hypertension by preventing the actions of angiontensin II on the adrenal gland and thereby prevent the release of aldosterone. The angiotensin II receptor blocker, **losartan,** prevents angiotensin II from constricting the efferent arteriole.

● **Hormones and the Nephron (Figure 5-4)**

FIGURE 5-4   **Hormones and the nephron**

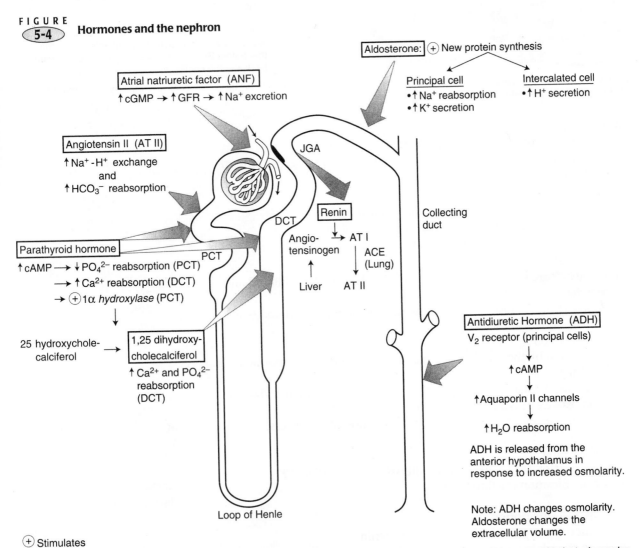

⊕ Stimulates

cGMP=cyclic guanosine monophosphate; *GFR*=glomerular filtration rate; *Na⁺*=sodium; *K⁺*=potassium; *HCO₃⁻*=bicarbonate; *JGA*=juxtaglomerular apparatus; *DCT*=distal convoluted tubule; *cAMP*=cyclic adenosine monophosphate; *PO₄²⁻*=phosphate; *PCT*=proximal convoluted tubule; *Ca²⁺*=calcium; *V₂*=vasopressin receptor, type 2; *H₂O*=water

● **Effects of volume change on fluid levels (Table 5-2)**

A variety of hormones, such as ADH, aldosterone, and atrial natriuretic factor, seek to regulate extracellular and intracellular volumes. Intake and output, as well as hormonal imbalance, can significantly alter the homeostatic fluid balance in the body.

TABLE 5-2	Effects of Volume Change on Fluid Levels				
Type	**Key Examples**	**ECF Volume**	**ICF Volume**	**ECF Osmolarity**	**Hct and Serum [Na$^+$]**
Isosmotic volume expansion	Isotonic NaCl infusion	↑	No change	No change	↓Hct — [Na$^+$]
Isosmotic volume contraction	Diarrhea	↓	No change	No change	↑ Hct — [Na$^+$]
Hyperosmotic volume expansion	High NaCl intake	↑	↓	↑	↓ Hct ↑ [Na$^+$]
Hyperosmotic volume contraction	Sweating Fever Diabetes insipidus	↓	↓	↑	— Hct ↑ [Na$^+$]
Hyposmotic volume expansion	SIADH	↑	↑	↓	— Hct ↓ [Na$^+$]
Hyposmotic volume contraction	Adrenal insufficiency	↓	↑	↓	↑ Hct ↓ [Na$^+$

— = no change; ECF = extracellular fluid; Hct = hematocrit; ICF = intracellular fluid; SIADH = syndrome of inappropriate secretion of antidiuretic hormone.

From Costanzo LS: *BRS Physiology, 2nd edition.* Baltimore, Williams & Wilkins, 1998, p. 139.

● Electrolyte balance in the nephron (Figure 5-5)

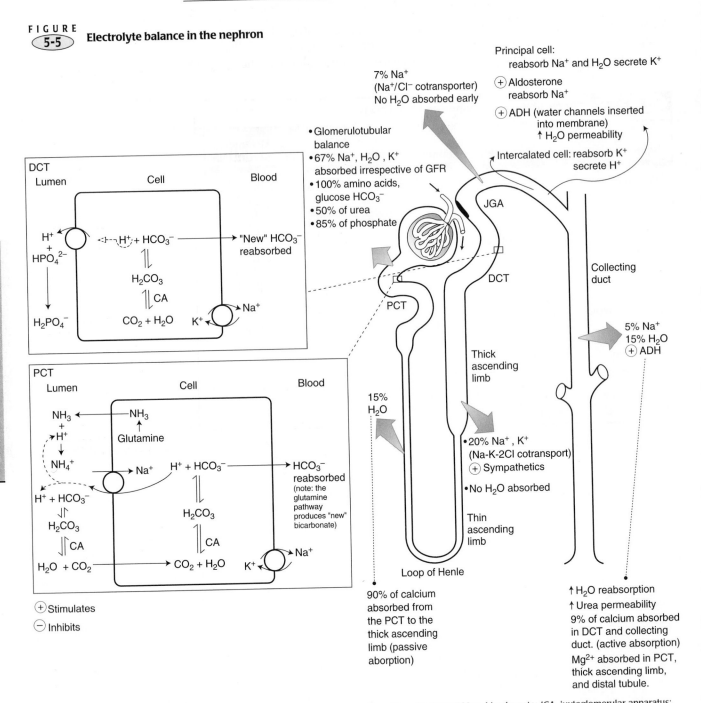

FIGURE 5-5 Electrolyte balance in the nephron

Principal cell:
reabsorb Na^+ and H_2O secrete K^+

⊕ Aldosterone
reabsorb Na^+

⊕ ADH (water channels inserted into membrane)
↑ H_2O permeability

7% Na^+
(Na^+/Cl^- cotransporter)
No H_2O absorbed early

Intercalated cell: reabsorb K^+
secrete H^+

• Glomerulotubular balance
• 67% Na^+, H_2O , K^+ absorbed irrespective of GFR
• 100% amino acids, glucose HCO_3^-
• 50% of urea
• 85% of phosphate

JGA

DCT

DCT		
Lumen	Cell	Blood

H^+
+
HPO_4^{2-}

⟵--[--H^++ HCO_3^- ⟶ → "New" HCO_3^- reabsorbed

H_2CO_3

↕ CA

$H_2PO_4^-$ $CO_2 + H_2O$ K^+ ← ○ ← Na^+

Collecting duct

5% Na^+
15% H_2O
⊕ ADH

PCT		
Lumen	Cell	Blood

NH_3 ← NH_3
+
↗H^+ Glutamine
↓
NH_4^+ ○ → Na^+ H^+ + HCO_3^- ⟶ → HCO_3^- reabsorbed
(note: the glutamine pathway produces "new" bicarbonate)
H^+ + HCO_3^-
↕ H_2CO_3
H_2CO_3
↕CA   ↕ CA
$H_2O + CO_2$ ⟶ → $CO_2 + H_2O$ K^+ ← ○ ← Na^+

Thick ascending limb

15% H_2O

• 20% Na^+ , K^+
(Na-K-2Cl cotransport)
⊕ Sympathetics

• No H_2O absorbed

Thin ascending limb

⊕ Stimulates
⊖ Inhibits

Loop of Henle

90% of calcium absorbed from the PCT to the thick ascending limb (passive aborption)

↑ H_2O reabsorption
↑ Urea permeability
9% of calcium absorbed in DCT and collecting duct. (active absorption)
Mg^{2+} absorbed in PCT, thick ascending limb, and distal tubule.

cGMP=cyclic guanosine monophosphate; *GFR*=glomerular filtration rate; *Na⁺*=sodium; *K⁺*=potassium; *HCO₃⁻*=bicarbonate; *JGA*=juxtaglomerular apparatus; *DCT*=distal convoluted tubule; *cAMP*=cyclic adenosine monophosphate; *PO₄²⁻*=phosphate; *PCT*=proximal convoluted tubule; *Ca²⁺*=calcium; *V₂*=vasopressin receptor, type 2; *H₂O*=water

Acidosis or alkalosis is determined by evaluating blood pH, arterial pCO_2 content, and bicarbonate concentration. Anion gap (AG) is calculated using the following equation: $AG = Na^+ - (Cl^- + HCO_3^-)$. A normal anion gap is between 10 and 16. Certain acidotic conditions result in an elevated anion gap by altering the concentration of anions not considered in the above formula (lactate, β-OH butyrate, formate). A comparison of acidosis versus alkalosis is made in Table 5-3. The effects of metabolic and respiratory acid–base disturbances are outlined in Table 5-4.

THE RENAL SYSTEM

TABLE 5-3 **Acidosis and Alkalosis**

Metabolic Disturbance	Presentation	Causes
Metabolic acidosis	• Rapid onset • Fatigue • Shortness of breath • Abdominal pain • Vomiting • **Kussmaul respirations** • Hypotension • Tachycardia	• Chronic renal failure • Lactic acidosis • Uremia • **Ketoacidosis** • Intoxication (aspirin, methanol, ethylene glycol) • *****Diarrhea** • *****Renal tubular acidosis** • *****Acetazolamide
Respiratory acidosis	• **Hypercapnia** • Confusion • Blunted sensation and pain response • **Asterixis** • Papilledema	• Respiratory depression by drugs • Cerebral disease • Cardiopulmonary arrest • Neuromuscular disease (e.g., myasthenia gravis) • Poor ventilation secondary to disease (e.g., asthma, pneumonia, bronchitis, emphysema)
Metabolic alkalosis	• No specific signs or symptoms • Can cause apathy, stupor, and confusion • If coupled with low calcium, can cause tetany	• Diuretics • Vomiting • Milk alkali syndrome • Large intake of alkaline substance • **Cushing's syndrome** • Primary aldosteronism
Respiratory alkalosis	• **Hyperventilation** • Numbness • Tingling • Paresthesia • Tetany, if severe	• Asthma • Pneumonia • Pulmonary edema • Heart disease with cyanosis • Pulmonary fibrosis • Aspirin intoxication • **Gram-negative sepsis** • Fever • Anxiety • Pregnancy • Drugs • Diseases that stimulate the medullary respiratory center

*=Normal anion gap acidosis (acidosis items not starred have an increased anion gap)

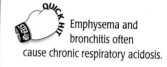

QUICK HIT Kussmaul respiration is not the same as Kussmaul's sign which is found in pericarditis.

QUICK HIT Emphysema and bronchitis often cause chronic respiratory acidosis.

QUICK HIT Renal tubular acidosis (RTA) is characterized by a normal anion gap. Type 1 (distal) RTA is caused by a failure to excrete titratable acid and NH_4^+. Type 2 RTA is caused by renal loss of HCO_3^-. Type 4 RTA is caused by hypoaldosteronism, which leads to poor excretion of NH_4^+ and hyperkalemia.

THE RENAL SYSTEM

TABLE 5-4 **Effects of Metabolic and Respiratory Acid-Base Disturbances**

Primary Disorder	pH	[H+]	[HCO_3^-]	PCO_2
Metabolic acidosis	↓	↑	↓ *	↓
Metabolic alkalosis	↑	↓	↑ *	↑
Acute respiratory acidosis	↓	↑	↑	↑ *
Chronic respiratory acidosis	↓	↑	↑↑	↑ *
Acute respiratory alkalosis	↑	↓	↓	↓ *
Chronic respiratory alkalosis	↑	↓	↓↓	↓ *

* = primary disorder; ↑ = increased; ↓ = decreased

GLOMERULAR DISEASES

I. Nephrotic Syndrome
  A. **Features**
   1. **Proteinuria** of more than 3.5–4.0 gm of protein/day
   2. Hypoalbuminemia
   3. Edema
   4. Hyperlipidemia
  B. **Etiology**
   1. Idiopathic—75%
   2. Systemic disease—25%
  C. Common types (see Table 5-5)

● **Nephrotic Glomerular Diseases (Table 5-5)**

TABLE 5-5 Nephrotic Glomerular Diseases

Glomerular Disease	Etiology	Clinical Features	Notes
Minimal change disease (lipoid nephrosis)	Fusion of foot processes on the basement membrane leads to loss of negative charge and changes the protein selectivity; altered appearance of villi on epithelial cells	Electron microscopy shows **fusion of podocyte foot processes,** and lipid-laden renal cortices	**Common in young children** (usually under 5 years of age); responds well to steroids; albumin usually selectively secreted
Membranous glomerulonephritis	Idiopathic; secondarily caused by SLE, hepatitis B, syphilis, gold, penicillamine, malignancy	Basement membrane thickening; **"spike and dome"** with **subepithelial IgG and C3 deposits**	Common in young adults
Diabetic nephropathy	Microangiopathy leading to thickening of basement membrane	Basement membrane thickening	Two types: diffuse and nodular glomerulosclerosis; nodular has **Kimmelstiel-Wilson nodules;** usually leads to renal failure
Renal amyloidosis	Subendothelial / mesangial amyloid deposits; associated with multiple myeloma	Stains: periodic acid-Schiff (PAS) (−); **Congo Red (+)**	Increasing severity leads to renal failure
Lupus nephropathy	**Anti ds-DNA**	WHO Classifications: • WHO I: normal • WHO II: mesangial proliferation; little clinical relevance • WHO III (focal proliferative): < ½ of glomeruli affected	Degree of kidney involvement correlates to SLE prognosis; may have nephritic qualities

(continued)

TABLE 5-5 **Nephrotic Glomerular Diseases** *(Continued)*

Glomerular Disease	Etiology	Clinical Features	Notes
		• **WHO IV (diffuse proliferative):** worst prognosis; **wire-loop lesions;** (subendothelial immune complex deposition of IgM and IgG+C3) • WHO V: membranous glomerulonephritis	
Focal and segmental glomerulosclerosis	Has four possible etiologies: idiopathic; superimposed on pre-existing pathology; associated with loss of renal mass; secondary to other disorders (e.g., heroine abuse or HIV)	Sclerosis of some glomeruli; only capillary tuft is involved in affected glomeruli	Clinically similar to minimal change disease, but affects older population

HIV=human immunodeficiency virus; *IgG*=immunoglobulin G; *C₃*=third component of complement; *SLE*=systemic lupus erythematosus; *ds-DNA*=double-stranded deoxyribonucleic acid; *WHO*=World Health Organization

II. Nephritic Syndrome
A. Features
1. **Hematuria**
2. Hypertension
3. Oliguria
4. Azotemia
B. Common types of nephritic glomerular diseases are described in Table 5-6.

TABLE 5-6 **Nephritic Glomerular Diseases**

Disease	Etiology	Special Features	Notes
Post-streptococcal glomerulonephritis	Post-streptococcal pharyngitis or impetigo; hepatitis B; high ASO-titer; low C3; type III hypersensitivity	**"Lumpy bumpy"** deposits of IgG and C3; subepithelial humps on electron microscopy	Common in children; self-resolving; most common organism is group A-hemolytic streptococci; red cell casts in urine
Rapidly progressive (**crescenteric**) glomerulonephritis	**ANCA positive;** poststrep etiology 50%; renal failure within weeks or months	Accumulation of fibrin, macrophages, and PMN's in Bowman's capsule; wrinkling of basement membrane on electron microscopy (**crescents**)	If also involves upper respiratory system, then termed **Wegener's**
Goodpasture's syndrome	**Anti-glomerular basement membrane and alveolar basement membrane antibodies**	**Linear pattern** of IgG on fluorescence microscopy; may be associated with hemoptysis and pulmonary hemorrhage	Usually **males in their mid-20s**

(continued)

TABLE 5-6 Nephritic Glomerular Diseases *(Continued)*

Disease	Etiology	Special Features	Notes
Alport's syndrome	Hereditary structural defect in collagen IV leads to leaky basement membrane	Glomerular basement membrane splitting on electron microscopy	Appears before age 20; associated with deafness and ocular problems

ASO=antistreptolysin O; C_3=third component of complement; *ANCA*=antineutrophil cytoplasmic antibody; *PMN*=polymorphonuclear leukocyte; *IgG*=immunoglobulin G

III. Non-nephritic, non-nephrotic glomerular diseases are described in Table 5-7.

TABLE 5-7 Non-nephritic, Non-nephrotic Glomerular Diseases

Disease	Etiology	Clinical Features	Notes
IgA nephropathy (Berger's disease)	IgA deposits in mesangium; hematuria; usually follows infection	Mesangial cell proliferation on electron microscopy	Minimal clinical significance; common
Membranoproliferative glomerulonephritis	Type 2 has IgG autoantibody; C_3 is reduced in both types	Basement membrane thickens and appears as two layers; **"tram-track"** appearance on electron microscopy	Two types: Type 1 and Type 2 (dense deposit disease); may lead to either nephrotic or nephritic syndromes

IgA=immunoglobulin A

● Glomerular Deposits in Disease (Figure 5-6)

FIGURE
5-6 Glomerular deposits in disease

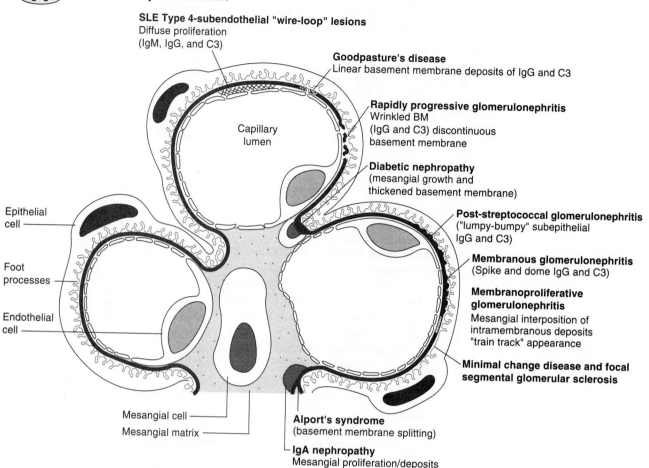

SLE Type 4-subendothelial "wire-loop" lesions
Diffuse proliferation
(IgM, IgG, and C3)

Goodpasture's disease
Linear basement membrane deposits of IgG and C3

Rapidly progressive glomerulonephritis
Wrinkled BM
(IgG and C3) discontinuous
basement membrane

Capillary lumen

Diabetic nephropathy
(mesangial growth and
thickened basement membrane)

Epithelial cell

Post-streptococcal glomerulonephritis
("lumpy-bumpy" subepithelial
IgG and C3)

Foot processes

Membranous glomerulonephritis
(Spike and dome IgG and C3)

Membranoproliferative glomerulonephritis
Mesangial interposition of
intramembranous deposits
"train track" appearance

Endothelial cell

Minimal change disease and focal segmental glomerular sclerosis

Mesangial cell

Mesangial matrix

Alport's syndrome
(basement membrane splitting)

IgA nephropathy
Mesangial proliferation/deposits
(IgG and C3)

SLE=systemic lupus erythematosus; *Ig*=immunoglobulin; *C₃*=third component of complement

URINARY TRACT INFECTIONS (UTIs)

I. Cystitis
A. Characteristic clinical features
   1. **Dysuria**
   2. **Frequency**
   3. **Urgency**
   4. Suprapubic pain
B. Etiology and pathogenesis
   1. Bacteria gain access to the urinary tract via the urethra.
   2. Cystitis most frequently involves normal colonic flora.
      a. *Escherichia coli* is the most common cause (approximately 80%).
      b. Proteus, Klebsiella, and Enterobacter have also been implicated.
      c. *Staphylococcus saprophyticus* causes 10%–15% of infections in young women.
   3. **Women** have a higher incidence of infection because they have shorter urethras.

   4. Other risk factors include sexual activity, pregnancy, urinary obstruction, neurogenic bladder, and vesicoureteral reflux.
  C. Diagnostic findings
   1. Characteristic clinical features are present.
   2. **Pyuria** (more than 8 leukocytes/high power field)
   3. Bacterial culture yields **greater than 10^5 organisms/mL.**
  D. Treatment
   1. Cystitis is treated empirically with antibiotics.
   2. Recurrent cystitis may require prophylactic antibiotics.

II. Acute Pyelonephritis

  A. **Characteristic clinical features**
   1. **Flank pain** or **costovertebral angle** (CVA) **tenderness**
   2. **Dysuria**
   3. **Fever**
   4. Chills
   5. Nausea and vomiting
   6. Diarrhea
  B. Etiology and pathogenesis
   1. Bacteria **ascend** from an infected urinary bladder to the kidney via **vesicoureteral** reflux.
   2. Infection may also spread **hematogenously** to the kidney (may not necessarily be preceded by acute cystitis).
   3. Causative organism is usually *E. coli.*
  C. **Diagnostic findings**
   1. Characteristic clinical features are present.
   2. Bacteriuria, pyuria, and **white blood cell casts** are seen on urine microscopy.
   3. Urine and blood cultures are performed to determine infection.
  D. Treatment
   1. Treatment is with **intravenous antibiotics.**
   2. Recurrent infection can lead to chronic pyelonephritis. This condition has several complications:
    a. **Scarring and deformity of the renal pelvis and calyces**
    b. Interstitial fibrosis and tubular atrophy
    c. Atrophy of the tubules leads to microscopic **"thyroidization"** of the kidney.

MAJOR CAUSES OF ACUTE
RENAL FAILURE (Figure 5-7)

FIGURE
5-7   **Etiology of acute renal failure**

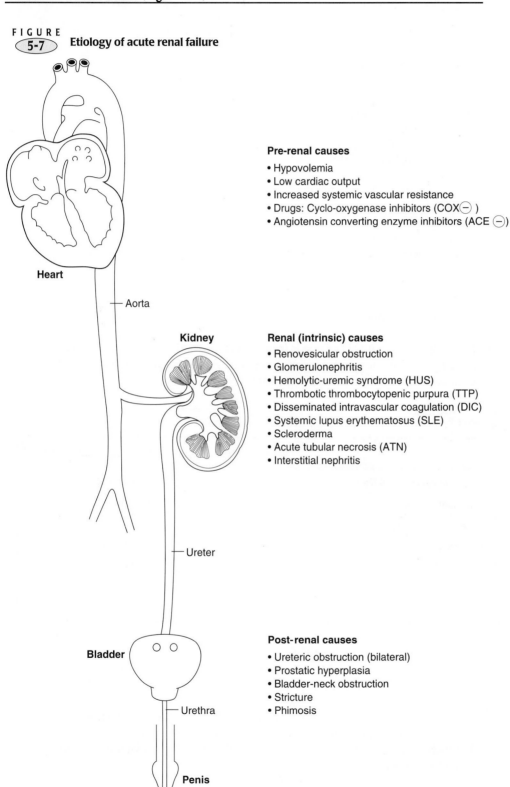

Heart

Aorta

Kidney

Bladder

Ureter

Urethra

Penis

Pre-renal causes

- Hypovolemia
- Low cardiac output
- Increased systemic vascular resistance
- Drugs: Cyclo-oxygenase inhibitors (COX⊖)
- Angiotensin converting enzyme inhibitors (ACE ⊖)

Renal (intrinsic) causes

- Renovesicular obstruction
- Glomerulonephritis
- Hemolytic-uremic syndrome (HUS)
- Thrombotic thrombocytopenic purpura (TTP)
- Disseminated intravascular coagulation (DIC)
- Systemic lupus erythematosus (SLE)
- Scleroderma
- Acute tubular necrosis (ATN)
- Interstitial nephritis

Post-renal causes

- Ureteric obstruction (bilateral)
- Prostatic hyperplasia
- Bladder-neck obstruction
- Stricture
- Phimosis

I. Pre-renal failure is defined as oliguria and increase in BUN and creatinine with inherently normal renal function.

   A. Hypovolemic states

      1. Hemorrhage

      2. Burns

      3. Dehydration

      4. Vomiting

      5. Diarrhea

      6. Diuretics

      7. Pancreatitis

   B. Low cardiac output states

      1. Arrhythmias

      2. Pulmonary embolus

      3. Myocardial or valvular disease

      4. Tamponade

      5. Pulmonary hypertension

   C. **Renal vasoconstrictive states** resulting in ischemia may be caused by the following:

      1. Cirrhosis with ascites

      2. Vasoconstrictive drugs: epinephrine, norepinephrine, cyclosporine, amphotericin B

   D. Intrinsic decrease of renal perfusion

      1. Cyclo-oxygenase (COX) inhibitors

      2. ACE inhibitors

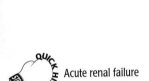 COX is inhibited by aspirin and other NSAIDs, but not by acetaminophen.

II. Acute intrinsic renal failure is inherent malfunction of the renal tissue. It may be glomerular, tubular, or interstitial. For a comparison of pre-renal versus intrinsic renal failure, see Table 5-8.

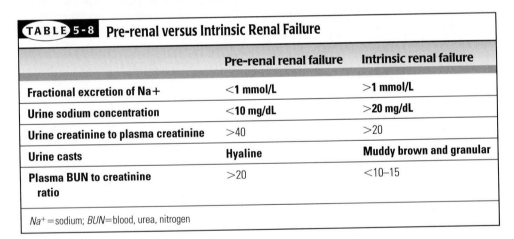

TABLE 5-8	Pre-renal versus Intrinsic Renal Failure	
	Pre-renal renal failure	**Intrinsic renal failure**
Fractional excretion of Na+	<1 mmol/L	>1 mmol/L
Urine sodium concentration	<10 mg/dL	>20 mg/dL
Urine creatinine to plasma creatinine	>40	>20
Urine casts	Hyaline	Muddy brown and granular
Plasma BUN to creatinine ratio	>20	<10–15

Na^+=sodium; *BUN*=blood, urea, nitrogen

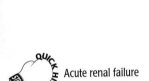 Acute renal failure and acute tubular necrosis are often used synonymously. However, acute renal failure can occur without acute tubular necrosis.

   A. Acute tubular necrosis (ATN):

      1. Drugs that may lead to ATN are: exogenous toxins (contrast, cyclosporine, aminoglycosides, ethylene glycol, acetaminophen, heavy metals); endogenous toxins (myoglobin, uric acid, oxalate).

      2. Ischemia can result in ATN via: abruptio placentae, postpartum hemorrhage, and similar causes related to pre-renal failure.

   B. Obstruction of renal vasculature from atherosclerosis, vasculitis, or other factors may also cause acute intrinsic renal failure.

   C. Diseases that affect the glomeruli or microvasculature include

      1. Disseminated intravascular coagulopathy (DIC)

      2. Glomerulonephritis

      3. Hemolytic uremic syndrome (HUS)

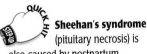 **Sheehan's syndrome** (pituitary necrosis) is also caused by postpartum hemorrhage and leads to loss of gonadotropins, thyroid-stimulating hormone (TSH), and ACTH, which clinically manifests itself as fatigue, weight loss, and amenorrhea.

THE RENAL SYSTEM

4. Thrombotic thrombocytopenic purpura (TTP)
5. Pregnancy
6. Scleroderma
7. Systemic lupus erythematosus (SLE)

D. **Interstitial nephritis** can have many causes.
   1. β-lactams
   2. Sulfonamides
   3. Trimethoprim (TMP)
   4. Rifampin
   5. COX inhibitors
   6. Diuretics
   7. Captopril
   8. Infection
   9. Idiopathic

E. Acute renal transplant rejection is a cause of ATN.

III. **Post-renal failure is bilateral obstruction of the ureters or obstruction of the urethra. It accounts for less than 5% of acute renal failure (ARF) and has a variety of causes:**

A. Urolithiasis (see section on stone formation)
B. Prostatic hyperplasia
C. Tumor obstructing the bladder or the ureters bilaterally
D. Neurogenic bladder

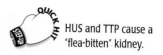 HUS and TTP cause a "flea-bitten" kidney.

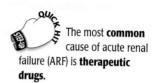 The most **common** cause of acute renal failure (ARF) is **therapeutic drugs.**

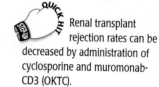 Renal transplant rejection rates can be decreased by administration of cyclosporine and muromonab-CD3 (OKTC).

 Finesteride, a 5-α-reductase inhibitor, is used to treat benign prostatic hyperplasia (BPH). Cold medicines and α-agonists exacerbate BPH.

THE RENAL SYSTEM

● Chronic Renal Failure (CRF) and Uremia (Figure 5-8)

FIGURE
5-8   Manifestations of chronic renal failure and uremia

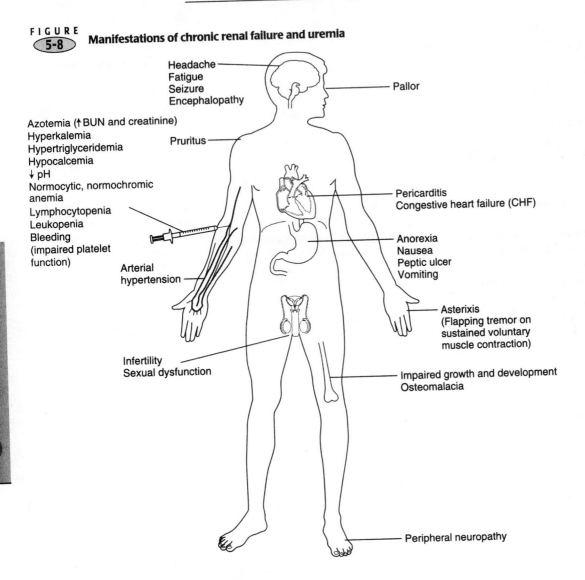

I. Major causes of CRF
A. Hypertension
B. Diabetes mellitus

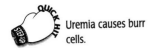
Uremia causes burr cells.

II. Profound loss of renal function leads to uremia
A. GFR reduced to 50%–65% of normal
B. Byproducts of amino acid and protein metabolism (especially urea) cause a variety of signs and symptoms
1. **Endocrine / electrolyte symptoms**
   – Hyperkalemia
   – Hypertriglyceridemia
   – Hyperuricemia
   – Hypocalcemia
   – Impaired growth and development
   – Infertility and sexual dysfunction
   – Metabolic acidosis
   – Osteomalacia
2. **Gastrointestinal Symptoms**
   – Anorexia
   – Nausea

THE RENAL SYSTEM ● 125

– Peptic ulcer
– Vomiting
3. **Renal Symptoms**
  – Azotemia
4. **Cardiovascular and Pulmonary Symptoms**
  – Arterial hypertension
  – CHF
  – Pericarditis
5. **Dermatological Symptoms**
  – Pallor
  – Pruritus
6. **Neuromuscular Symptoms**
  – Asterixis
  – Headache and fatigue
  – Peripheral neuropathy
7. **Hematologic Symptoms**
  – Increased susceptibility to infection
  – Lymphocytopenia and leukopenia
  – Normocytic, normochromic anemia

KIDNEY STONE FORMATION (Figure 5-9)

FIGURE
5-9 **Comparison of different types of kidney stones**

Calcium Stones
A. Calcium Oxalate (CO)   B. Calcium Phosphate (CP)

80% of stones
Men
20–30 years of age
Multiple (every 2–3 years)
Familial predisposition
Radiopaque
May be caused by primary hyperthyroidism

Struvite
12% of stones
Women
Risk factors:
Catheter, UTI's (especially Proteus)
May fill renal pelvis and calyces ("staghorn")
Radiopaque

Uric acid
7% of stones
Men
Risk factors:
50% have gout
Strong negative birefringence
Radiolucent
Associated with cell lysis (e.g., chemotherapy, leukemia)

Cystine
1% of stones
Uncommon
Hereditary
Radiopaque (due to sulfur component)

Clinical manifestations of kidney stones include hematuria and flank pain. *UTI*=urinary tract infection

ADULT POLYCYSTIC KIDNEY DISEASE (APKD) VERSUS NORMAL KIDNEY (Figure 5-10)

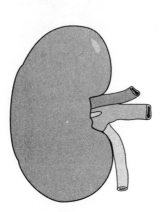
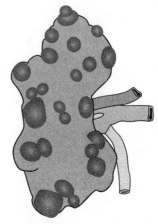

FIGURE 5-10 Adult polycystic kidney disease versus normal kidney

Normal kidney   Kidney with adult polycystic kidney disease

I. Etiology of APKD
  A. **Autosomal dominant**
  B. Occurs in mid-life

II. Clinical features of APKD
  A. Bilateral
  B. Kidney parenchyma is partially replaced with cysts
  C. **Hematuria**
  D. Hypertension
  E. **Large palpable kidneys**
  F. Progressively worsening renal function leading to renal failure

III. APKD is associated with berry aneurysms of **circle of Willis** and cystic disease in other organs, especially the liver.

RENAL CANCERS (Table 5-9)

TABLE 5-9 Renal Cancers

Malignancy	Etiology	Clinical Features	Notes
Renal cell carcinoma	**Smoking;** alteration of chromosome 3 (as seen in **von Hippel Lindau disease)**	Afflicts men 45–65 years of age; hematuria; mass; pain; fever; **secondary polycythemia;** paraneoplastic syndrome; usually extends from renal poles; with **clear cells**	Most common renal malignancy; may be associated with increased erythropoietin (EPO)

(continued)

TABLE 5-9 **Renal Cancers** *(Continued)*

Malignancy	Etiology	Clinical Features	Notes
Wilms' tumor (nephroblastoma)	Chromosome 11 abnormality; **WAGR**	**Palpable flank mass** in children 2–5 year olds; hematuria	Most common renal malignancy of childhood
Transitional cell carcinoma	Cyclophosphamide treatment; **smoking;** aniline dye exposure; **phenacetin** abuse	Hematuria	Most common tumor of the collecting system

WAGR=Wilms' tumor, aniridia, genitourinary abnormalities, and mental retardation

I. **The classic triad of hematuria, flank pain, and a flank mass is seen only in 10%–20% of renal cancer patients. Most are sporadic; however, smoking accounts for 20%–30% of cases.**

II. **Nephroblastoma (Wilms' tumor)**
  A. **Most common malignant renal tumor in children**
  B. Malignant tissue is derived from embryonic nephrogenic tissue.
  C. Peak incidence is between 2–4 years of age.
  D. The **two-hit theory** of oncogenesis, which explains the etiology of Wilms', requires a mutation of both copies of the Wilms' tumor-1 (WT-1) tumor suppressor gene on chromosome 11p.
  E. **Characteristic clinical features**
    1. Hematuria
    2. Hypertension
    3. Large abdominal mass
    4. Intestinal obstruction
  F. Part of **WAGR syndrome** (**W**ilms' tumor, **A**niridia, **G**enital anomalies, **M**ental **R**etardation)

THERAPEUTICS

● **Effects of Diuretics on the Nephron (Figure 5-11)**

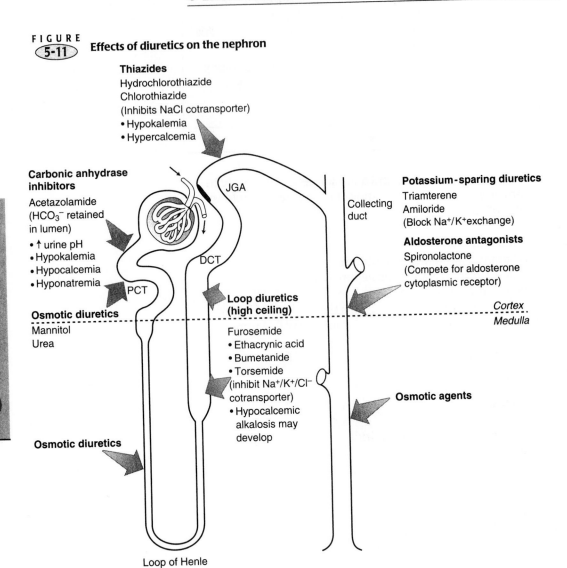

FIGURE 5-11 Effects of diuretics on the nephron

Thiazides
Hydrochlorothiazide
Chlorothiazide
(Inhibits NaCl cotransporter)
• Hypokalemia
• Hypercalcemia

Carbonic anhydrase inhibitors
Acetazolamide
(HCO_3^- retained in lumen)
• ↑ urine pH
• Hypokalemia
• Hypocalcemia
• Hyponatremia

Osmotic diuretics
Mannitol
Urea

JGA

DCT

PCT

Potassium-sparing diuretics
Triamterene
Amiloride
(Block Na^+/K^+ exchange)

Aldosterone antagonists
Spironolactone
(Compete for aldosterone cytoplasmic receptor)

Collecting duct

Cortex
Medulla

Loop diuretics (high ceiling)
Furosemide
• Ethacrynic acid
• Bumetanide
• Torsemide
(inhibit $Na^+/K^+/Cl^-$ cotransporter)
• Hypocalcemic alkalosis may develop

Osmotic agents

Osmotic diuretics

Loop of Henle

DCT=distal convoluted tubule; *JGA*=juxtaglomerular apparatus; *PCT*=proximal convoluted tubule

Anti-Diuretics
Desmopressin

Vasopressin
[also called antidiuretic hormone(ADH)]

Anti-microbials for UTI
Ciprofloxacin
Doxycyline
Methenamine

Nalidixic acid
Nitrofurantoin

Trimethoprim-sulfamethoxazole

Diuretics

Acetazolamide
Amiloride
Bumetanide
Chlorothiazide

Ethacrynic Acid
Furosemide
Hydrochlorothiazide
Mannitol

Spironolactone
Torsemide
Triamterene
Urea

Gout

Allopurinol
Colchicine

Indomethacin
Phenylbutazone

Probenecid
Sulfinpyrazone

QUICK HIT Mannitol (an osmotic diuretic) is used in acute renal failure to maintain urine flow.

QUICK HIT **Corticosteroids** are often used to help resolve nephritic and nephrotic syndromes.

THE RENAL SYSTEM

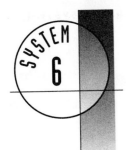

The Endocrine System

DEVELOPMENT

I. Hypothalamus
A. A division of the **diencephalon**
B. Forms from the embryological forebrain (see System 1 "The Nervous System")

II. Pituitary gland consists of two lobes:
A. Anterior lobe: forms from **Rathke's pouch,** an ectodermal diverticulum of the primitive mouth that invaginates upward
B. Posterior lobe: forms from an invagination of the **hypothalamus**

III. Thyroid gland
A. Forms from the endoderm of the floor of the pharynx
B. Begins as a diverticulum that migrates caudally
C. Thyroid follicular cells are derived from endoderm
D. The calcitonin-producing **parafollicular cells (C-cells)** originate from the ultimobranchial bodies of the fourth pharyngeal pouch.

IV. Parathyroid glands
A. **Inferior parathyroid glands** develop from the **third pharyngeal pouch.**
B. **Superior parathyroid glands** develop from the **fourth pharyngeal pouch.**
C. The parathyroid glands migrate caudally and come to lie on the dorsal surface of the thyroid gland.

IV. Adrenal glands
A. **Gross description**
    1. Paired adult adrenal glands weigh 4 g each.
    2. They are located immediately anterosuperior to the superior renal poles.
    3. They are enclosed in renal fascia.
B. **Adrenal cortex**
    1. Forms from the mesoderm
    2. Includes 3 major parts:
        a. **Zona glomerulosa** and **zona fasciculata** are present at birth.
        b. **Zona reticularis** is not completely formed until 3 years of age.
C. Medulla of adrenal gland: **Chromaffin cells** form from neural crest cells that invade the adrenal glands during development.

V. Pancreas
A. Forms from a ventral and dorsal bud of endoderm from the foregut
    1. The ventral bud forms the uncinate process and part of the pancreatic head.

2. The dorsal bud forms part of the head, body, and tail.

B. Exocrine pancreas: acinar cells and ducts form from endoderm surrounded by mesoderm.

C. Endocrine pancreas: mesodermal cells aggregate to form **pancreatic islet cells.**

VI. Gonads (see System 7 "Reproductive System")

CONGENITAL MALFORMATIONS (Table 6-1)

There is a wide spectrum of developmental abnormalities involving the endocrine system. Some of these malformations are anatomical, while others are biochemical.

TABLE 6-1 Congenital Malformations

Malformation	Description
Craniopharyngioma	-Cystic tumor of the pituitary that forms from the remnants of **Rathke's pouch**
Thyroglossal duct cysts	-A remnant of the descending migratory path of the thyroid that persists into adult life -Most are asymptomatic, but an infection may cause swelling and produce a progressively enlarging moveable mass
Absence of parathyroid glands	-Occurs in **DiGeorge syndrome** (thymic aplasia) (see System 9 "Hematopoietic and Lymphoreticular System") -Inability to produce parathyroid hormone leads to hypoparathyroidism
Congenital adrenal hyperplasia	-See Figure 6-8
Annular pancreas	-Ventral and dorsal pancreatic buds form a ring around the duodenum -May cause **duodenal obstruction**
Accessory pancreatic tissue	-Normal pancreatic tissue found within the wall of the stomach -Most common type of choristoma (normal tissue found misplaced within another organ)

Thyroglossal duct cysts are **midline** cysts of the neck. Branchial cleft cysts lie laterally, anywhere along the anterior border of the sternocleidomastoid muscle.

Hormones are biologically active chemicals formed in an organ and carried through the blood to act on adjacent cells of the same organ or on a different body part.

HORMONES (Table 6-2)

TABLE 6-2 Hormones

Hormone	Secreted by	End-organ effects of hormones	Stimulated by	Inhibited by
GnRH	Hypothalamus	LH/FSH secretion	Puberty	Progesterone; testosterone
FSH	Anterior pituitary gland	Growth of follicles and estrogen secretion (acts on granulosa cells); maturation of sperm (acts on Sertoli's cells)	Pulsatile release of GnRH	Constant GnRH release; Inhibin

(continued)

THE ENDOCRINE SYSTEM

QUICK HIT
Finasteride, a 5α-reductase inhibitor, is used in the treatment of benign prostatic hypertrophy. Flutamide, a competitive androgen receptor blocker, is used to treat prostatic carcinoma.

QUICK HIT
The hormone hCG is increased in normal pregnancy, hydatidiform moles, choriocarcinomas, gestational tumors, ectopic pregnancy, and pseudocyesis.

QUICK HIT
The anti-inflammatory effect of cortisol is mediated by its induction of **lipocortin**, which inhibits phospholipase A$_2$ and prostaglandin synthesis. Cortisol also inhibits the production of IL-2.

QUICK HIT
Somatostatin is also secreted in the brain, GI tract, and delta cells of the pancreas. It functions to systemically decrease secretion of insulin, glucagon, and gastrin.

TABLE 6-2 Hormones *(Continued)*

Hormone	Secreted by	End-organ effects of hormones	Stimulated by	Inhibited by
LH	Anterior pituitary gland (basophils)	Ovulation; formation of corpus luteum; estrogen/progesterone synthesis (acts on theca leutin cells); synthesis/secretion of testosterone (acts on Leydig's cells)	Pulsatile release of GnRH	Constant GnRH release; Progesterone; testosterone
Estrogen	Ovary (granulosa cells)	Proliferative phase of menstrual cycle; development of female reproductive organs	FSH	Estrogen
Progesterone	Ovary (granulosa lutein cells)	Breast development; secretory activity during luteal phase	LH	Progesterone
Testosterone	Testes (Leydig's cells)	Spermatogenesis; conversion of testosterone to dihydrotestosterone via 5α-reductase stimulates development of secondary male sex characteristics	LH	Testosterone
hCG	Placenta (syncytiotrophoblast)	Increased estrogen/progesterone synthesis		
ACTH	Anterior pituitary	Synthesis and secretion of adrenal cortical hormones	CRH; stress	Cortisol
Cortisol (glucocorticoids)	Adrenal cortex (zona fasiculata)	Anti-inflammatory effects (via inhibition of phospholipase A$_2$); immunosuppressive effects; stimulation of gluconeogenesis; increased blood sugar	ACTH	Cortisol
Aldosterone	Adrenal cortex (zona glomerulosa)	Increased renal sodium reabsorption and potassium secretion; increased in blood volume	Decrease in blood volume; angiotensin II; hyperkalemia; hyponatremia	Hypernatremia; hypokalemia; fluid overload
TSH	Anterior pituitary	Synthesis and secretion of thyroid hormone (T$_4$, T$_3$)	TRH	T4, T3
T4, T3	Thyroid	Growth; maturation of CNS; increased basal metabolic rate, cardiac output, and nutrient utilization	TSH; estrogen	Somatostatin; dopamine
Somatostatin (somatotropin inhibiting hormone)	Hypothalamus	Inhibited secretion of growth hormone	Growth hormone; somatomedins (IGF)	

(continued)

TABLE 6-2 **Hormones** *(Continued)*

Hormone	Secreted by	End-organ effects of hormones	Stimulated by	Inhibited by
GH (somato-tropin)	Anterior pituitary (acidophils)	Decreased glucose uptake; increased protein synthesis, growth, organ size, and lean body mass	GHRH; exercise; sleep; puberty; hypoglycemia; estrogen; stress; endogenous opiates	Somatomedins (IGF); somatostatin; obesity; pregnancy; hyperglycemia
Prolactin	Anterior pituitary (acidophils)	Stimulation of milk production and secre-tion; breast development; inhibition of ovulation	Prolactin-stimulating factor; TRH	Prolactin-inhibiting factor (dopamine)
Oxytocin	Hypothalamus via posterior pituitary	Milk ejection from breast (milk letdown); uterine contraction	Suckling; dilation of the cervix	Alcohol; stress
PTH	Parathyroid gland (chief cells)	Increased serum calcium; increased renal calcium absorption; inhibition of phosphate reabsorption; activates Vitamin D to increase intestinal calcium absorption	Decreased serum calcium; mild decreased serum magnesium	Severe decrease in serum magnesium
Vitamin D (1,25 dihy-droxychole-calciferol)	Kidney (active form produced by activity of 1α-12-hydroxylase); sun-exposed skin	Increased intestinal calcium and phosphorus absorp-tion; increased bone cal-cium resorption; increased kidney phosphate and calcium resorption	Decreased serum calcium; increased PTH; decreased serum phosphate	
ADH (Vaso-pressin)	Hypothalamus via posterior pituitary	Increased water perme-ability in distal tubules and collecting duct to reg-ulate osmolarity (V2 receptor); constriction of vascular smooth muscle (V1 receptor)	Volume contraction; nicotine; opiates; increased serum osmolarity	Ethanol; ANF; decreased serum osmolarity
Glucagon	Pancreatic islet cells (α- cells)	Increased blood glucose; increased glycogenolysis and gluconeogenesis in the liver; increased lipolysis and ketone production	Decreased blood glucose; increased amino acids, ACh	Increased blood glucose; insulin; somatostatin
Insulin	Pancreatic islet cells (β-cells)	Decreased blood glucose caused by increased uptake into muscle and fat; decreased glyco-genolysis and gluconeo-genesis; increased protein synthesis; increased fat deposition; inhibition of lipolysis	Increased blood glucose, amino acids; glucagon; ACh	Decreased blood glucose; somatostatin

ACh=acetylcholine; *ACTH*=adrenocorticotropic hormone; *ADH*=antidiuretic hormone; *ANF*=atrial natriuretic factor; *CNS*=central nervous system; *CRH*=corticotropin-releasing hormone; *FSH*=follicle stimulating hormone; *GH*=growth hormone; *GHRH*=growth hormone-releasing factor; *GnRH*=gonadotropin-releasing hormone; *hCG*=human chorionic gonadotropin; *IGF*=insulin-like growth factor; *LH*=luteinizing hormone; *PTH*=parathyroid hormone; T_3=triiodothyronine; T_4=thyroxine; *TRH*=thyrotropin-releasing hormone; *TSH*=thyroid stimulating hormone

THE ENDOCRINE SYSTEM

QUICK HIT Glucose enters cells through facilitated transporters designated GLUT-1 through GLUT-5. GLUT-4 is abundant in skeletal muscle and adipocytes, while GLUT-1 is found on erythrocytes.

QUICK HIT T_4 is converted to the T_3 in the periphery, as T_3 is 3–5 times more potent than T_4. T_4 has a half-life of 5–7 days, while T_3 has a half-life of 1 day.

Hormone function can be localized or systemic. Hormones can alter the activity or structure of the target organ(s) depending on the specificity of the hormone's effects. Hormones play an essential role in homeostasis, reproductive function, and metabolism, but are vital in nearly every other body system as well.

● Hormones of the Hypothalamo-Pituitary Axis (Figure 6-1)

FIGURE 6-1 **Hypothalamo-Pituitary Axis**

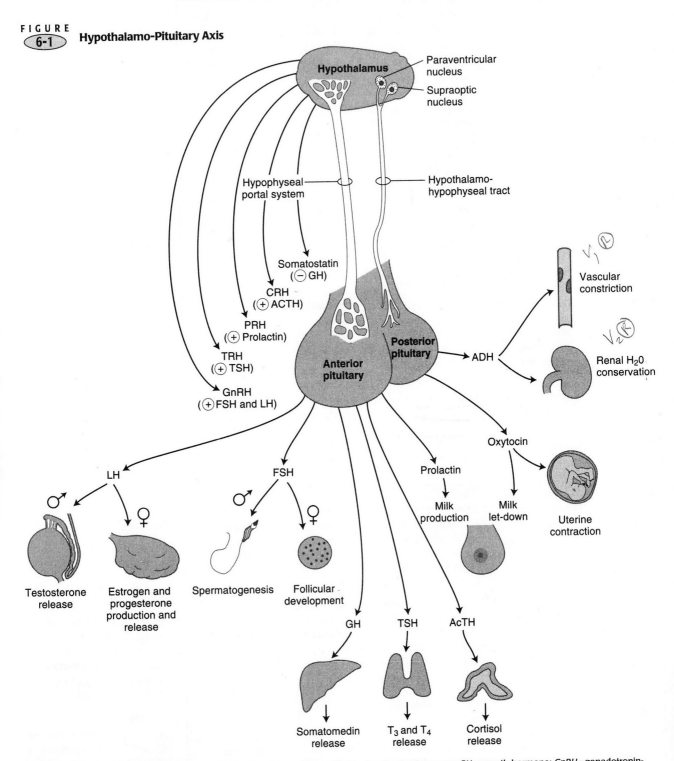

ACTH=adrenocorticotropic hormone; ADH=antidiuretic hormone; CRH=corticotropin-releasing hormone; GH=growth hormone; GnRH=gonadotropin-releasing hormone; FSH=follicle-stimulating hormone; LH=luteinizing hormone; PRH=prolactin-releasing hormone; T_3=triiodothyronine; T_4=thyroxine; TRH=thyrotropin-releasing hormone; TSH=thyroid-stimulating hormone

● Hormones of the Adrenal Gland (Figure 6-2)

FIGURE
6-2 **Hormones of the Adrenal Gland**

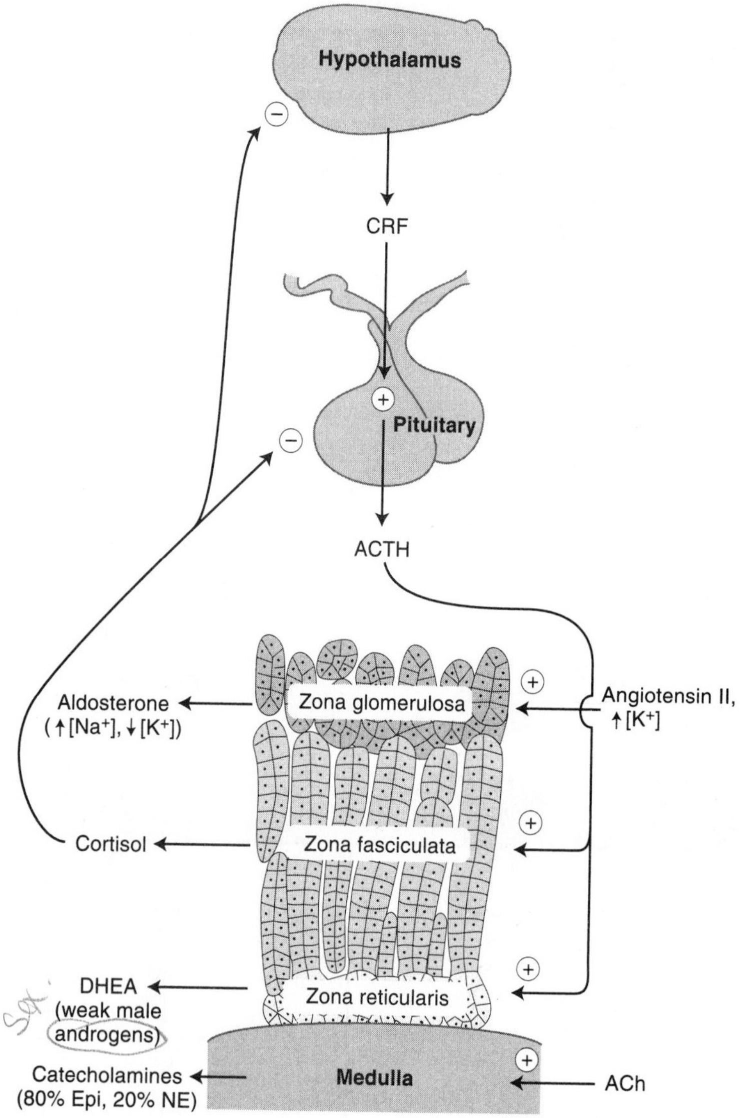

ACh=acetylcholine; ACTH=adrenocorticotropic hormone; AT II=angiotensin II; CRF=corticotropin-releasing factor;
DHEA=dehydroepiandrosterone; Epi=epinephrine; K$^+$=potassium; Na$^+$=sodium; NE=norepinephrine

● **Hormone Second-Messenger Systems**

Second-messenger systems are the process by which extracellular signals are translated into cellular responses. Biologically active chemicals, such as hormones, bind to receptor sites on the cell membrane, resulting in phosphorylation of intracellular proteins or changes in ion channel conductivity and subsequent cellular modulation. (Table 6–3) (Figure 6-3)

(text continues on page 138)

TABLE 6-3	Hormone Second-Messenger Systems				
cAMP	**cGMP**	**IP3**	**Steroid**	**Tyrosine Kinase**	
• β-1 agonists • β-2 agonists • LH • FSH • TSH • ADH (V2) • hCG • CRH • PTH • Calcitonin • Glucagon • ∝-2 agonists (decrease cAMP)	• ANP • EDRF	• α-1 agonists • GnRH • TRH • GHRH • Angiotensin II • ADH (V1) • Oxytocin	• Aldosterone • Estrogen • Glucocorticoids • Testosterone • Progesterone • Thyroid • Vitamin D	• Insulin • IGF-1 • Prolactin • GH	

(see also abbreviation key to Table 6-2) *cAMP*=cyclic adenosine monophosphate; *cGMP*=cyclic guanine monophosphate; *IGF*=insulin growth factor; *IP₃*=inositol-1,4,5-triphosphate

QUICK HIT

LH, FSH, and TSH are hormones consisting of 2 subunits: α and β. The α subunits in these hormones are identical, while the β subunit is unique for each hormone.

THE ENDOCRINE SYSTEM

FIGURE 6-3 **Hormone Second Messenger Systems**

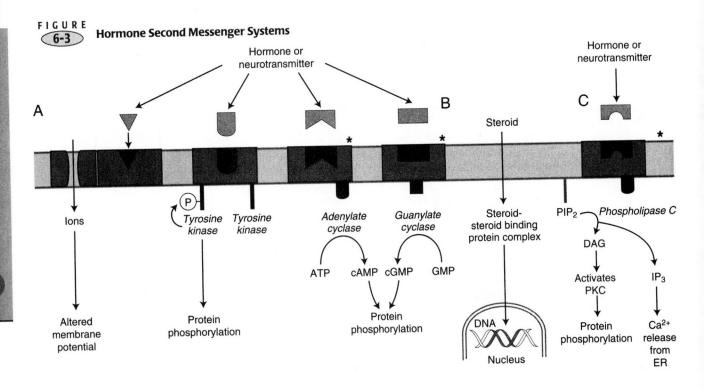

AMP=adenosine monophosphate; *ATP*=adenosine triphosphate; *Ca²⁺*=calcium; *cAMP*=cyclic adenosine monophosphate; *cGMP*=cyclic guanosine monophosphate; *DAG*=diacylglycerol; *DNA*=deoxyribonucleic acid; *ER*=endoplasmic reticulum; *GDP*=guanosine diphosphate; *GMP*=glucose monophosphate; *GTP*=guanosine triphosphate; *IP₃*=inositol-1,4,5-triphosphate; *P*=phosphate; *P [enclosed in circle]*=phosphorylated; *PIP₂*=phosphatidylinositol biphosphate; *PKC*=protein kinase C

FIGURE 6-3 *(Continued)*

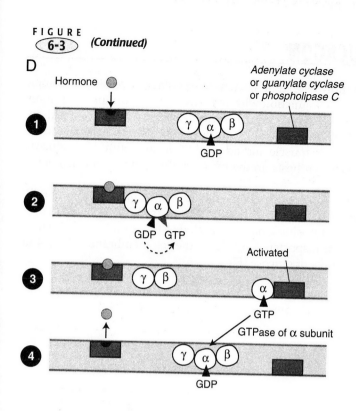

D

Hormone

Adenylate cyclase or *guanylate cyclase* or *phospholipase C*

γ α β GDP

① ② ③ ④

GDP GTP

Activated

α GTP

GTPase of α subunit

γ α β GDP

A. Peptide mechanism. Peptide binds to hormone receptor site and influences various second messenger systems. These hormones are typically short-acting and do not involve gene regulation, in contrast to steroid hormones, which have a slower onset of action.

B. Steroid mechanism. Lipid-soluble steroid penetrates cell membrane and binds to steroid binding protein. This complex enters the nucleus and influences DNA synthesis.

C. Phospholipase C mechanism.

D. G protein mechanism.

1. Messenger system prior to hormone binding.

2. After hormone binding, GTP replaces GDP on G protein.

3. GTP, attached to α-subunit, dissociates from the β-γ complex and converts ATP to cAMP.

4. Hormone is released from binding site and complex returns to inactive state when GTPase cleaves GTP to GDP.

★ Mechanism utilizing a G protein, as shown in D

CALCIUM HOMEOSTASIS (Figure 6-4)

FIGURE 6-4 **Calcium Homeostasis**

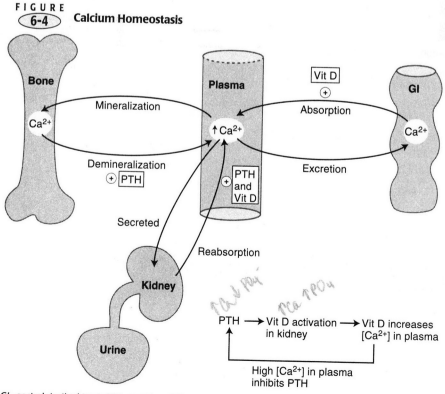

GI=gastrointestinal tract; PTH=parathyroid hormone

INSULIN AND GLUCAGON

Insulin is a polypeptide hormone that serves to regulate several physiologic processes. Its primary role, in conjunction with the polypeptide hormone glucagon, is to **maintain blood glucose levels.** When blood glucose levels rise after a meal, insulin is released from the **β-cells** of the pancreatic islets of Langerhans'. Insulin interacts with surface receptors on muscle and adipose tissue and stimulates glucose absorption and triacylglycerol synthesis. In the liver, insulin inhibits gluconeogenesis and glycogen breakdown.

Insulin is formed from two polypeptides linked by disulfide bridges (Figure 6-5). The insulin receptor is **tyrosine kinase** linked; binding of insulin to the α subunit causes phosphorylation of the tyrosine kinase connected to the β subunit. This stimulates recruitment of glucose transporters (GLUTs) to the cell membrane (GLUT 4 in muscle) and increases the uptake of glucose (Figure 6-6).

THE ENDOCRINE SYSTEM

FIGURE 6-5 **Formation of Insulin**

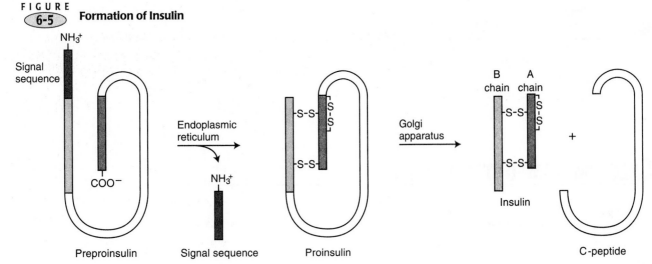

C=carbon; *O*=oxygen; *S*=sulfur (Adapted from Champe PC and Harvey RA: *Lippincott's Illustrated Reviews: Biochemistry, 2nd edition.* Philadelphia, Lippincott-Raven Publishers, 1994, p. 270. Used by permission of Lippincott Williams & Wilkins.)

FIGURE
6-6

FIGURE
6-6 **Insulin Recruitment of Glucose Transporters**

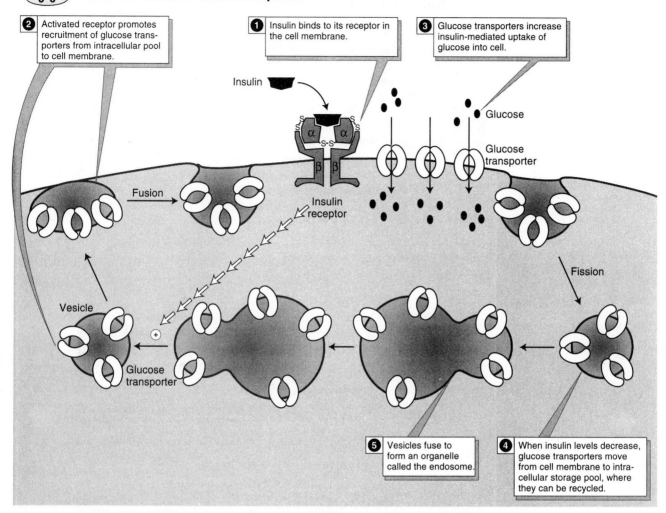

2 Activated receptor promotes recruitment of glucose transporters from intracellular pool to cell membrane.

1 Insulin binds to its receptor in the cell membrane.

3 Glucose transporters increase insulin-mediated uptake of glucose into cell.

Insulin

Glucose

Glucose transporter

Insulin receptor

Fusion

Fission

Vesicle

Glucose transporter

5 Vesicles fuse to form an organelle called the endosome.

4 When insulin levels decrease, glucose transporters move from cell membrane to intracellular storage pool, where they can be recycled.

(Adapted from Champe PC and Harvey RA: *Lippincott's Illustrated Reviews: Biochemistry, 2nd edition.* Philadelphia, Lippincott-Raven Publishers, 1994, p. 274. Used by permission of Lippincott Williams & Wilkins.)

Glucagon counteracts the actions of insulin. It is a single polypeptide secreted by the **α-cells** of the islets of Langerhans'. Glucagon is secreted in response to low blood glucose, increased amino acids in the blood, and epinephrine, and leads to a rise in blood glucose concentration via **gluconeogenesis** and **glycogenolysis.** Glucagon is also responsible for the formation of ketone bodies and increased uptake of amino acids by the liver.

● **Blood Levels of Insulin and Glucagon after a High Carbohydrate Meal (Figure 6-7)**

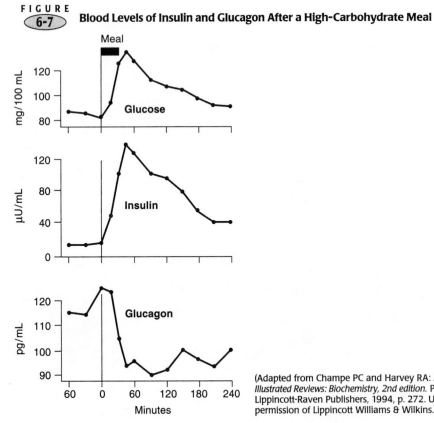

FIGURE
6-7 **Blood Levels of Insulin and Glucagon After a High-Carbohydrate Meal**

(Adapted from Champe PC and Harvey RA: *Lippincott's Illustrated Reviews: Biochemistry, 2nd edition.* Philadelphia, Lippincott-Raven Publishers, 1994, p. 272. Used by permission of Lippincott Williams & Wilkins.)

BLOOD GLUCOSE LEVELS

I. Hypoglycemia
  A. **Causes**
    1. Excess insulin administration (in a diabetic patient)
    2. Sulfonylurea administration
    3. Alcohol ingestion
    4. Insulinoma
    5. Factitious hyperinsulinism
  B. **Symptoms**
    1. Sweating
    2. Palpitations
    3. Anxiety
    4. Tremor
  C. Whipple's triad (required for diagnosis)
    1. Low blood glucose
    2. Hypoglycemic symptoms
    3. Improvement of symptoms with glucose administration
  D. In diabetic patients, these symptoms may not be present, and blood glucose may be allowed to drop to dangerous levels, and coma or death may result.
  E. Therapy
    1. Glucose or intravenous (IV) dextrose should be given after measuring blood glucose levels.

2. Glucagon should be administered.

3. Epinephrine is sometimes appropriate therapy.

II. Hyperglycemia

A. Causes

    1. Diabetes mellitus

    2. Chronic pancreatitis

    3. Acromegaly

    4. Cushing's syndrome

    5. Adverse drug reactions due to:

        a. Furosemide

        b. Glucocorticoids

        c. Growth hormone

        d. Oral contraceptives

        e. Thiazides

B. Acute symptoms

    1. Ketoacidosis or hyperosmolar nonketotic coma

    2. Polyuria

    3. Polydipsia

    4. Polyphagia

    5. Weight loss

    6. Encephalopathy

        a. Tremulousness

        b. Convulsions

        c. Coma

C. The chronic symptoms of hyperglycemia mimic the chronic complications of diabetes (Table 6-4).

DIABETES MELLITUS

Diabetes mellitus (or simply, diabetes) refers to a group of disorders that are characterized by hyperglycemia and affect 1%–2% of the United States population. While the pathogenesis of these disorders are varied, individuals with diabetes lack the ability to produce sufficient insulin to meet their metabolic needs. Furthermore, all diabetic patients are vulnerable to complications such as nephropathy, neuropathy, and retinopathy. Monitoring and control of blood sugar, insulin replacement, and proper diet can significantly reduce the morbidity and mortality of this disease.

● **Diagnosis of Diabetes Mellitus (see Table 6-4)**

TABLE 6-4	Diagnosis of Diabetes Mellitus		
	Normal	**Impaired Glucose Tolerance**	**Diabetes Mellitus**
Fasting blood glucose level	< 115 mg/dL	<140 mg/dL	126 mg/dL
Blood glucose level following oral glucose tolerance test (OGTT)	< 140 mg/dL	or 140–199 mg/dL	or 200 mg/dL

Type I versus Type II diabetes mellitus is compared in Table 6-5.

THE ENDOCRINE SYSTEM

Rubella, mumps, and coxsackie are viral agents which can trigger the autoimmune response of the body to pancreatic β cells and cause Type I diabetes (also called juvenile onset diabetes).

TABLE 6-5 Type I versus Type II Diabetes Mellitus		
	Type I Diabetes (IDDM) 15%	**Type II Diabetes (NIDDM)** 85%
Cause	Possible **autoimmunity** to beta cells triggered by viral cause	Increased **insulin resistance,** decreased receptors, or decreased conversion of proinsulin to insulin
Chromosomal association	6 (HLA DQ)	Unknown
Family history	Weak predictor	Strong predictor
Age of onset	Under 25 years of age	Over 40 years of age
Body habitus	Normal to thin	Obese
Plasma insulin	Low	Normal to high
Plasma glucagon	High but suppressible	High and resistant to suppression
Pancreas morphology	Atrophy and fibrosis; beta cell depletion	Atrophy and amyloid deposits; variable beta cell population
Acute complication (see Table 6-6)	Ketoacidosis	Hyperosmolar coma
Common symptoms	**Polydipsia, polyuria, polyphagia (symptoms of hyperglycemia)**	Variable: from asymptomatic to polydipsia, polyuria, polyphagia
Response to insulin therapy	Responsive	Variable
Response to sulfonylurea therapy	Unresponsive	Responsive

IDDM=insulin-dependent diabetes mellitus; *NIDDM*=non-insulin-dependent diabetes mellitus

Sulfonylureas, used in the treatment of NIDDM, reduce K^+ efflux and increase $Ca_2{}^+$ influx, thus increasing secretion of insulin from β-cells.

● **Diabetic Ketoacidosis (DKA) and Nonketotic Hyperosmolar (NKH) State (Table 6-6)**

The ketone bodies (**acetoacetate, β-hydroxybutyrate**) are produced by the liver from acetyl CoA in the fasting state. The body (including the brain after 4–5 days) utilizes the ketone bodies for energy instead of glucose and amino acids. RBCs, however, can only use glucose.

DKA and NKH are not mutually exclusive. Patients may present with features of both.

TABLE 6-6 Diabetic Ketoacidosis (DKA) and Nonketotic Hyperosmolar (NKH) State		
	DKA	**NKH**
Pathology	Increased serum **ketone bodies** (> 2 mMol/L); anion gap metabolic acidosis (pH < 7.2); **hyperglycemia** (glucose > 300 mg/dL due to increased production and decreased uptake)	**Hyperglycemia** (> 600 mg/dL); **hyperosmolarity** (> 320 mg/dL); pH > 7.3
Patient	Type I (IDDM)	An older Type II (NIDDM)
Precipitating event	50% **infection** (look for fever); 25% insufficient insulin	**Decreased ability to sense thirst or obtain enough water;** infection; vascular event (CVA, MI)
Fluid loss	5–7 Liters	9 Liters

(continued)

TABLE 6-6 Diabetic Ketoacidosis (DKA) and Nonketotic Hyperosmolar (NKH) State (Continued)

	DKA	NKH
Clinical presentation	Nausea and vomiting; **Kussmaul respiration;** osmotic diuresis; shock; coma	Usually **coma** if serum osmolarity > 350 mg/dL
Mortality	10%	17%
Treatment	Insulin; saline; K+ replacement	Saline (essential); insulin
Complications	**Cerebral edema;** hyperchloremic (non-gap) metabolic acidosis	Dehydration is more severe (older patients have lower body water stores)

● Chronic Symptoms of Diabetes (Table 6-7)

TABLE 6-7 Chronic Symptoms of Diabetes Mellitus

Anatomical Location	Clinical Features
Red blood cells	Glycosylation (**HbA1c**); measure of long-term control of diabetes (reflects past 3 months)
Blood vessels	**Atherosclerosis;** coronary artery disease; gangrene; peripheral vascular disease
Eyes	**Retinopathy;** hemorrhage; hard exudates; cotton-wool spots; cataracts; glaucoma
Gastrointestinal tract	Constipation, gastroparesis
Kidneys	Nephropathy; **nodular sclerosis; Kimmelstiel-Wilson nodules;** chronic renal failure; azotemia
Penis	Impotence due to autonomic neuropathy
Feet	**Stocking–glove peripheral neuropathy;** ulcers

PITUITARY DISORDERS (Table 6-8)

The pituitary gland sits in the sella turcica. The anterior portion is regulated by the hypothalamus. The posterior portion contains extensions of hypothalamic neurons.

QUICK HIT
Excess prolactin can result from estrogen therapy or drugs such as antipsychotics that interfere with dopamine (prolactin-inhibiting hormone).

TABLE 6-8 Pituitary Disorders

Disorder	Etiology	Clinical Features	Laboratory Diagnosis	Treatment
Prolactinoma	Lactotrophic (chromophobic) anterior pituitary tumor; **most common** pituitary tumor	Decreased libido; amenorrhea; gynecomastia; galactorrhea; virilization	Minimal or no increase in serum prolactin after TRH given	Bromocriptine and/or surgery
Acromegaly (adults)/Gigantism (children)	Somatotrophic (acidophilic) anterior pituitary adenoma	Prominent forehead, jaw; **large hands, feet; enlargement of viscera;** hyperglycemia; renal failure; hypertension; mental disturbances	Excess growth hormones and somatomedins (IGF-1)	Transphenoidal surgery, bromocriptine, radiation, and/or octreotide

(continued)

TABLE 6-8 **Pituitary Disorders** (*Continued*)

Disorder	Etiology	Clinical Features	Laboratory Diagnosis	Treatment
Cushing's disease	Hypersecretion of ACTH from basophilic adenoma of pituitary	(see Table 6-10)	Suppression of ACTH secretion during high-dose dexamethasone test	Surgery or pituitary irradiation
Simmond's disease	Pituitary tumors, ischemia, trauma; DIC; sickle cell anemia	Marked wasting; **panhypopituitarism;** headache; vomiting	Decreased levels of FSH, LH, ACTH, TSH	Hormone replacement
SIADH	Pituitary hypersecretion; ectopic production of ADH (**small cell lung cancer**); water retention	Decreased urinary output; fatigue; mental disturbances	Hyponatremia; high urine osmolality	Fluid restriction *demeclocycline*
Diabetes insipidus	**Neurogenic** (central): ADH insufficiency **Nephrogenic:** lack of end-organ (kidney) response	Dehydration; thirst; polyuria; recent trauma to the head or anoxia	See Table 6-9; hypernatremia	Neurogenic: desmopressin (DDAVP) acts as ADH; Nephrogenic: fluid restriction and thiazide diuretics (works by a paradoxical effect)

(see also Table 6-2 abbreviation key) *DDAVP*=1-deamino-8-D-arginine vasopressin; *DIC*=disseminated intravascular coagulation; *SIADH*=syndrome of inappropriate secretion of antidiuretic hormone

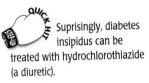

Sheehan's syndrome is a form of Simmond's disease caused by postpartum pituitary necrosis resulting from blood loss and ischemia during childbirth.

Suprisingly, diabetes insipidus can be treated with hydrochlorothiazide (a diuretic).

Primary polydipsia, a psychological condition of drinking excess water, causes a decrease in plasma osmolality and therefore can be differentiated from diabetes insipidus, which causes an increase in plasma osmolality. Patients who present with primary polydipsia are generally young or middle-aged women with a history of neurosis.

DIABETES INSIPIDUS (Table 6-9)

Diabetes insipidus is a disease characterized by excessive, low osmolality urine output. There are two forms: central and nephrogenic.

TABLE 6-9 **Diabetes Insipidus**

	Urine osmolarity greater than 280 mOsm/kg with dehydration	Response to ADH after dehydration
Normal	+	−
Central diabetes insipidus	−	+
Partial diabetes insipidus	+	+
Nephrogenic diabetes insipidus	−	−
Primary polydipsia	+	+

ADH=antidiuretic hormone

THE ADRENALS

● Congenital Adrenal Hyperplasia (Figure 6-8)

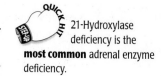

21-Hydroxylase deficiency is the **most common** adrenal enzyme deficiency.

FIGURE
6-8 Congenital Adrenal Hyperplasia (CAH)

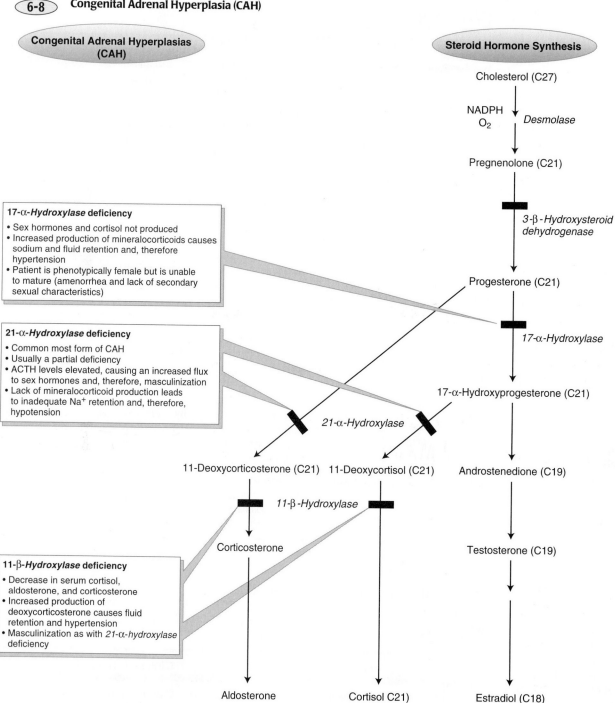

Congenital Adrenal Hyperplasias (CAH)

Steroid Hormone Synthesis

Cholesterol (C27)

NADPH O₂ → *Desmolase*

Pregnenolone (C21)

3-β-Hydroxysteroid dehydrogenase

Progesterone (C21)

17-α-Hydroxylase

17-α-Hydroxyprogesterone (C21)

21-α-Hydroxylase

11-Deoxycorticosterone (C21)   11-Deoxycortisol (C21)   Androstenedione (C19)

11-β-Hydroxylase

Corticosterone

Testosterone (C19)

Aldosterone   Cortisol C21)   Estradiol (C18)

17-α-Hydroxylase deficiency
• Sex hormones and cortisol not produced
• Increased production of mineralocorticoids causes sodium and fluid retention and, therefore hypertension
• Patient is phenotypically female but is unable to mature (amenorrhea and lack of secondary sexual characteristics)

21-α-Hydroxylase deficiency
• Common most form of CAH
• Usually a partial deficiency
• ACTH levels elevated, causing an increased flux to sex hormones and, therefore, masculinization
• Lack of mineralocorticoid production leads to inadequate Na⁺ retention and, therefore, hypotension

11-β-Hydroxylase deficiency
• Decrease in serum cortisol, aldosterone, and corticosterone
• Increased production of deoxycorticosterone causes fluid retention and hypertension
• Masculinization as with *21-α-hydroxylase* deficiency

(Adapted from Champe PC and Harvey RA: *Lippincott's Illustrated Reviews: Biochemistry, 2nd edition.* Philadelphia, Lippincott-Raven Publishers, 1994, p. 224. Used by permission of Lippincott Williams & Wilkins.)

THE ENDOCRINE SYSTEM

The adrenal glands are anatomically divided into a medulla and a cortex. The cortex is itself divided into three anatomic layers. The four anatomic layers of the adrenal glands are responsible for a variety of metabolic functions in the body.

● **Adrenal Cortex Pathology (Table 6-10)**

TABLE 6-10 Adrenal Cortex Pathology

Disease	Etiology	Clinical Features
Cushing's syndrome	Excess cortisol due to **iatrogenic corticosteroid therapy (most common cause)**, adrenal adenoma (more common than carcinoma); ectopic ACTH from neoplasm (especially **small cell lung carcinoma**)	Peripheral muscle wasting and weakness; **central obesity** with "moon face" and "buffalo hump"; easy bruising with abdominal striae; bone demineralization, osteoporosis, psychosis, acne; hirsutism; hyperglycemia; hypertension
Cushing's disease	Excess cortisol due to **pituitary hypersecretion of ACTH;** bilateral hyperplasia of adrenal cortex; **second most common** cause of Cushing's syndrome	Identical to Cushing's syndrome
Conn's syndrome (primary hyperaldosteronism)	Adrenal cortex **adenoma** (more common than hyperplasia, which is more common than carcinoma); sodium retention; **low plasma renin**	**Hypertension;** hypokalemic alkalosis
Secondary hyperaldosteronism	Renal tumors; renal ischemia; edematous conditions (cirrhosis, nephrotic syndromes, CHF); **increased plasma renin**	**Hypertension;** hypokalemic alkalosis
Addison's disease	Most commonly **idiopathic** cortisol deficiency; possibly auto-immune; may be due to tumor, infections (i.e., tuberculosis)	**Hypotension** (low serum sodium); **hyperpigmentation;** increased serum potassium
Waterhouse-Friderichsen syndrome	***Neisseria meningitides*** infection (meningitis) leads to DIC; hemorrhagic adrenal **necrosis** and collapse	Acute hypotension and salt wasting; **shock;** more common in children; death within hours if not treated

ACTH=adrenocorticotropic hormone; *CHF*=congestive heart failure; *DIC*=disseminated intravascular coagulation

● **Adrenal Medulla Pathology (Table 6-11)**

TABLE 6-11 Adrenal Medulla Tumors

Tumor	Pathology	Clinical Manifestation
Neuroblastoma	**Malignant;** excess catecholamine secretion; **N-myc** (oncogene) amplification	**Children;** degree of N-myc amplification related to prognosis
Pheochromocytoma	**Benign** (10% malignant); tumor of chromaffin cells; seen in MEN IIa and IIb	**Adults;** hypertension (usually paroxys-mal); palpitations, sweating, and headache; urinary vanillylmandelic acid (**VMA**)

MEN=multiple endocrine neoplasia

THE ENDOCRINE SYSTEM

QUICK HIT Hyperpigmentation in Addison's disease is caused by increased production of pro-opiomelanocortin (POMC) by the pituitary. POMC is enzymatically split to yield ACTH and melanocyte-stimulating hormone (**MSH**).

QUICK HIT Extra-adrenal chromaffin cell tumors are called paragangliomas (e.g., tumors originating in the organ of Zuckerkandl).

QUICK HIT The pheochromocy-toma rule of tens: 10% malignant, 10% multiple, 10% bi-lateral, 10% familial, 10% extra-adrenal, 10% children.

THYROID

● Formation of Thyroid Hormone (Figure 6-9)

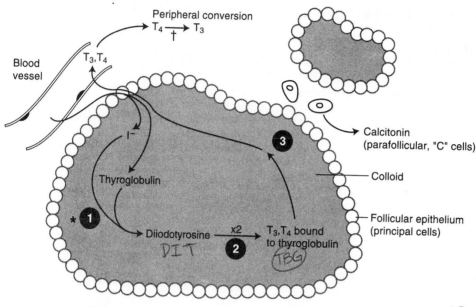

FIGURE
6-9   **Formation of Thyroid Hormone**

Peripheral conversion
$T_4 \rightleftharpoons T_3$ †

Blood vessel

T_3, T_4

I^-

Thyroglobulin

* 1

Diiodotyrosine
DIT

x2   2

T_3, T_4 bound to thyroglobulin
(TBG)

3

Calcitonin (parafollicular, "C" cells)

Colloid

Follicular epithelium (principal cells)

$T_4 = 2\,DIT$
$(+)\ T_3 = 1\,DIT + 1\,MIT$

1 Oxidation of I^- by peroxidase followed by iodination of thyroglobulin

2 Condensation

3 Proteolytic release of hormone from follicle

* Inhibited by propylthiouracil and methimazole

† Inhibited by propylthiouracil

● Myxedema

I. Can be described as hypothyroidism of the **adult**

II. Causes
A. **Hashimoto's thyroiditis** (see below)
B. Idiopathic causes
C. Iodine deficiency
  1. A problem in geographic areas with poor nutrition
  2. Deficiency in pregnant women can lead to cretinism in the child (see below)
D. High doses of iodine, paradoxically, lead to a decrease in thyroid hormone production.
E. **Over-irradiation** of the thyroid using I_{131} for treatment of hyperthyroidism

III. Clinical features of the hypothyroid state
A. Cold intolerance
B. Weight gain
C. Constipation
D. Lowering of voice
E. Menorrhagia
F. Slowed mental and physical function

G. Dry skin with coarse and brittle hair
H. Reflexes showing slow return phase

IV. Treatment is usually with levothyroxine.

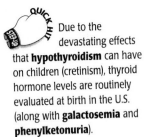 Due to the devastating effects that **hypothyroidism** can have on children (cretinism), thyroid hormone levels are routinely evaluated at birth in the U.S. (along with **galactosemia** and **phenylketonuria**).

● Cretinism

I. Can be described as hypothyroidism of the fetus or child

II. Causes
  A. **Iodine-deficient diet** in the mother, or during the early life of the child
  B. Thyroid-related enzyme deficiency
  C. Thyroid developmental defect
  D. Failure of thyroid descent during development
  E. Transfer of anti-thyroid antibodies from mother with autoimmune disease to fetus

III. Clinical features
  A. Impaired physical growth
  B. **Mental retardation**
  C. Enlarged tongue
  D. Enlarged, distended abdomen

● Hashimoto's Thyroiditis

I. An autoimmune disorder causing hypothyroidism and a painless goiter
  A. Dense infiltrate of lymphocytes into the thyroid gland
  B. Anti-thyroglobulin and anti-thyroid peroxidase (formerly anti-microsomal) antibodies
  C. **5:1 female predominance**
  D. Incidence increases with age
  E. Associated with human leukocyte antigen DR5 **(HLA-DR5)** and **HLA-B5**

II. Is the most common form of hypothyroidism in those with adequate iodine intake.

III. Clinical features
  A. Slowly progressing course with stages of euthyroid state, hyperthyroid state, and hypothyroid state.
  B. May lead to a scarred and shrunken gland in hypothyroid state.
  C. Microscopically, thyroid resembles lymph node.

IV. Associated with other autoimmune disorders
  A. Diabetes mellitus
  B. Pernicious anemia
  C. Sjögren's syndrome

● Subacute (De Quervain's) Thyroiditis

I. Transient hyperthyroidism with painful goiter
  A. Focal destruction of thyroid
  B. Granulomatous inflammation
  C. 3:1 female predominance
  D. Associated with HLA-B35

II. Causes—possibly due to recent viral infection with coxsackie virus, echovirus, adenovirus, measles, or mumps

III. Clinical features
   A. Acute febrile state
   B. Rapid painful enlargement of the thyroid
   C. Transient hyperthyroidism due to gland destruction

IV. Self-limited disease

● Graves' Disease

I. Autoimmune disorder causing hyperthyroidism and a goiter
   A. Thyroid stimulating immunoglobulin (**TSI**) is an immunoglobulin G (IgG) antibody to the thyroid-stimulating hormone (TSH) receptor
   B. Binding of TSI to the TSH receptor stimulates thyroid hormone production and hyperplasia of the thyroid gland
   C. Associated with **HLA-DR3 and B8**
   D. **4:1 female** predominance

II. Clinical features of Graves' disease
   A. Hyperthyroidism and goiter due to autoimmune immunoglobulins
      1. Increased total thyroxine (T_4)
      2. Increased triiodothyronine (T_3)
      3. Decreased TSH level
      4. Increased resin radioactive T_3 uptake
      5. Increased radioactive iodine
   B. **Exophthalmos**
   C. Warm, moist, and flushed skin
   D. Thin, fine hair
   E. Cardiovascular system
      1. Vasodilatation leading to decreased total peripheral resistance
      2. Increased heart rate and cardiac output
      3. **Palpitations** and **fibrillations**
      4. More readily occurs in a previously damaged heart
   F. Muscle atrophy
      1. Weakening of skeletal muscles occurs.
      2. Vital capacity of lungs decreases due to weakened respiratory muscles.
   G. **Weight loss** occurs despite an increased appetite.
   H. Diarrhea is common.
   I. Menstrual flow may decrease or stop.

III. Treatment
   A. Antithyroid drugs (i.e., propylthiouracil or methimazole)
   B. A **β-blocker** to reduce the cardiac effects
   C. Radioactive iodine (I_{131})
   D. Surgery

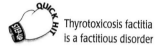 Thyrotoxicosis factitia is a factitious disorder (Munchausen's syndrome) in which the patient intentionally self-administers excess thyroid hormone (levothyroxine) to simulate the symptoms of hyperthyroidism.

Care must be taken when performing thyroid or parathyroid surgery as the recurrent laryngeal nerve runs directly posterior to these glands. Cutting the recurrent nerve leads to paralysis of the muscles used for speech (**except the cricothyroid**) and hoarseness on the affected side.

THE ENDOCRINE SYSTEM

● Thyroid Neoplasms (Table 6-12)

TABLE 6-12	**Thyroid Carcinomas**
Tumor	**Description**
Papillary tumor	• **Most common** thyroid cancer • **Best prognosis** of the thyroid cancers • **3:1 female predominance** • Usually occurs in third to fifth decade of life • "Ground glass" nuclei of neoplastic cells, also called "Orphan Annie Eyes" • **Psammoma bodies** may be present • Forms papillary projections covered with cuboidal epithelium within glandular spaces
Follicular tumor	• Worse prognosis than papillary • **3:1 female predominance** • Uniform cuboidal cells lining follicles • Lacks the distinctive nuclear features of papillary carcinoma
Medullary tumor	• Parafollicular cell neoplasm • **Secretes calcitonin** • Associated with MEN IIa and MEN IIb (MEN III)
Anaplastic thyroid carcinoma	• Anaplastic, undifferentiated neoplasm • More common in older patients • Rapidly fatal

MEN=multiple endocrine neoplasia

PARATHYROID PATHOLOGY (Table 6-13)

TABLE 6-13	**Parathyroid Disorders**	
Condition	**Etiology**	**Clinical Features**
Primary hyperparathyroidism	**Adenoma** (most common); hyperplasia more common than carcinoma; seen in MEN I and IIa; excess PTH; **hypercalcemia**	**Osteitis fibrosa cystica** (cystic "brown tumors" of bone); **renal calculi** and nephrocalcinosis; duodenal ulcers
Secondary hyperparathyroidism	**Hypocalcemia** due to **chronic renal failure** (loss of Vitamin D activation); parathyroid hyperplasia; excess PTH; high alkaline phosphatase; ectopic PTH (squamous cell lung carcinoma)	Cystic bone lesions; **metastatic calcification** of organs
Hypoparathyroidism	Most commonly secondary to **thyroidectomy;** seen in DiGeorge's syndrome; **hypocalcemia**	Tetany; positive **Chvostek's** and **Trousseau's** signs
Pseudohypoparathyroidism	Autosomal recessive; deficient organ response to PTH	**Short stature;** underdeveloped fourth and fifth digits

MEN=multiple endocrine neoplasia; *PTH*=parathyroid hormone

THE ENDOCRINE SYSTEM

QUICK HIT

Pancreatitis leads to fat necrosis due to release of pancreatic enzymes. The excess lipid binds calcium in a process called saponification and produces hypocalcemia.

MULTIPLE ENDOCRINE NEOPLASIA (MEN) SYNDROMES (Table 6-14)

The multiple endocrine neoplasia (MEN) syndromes are autosomal dominant conditions in which more than one endocrine organ is affected by either hyperplasia or neoplasia.

TABLE 6-14 Multiple Endocrine Neoplasia (MEN) Syndromes		
Type I (Wermer's syndrome)	**Type IIa (Sipple's syndrome)**	**Type IIb (or Type III)**
Hyperplasia or tumors of the thyroid, adrenal cortex, parathyroid, pancreas, or pituitary	Pheochromocytoma, medullary carcinoma of the thyroid, hyperparathyroidism	Pheochromocytoma, medullary carcinoma of the thyroid, multiple mucocutaneous neuromas (particularly of the GI tract)

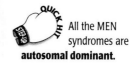

All the MEN syndromes are **autosomal dominant.**

Therapeutics

Adrenocorticoids	Fludrocortisone	Metyrapone
Dexamethasone	Hydrocortisone	Prednisone

Insulins and oral hypoglycemic drugs

Acarbose	Glipizide	Metformin
Acetohexamide	Glyburide	Troglitazone

Pituitary-hypothalamic drugs

Gonadotropin-releasing hormone (GnRH)	Human chorionic gonadotropin (hCG)	Bromocriptine
	Oxytocin	Desmopressin
	Octreotide	Growth hormone
		Leuprolide

Thyroid and parathyroid drugs

Levothyroxine	Propylthiouracil	Radioactive iodine (I_{131})
Potassium iodide		

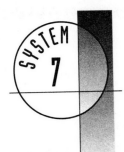

The Reproductive System

DETERMINATION OF SEX

Before the 7th week of gestation, the fetal gonads have not differentiated into either the male or female genotype. The presence or absence of the Y chromosome and the sex-determining region of the Y chromosome (SRY) determines gonadal differentiation. Gender determination, which occurs after the 7th week, depends on the type of gonads present.

FEMALE DEVELOPMENT

I. Ovaries and other female reproductive structures
   A. Primordial follicles contain **primary oocytes (XX genotype)** and follicular (granulosa) cells that form the ovaries.
   B. As the upper abdomen grows, the ovaries "descend" toward the perineum.
   C. The gubernaculum assists in this descent and then becomes the ovarian ligament and the round ligament of the uterus.
   D. The paramesonephric ducts develop into the uterine tubes and eventually into the uterus.

II. Vagina and Uterus (Figure 7-1)

FIGURE 7-1 Development of the Female Genital Tract

A. Reproductive system of the newborn female

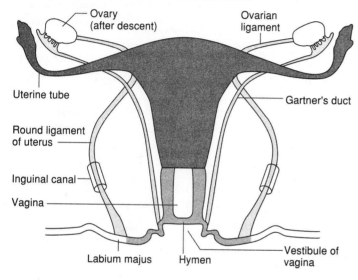

Structures arising from:
- ■ Paramesonephric duct
- ▨ Urogenital sinus
- □ Mesonephric duct

B. Stages of development of the female external genitalia

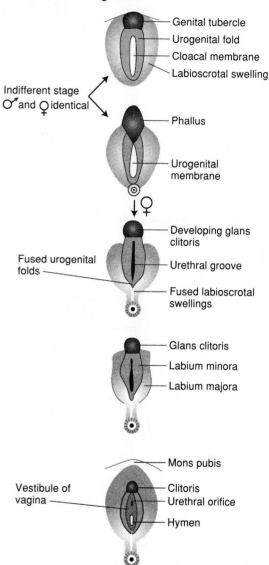

(Adapted from Moore KL, Persaud TVN. The Developing Human; Clinically Oriented Embryology, 6th edition. Philadelphia, W.B. Saunders, 1998.)

III. Breasts
A. Only the main lactiferous ducts develop during fetal life.
B. Glands enlarge during puberty due to increased levels of estrogens, progestins, prolactin, and growth hormone.

MALE DEVELOPMENT

I. Testes and other male reproductive organs
A. Primary sex cords contain primordial germ cells of **XY genotype**. The Y chromosome codes for the testes-determining factor (**TDF**) which allows for male gonadal differentiation.

B. Müllerian-inhibiting factor (**MIF**) is secreted by **Sertoli's cells**. MIF causes regression of the Müllerian (paramesonephric) ducts and their associated female genital structures.

C. The mesonephric ducts, under the influence of testosterone, become the ductus deferens, the seminal vesicles, and the ejaculatory ducts in the adult male.

II. The prostate gland forms from the urogenital sinus (Figure 7-2).

FIGURE 7-2 Development of the Male Genital Tract

A. **Reproductive system of the newborn male**

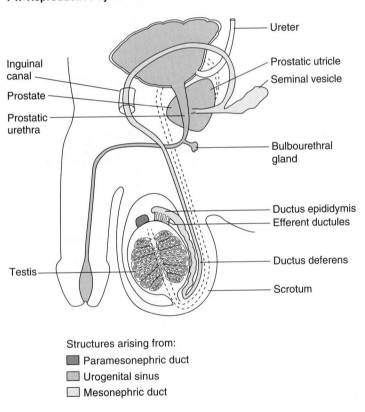

Structures arising from:
- ■ Paramesonephric duct
- ■ Urogenital sinus
- □ Mesonephric duct

B. **Stages of development of the male external genitalia**

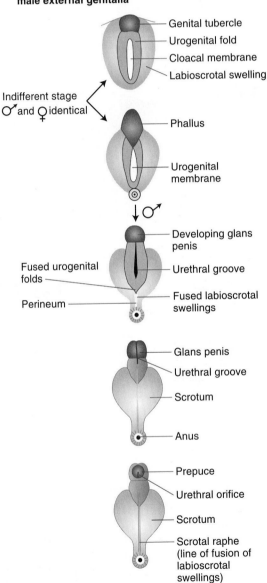

(Adapted from Moore KL, Persaud TVN. The Developing Human; Clinically Oriented Embryology, 6th edition. Philadelphia, W.B. Saunders, 1998.)

III. External genitalia

A. Testosterone is responsible for masculinization of genitalia.

B. The **genital tubercle** enlarges to become the glans penis.

C. The **urogenital fold** becomes the shaft of the penis.

D. The **labioscrotal swellings** fuse in the midline and become the scrotum.

(text continues on page 158)

SPERMATOGENESIS VERSUS OOGENESIS (Figure 7-3)

FIGURE 7-3 **Spermatogenesis versus Oogenesis**

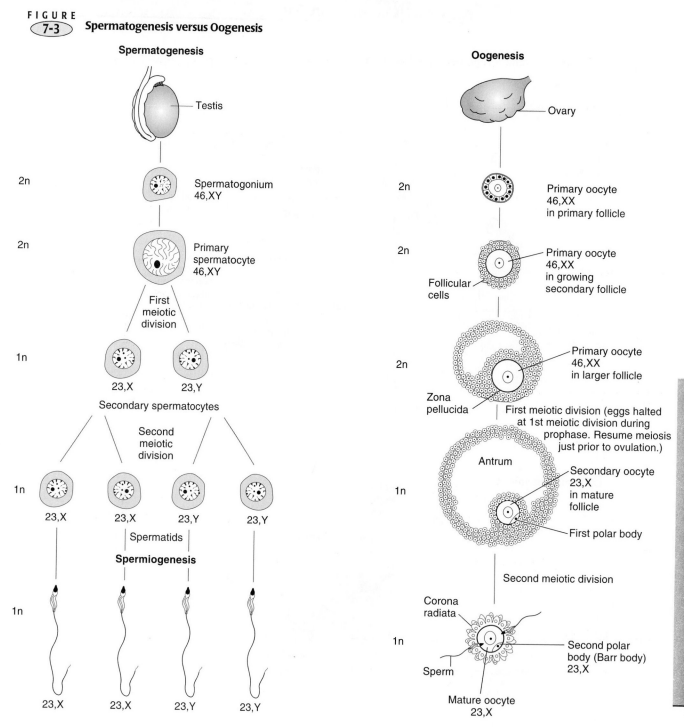

(Adapted from Moore KL, Persaud TVN. *The Developing Human; Clinically Oriented Embryology, 6th edition.* Philadelphia, W.B. Saunders, 1998.)

THE REPRODUCTIVE SYSTEM

IMPORTANT ANATOMICAL FEATURES OF THE PERINEUM (Figure 7-4)

FIGURE 7-4 Important Anatomical Features of the Perineum

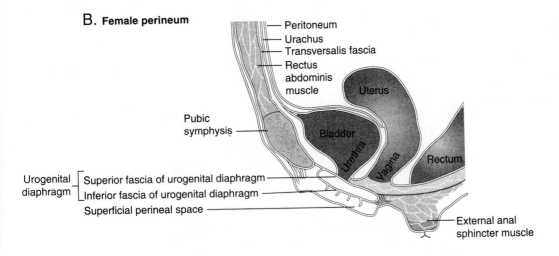

A. **Male perineum**

- Pubic symphysis
- Bladder
- Prostate gland
- Membranous layer of superficial fascia of abdomen (Scarpa's)
- Superior fascia of urogenital diaphragm
- Muscles within deep perineal space
- Inferior fascia of urogenital diaphragm
- Urogenital diaphragm
- Corpus cavernosum
- Urethra
- Corpus spongiosum
- Bulbospongiosus muscle
- Contents of superficial perineal space near midsagittal plane
- Membranous layer of superficial fascia of penis (Buck's)
- Membranous layer of superficial fascia of urogenital region (Colles')

B. **Female perineum**

- Peritoneum
- Urachus
- Transversalis fascia
- Rectus abdominis muscle
- Uterus
- Pubic symphysis
- Bladder
- Urethra
- Vagina
- Rectum
- Urogenital diaphragm
  - Superior fascia of urogenital diaphragm
  - Inferior fascia of urogenital diaphragm
- Superficial perineal space
- External anal sphincter muscle

THE REPRODUCTIVE SYSTEM

CONGENITAL MALFORMATIONS (Table 7-1)

Congenital malformations are most often caused by exposure to teratogens during the 3rd to 8th weeks of pregnancy, which is the period of organogenesis.

TABLE 7-1 Congenital Malformations

Malformation	Clinical Features
Hypospadias	• Urethra opens on the **ventral** side of the penis • Spongy urethra does not form properly or the **urogenital folds** do not fuse • The cause is a paucity of hormone receptors or too little hormone produced from the testes • More common than epispadias
Epispadias	• Urethra opens on the **dorsum** of the penis • **Genital tubercle** develops more dorsally than usual
Undescended testis (cryptorchidism)	• Most are of unknown cause • May be unilateral or bilateral • Most testes descend before one year of life • If testes remain undescended, **sterility or testicular cancer** can result
Congenital inguinal hernia (indirect hernia)	• A communication is formed between the **tunica vaginalis** (adjacent to the testis) and the peritoneal cavity • A loop of intestine may herniate into the opening and become entrapped, resulting in obstruction
True hermaphroditism	•**Both testicular** and **ovarian tissue** is present • External genitalia are ambiguous • Usually 46, XX
Female pseudohermaphroditism	• XX genotype with **virilization** of the external genitalia is present • The cause is **excess androgen exposure** • This malformation is most often due to congenital adrenal hyperplasia, a **21-hydroxylase deficiency** (autosomal recessive disease with low cortisol and high ACTH)
Male pseudohermaphroditism	• XY genotype with varying ambiguities of the external genitalia • The cause is a **lack of MIF and testosterone**
Androgen insensitivity syndrome (testicular feminization)	• **XY** genotype with female phenotype • Due to a **defective androgen receptor** • Vagina ends blindly (no uterus) • Normal female pubertal development occurs but pubic hair is scant and there are no menses
Double uterus	• The cause is failure of the **paramesonephric ducts** to completely fuse • The condition may appear in two forms: uterus divided internally by a thin septum; or a division of only the superior part of the uterus (bicornuate uterus)
Kallmann's syndrome	• A deficiency of GnRH results in decreased FSH and LH • No secondary sexual characteristics are present • Associated with hypoplasia of the olfactory bulbs (**anosmia**)

FSH=follicle stimulating hormone; GnRH=gonadotropin-releasing hormone; LH=luteinizing hormone; MIF=müllerian inhibiting factor

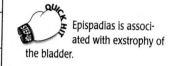

QUICK HIT Epispadias is associated with exstrophy of the bladder.

QUICK HIT Congenital inguinal hernia is associated with cryptorchidism.

THE REPRODUCTIVE SYSTEM

GENETIC ABNORMALITIES

The incidence of genetic abnormalities due to aberrant chromosomes significantly increases when the mother is over 35 years of age. In these patients, additional consideration should be given to genetic testing.

● **Genetic Abnormalities Caused by Abnormal Somatic Chromosomes (Table 7-2)**

QUICK HIT
Fragile X is the second most common cause of mental retardation in males. Down's syndrome is the most common cause.

QUICK HIT
There is an increased incidence of trisomy 21 in women over 35. The incidence of the Robertsonian translocation type of Down's syndrome is familial and does not increase with the age of the mother.

TABLE 7-2 Genetic Abnormalities Caused by Abnormal Somatic Chromosomes

Syndrome	Genotype	Description
Down's syndrome	Trisomy 21 (95%), or Robertsonian translocation of 14 and 21	• **Mental retardation** • Epicanthal folds • Large tongue • Brushfield's spots on iris • Simian crease in hands • Increased incidence of congenital heart disease, acute leukemia, and dementia of the Alzheimer type later in life
Edward's syndrome	Trisomy 18	• Mental retardation • Micrognathia • **Rocker bottom feet** • Second digit overlaps third and fourth • Increased incidence of congenital heart disease
Patau's syndrome	Trisomy 13	• Mental retardation • Microopthalmia • Polydactyly • Cleft lip and palate
Cri-du-chat syndrome	Deletion of 5p (5p−)	• Catlike cry • Mental retardation • Microcephaly • Hypertelorism

● **Genetic Abnormalities Caused by Abnormal Sex Chromosomes (Table 7-3)**

TABLE 7-3 Genetic Abnormalities Caused by Abnormal Sex Chromosomes

Syndrome	Genotype	Description
Turner's syndrome	45, X0	• **Monosomy** of the X chromosome • Absent Barr body • Short stature • Webbed neck

(continued)

THE REPRODUCTIVE SYSTEM

TABLE 7-3 **Genetic Abnormalities Caused by Abnormal Sex Chromosomes** *(Continued)*

Syndrome	Genotype	Description
		• Widely spaced nipples • Wide "shieldlike" chest • Wide carrying angle of arms • Lack of sexual maturity • Amenorrhea • Coarctation of the aorta
Klinefelter's syndrome	47, XXY	• Tall with long limbs • Often presents with gynecomastia • Hyalinization of seminiferous tubules • Lack of spermatogenesis leading to sterility • One Barr body
XYY syndrome	47, XYY	• Normal-appearing male, often tall • Often associated with **aggressive behavior** • May be over-represented in the population of incarcerated males
XXX syndrome	47,XXX	• Usually asymptomatic • Rarely associated with **menstrual irregularities** and mild mental retardation • Two Barr bodies
Fragile X syndrome	46, XY	• The end of the X chromosome appears delicate • **Macro-orchidism** • Common cause of **mental retardation** • Long face • Low-set, large ears
Prader-Willi syndrome	−15q12 (no paternal contribution, imprinting disorder)	• Obesity • **Hyperphagia** • **Hypogonadism** • Short stature • Mental retardation
Angelmans syndrome	−15q12 (no maternal contribution, imprinting disorder)	• Ataxia • Mental retardation • **Inappropriate laughter** • Patient appears to act like a **"happy puppet"**

QUICK HIT

Puberty in males, usually occurring at age 15, is marked by increased testosterone, leading to greater hair distribution, growth of genitalia, nocturnal emissions, deepening of the voice, and increased muscle mass. Precocious puberty in males has a similar pathology to that of females, with the exception that it has a later age of onset.

THE REPRODUCTIVE SYSTEM

MENARCHE, MENSTRUATION, AND MENOPAUSE (Figure 7-5)

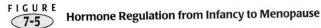

FIGURE 7-5 Hormone Regulation from Infancy to Menopause

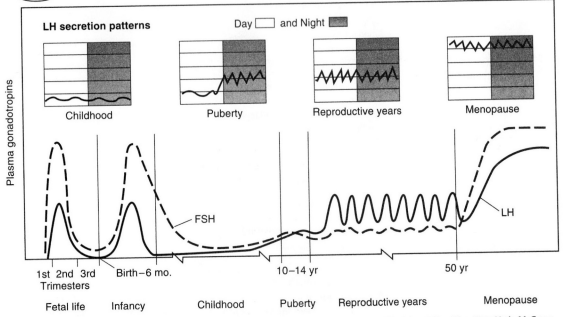

LH=luteinizing hormone (Adapted from Harrison TR, Fauci AS. *Harrison's Principles of Internal Medicine, 14th edition*. New York, McGraw-Hill, 1997.)

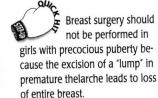

Breast surgery should not be performed in girls with precocious puberty because the excision of a 'lump' in premature thelarche leads to loss of entire breast.

I. Menarche
A. Is the final maturation of ovarian follicles
B. Is the first menstruation and usually occurs **between 11 and 14 years of age**
C. Follows thelarche (development of breast buds) by 2 years
D. Precocious puberty
  1. Pubertal changes before 9 years of age in boys and 8 years of age in girls.
  2. True precocious puberty
    a. Early, but normal pubertal development
    b. **Usually idiopathic**
    c. May cause emotional and social adjustment problems
  3. Incomplete precocious puberty
    a. Premature development of a single pubertal characteristic
    b. Types
      (1) Premature thelarche: breast budding prior to 8 years of age
      (2) Premature adrenarche: growth of axillary hair
      (3) Premature pubarche: growth of pubic hair
    c. Generally self-limiting
  4. Etiology
    a. Central—increased follicle stimulating hormone (FSH) and luteinizing hormone (LH)
    b. Peripheral—due to increased sex steroids

II. Menstruation and Fertilization

A. Hormone formation and function (Figure 7-6)

FIGURE
7-6   **Hormone Function within the Menstrual Cycle**

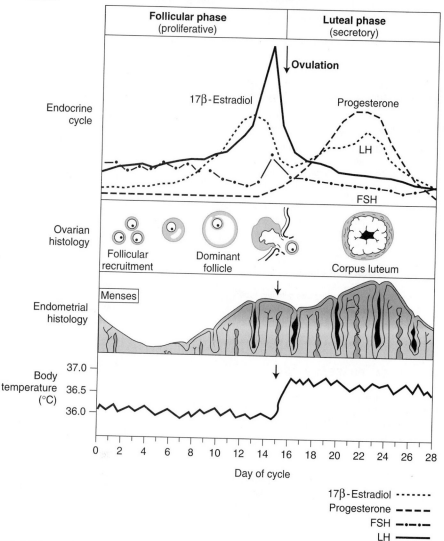

FSH=follicle stimulating hormone; LH=luteinizing hormone

1. Ovarian **steroids** are synthesized from **cholesterol**
2. LH regulates the conversion of cholesterol to pregnenolone (the first step in estrogen synthesis) in the theca cells
3. FSH regulates the final step in estrogen synthesis in the granulosa cells
4. Estrogen
   a. Secreted by the **ovary**
   b. Induces development of secondary sex characteristics
   c. Stimulates uterine growth and development
   d. Stimulates growth of endometrial spiral arteries
   e. Causes thickening of vaginal mucosa
   f. Induces development of the breast ductal system
   g. Bone growth (increased osteoblastic activity)
5. Progesterone
   a. Secreted by the **corpus luteum**
   b. Converts proliferative endometrium to secretory

  c. Induces proliferation of endometrium
  d. Inhibits uterine contractions
  e. Increases viscosity of cervical mucus
  f. Increases basal body temperature
  g. Induces development of breast glandular system
 B. The Menstrual Cycle (Figure 7-7)

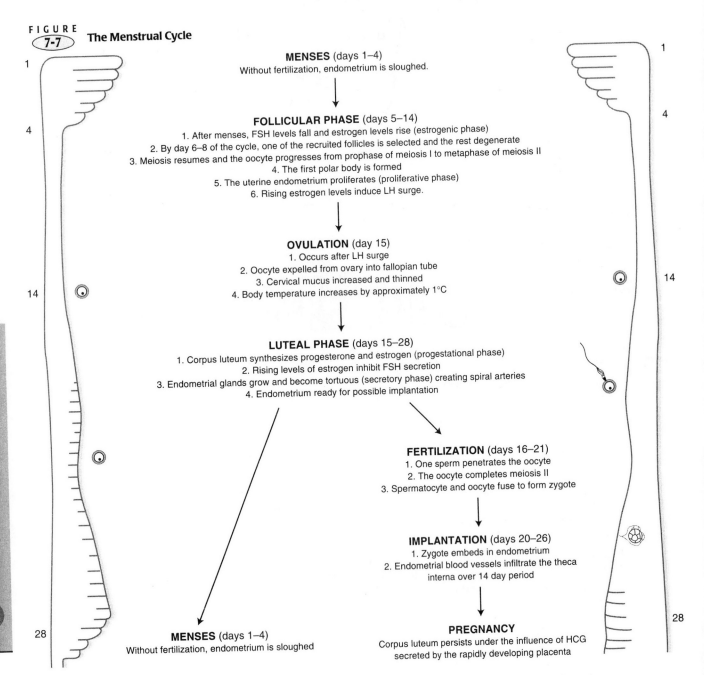

FIGURE 7-7   **The Menstrual Cycle**

MENSES (days 1–4)
Without fertilization, endometrium is sloughed.

FOLLICULAR PHASE (days 5–14)
1. After menses, FSH levels fall and estrogen levels rise (estrogenic phase)
2. By day 6–8 of the cycle, one of the recruited follicles is selected and the rest degenerate
3. Meiosis resumes and the oocyte progresses from prophase of meiosis I to metaphase of meiosis II
4. The first polar body is formed
5. The uterine endometrium proliferates (proliferative phase)
6. Rising estrogen levels induce LH surge.

OVULATION (day 15)
1. Occurs after LH surge
2. Oocyte expelled from ovary into fallopian tube
3. Cervical mucus increased and thinned
4. Body temperature increases by approximately 1°C

LUTEAL PHASE (days 15–28)
1. Corpus luteum synthesizes progesterone and estrogen (progestational phase)
2. Rising levels of estrogen inhibit FSH secretion
3. Endometrial glands grow and become tortuous (secretory phase) creating spiral arteries
4. Endometrium ready for possible implantation

FERTILIZATION (days 16–21)
1. One sperm penetrates the oocyte
2. The oocyte completes meiosis II
3. Spermatocyte and oocyte fuse to form zygote

IMPLANTATION (days 20–26)
1. Zygote embeds in endometrium
2. Endometrial blood vessels infiltrate the theca interna over 14 day period

MENSES (days 1–4)
Without fertilization, endometrium is sloughed

PREGNANCY
Corpus luteum persists under the influence of HCG secreted by the rapidly developing placenta

1. One cycle is defined as the time from the onset of one menses to the next, usually **28 days**
2. Some oocytes within the ovaries undergo developmental changes during the cycle (see Figure 7-8)

FIGURE
7-8

Developmental changes in the ovary

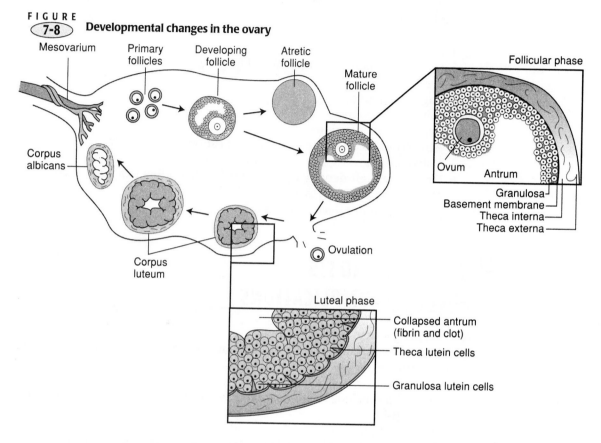

C. Disorders
1. Dysfunctional uterine bleeding
   a. A functional menstrual disorder with excessive bleeding during, or bleeding between, menstrual periods
   b. **Most common gynecological problem** during reproductive years
   c. Caused by
      (1) Leiomyoma
      (2) Anovulatory cycle
      (3) Organic lesions (tumors, polyps)
      (4) Complications of pregnancy (ectopic pregnancy, cesarean section, abortion)
      (5) Endometrial hyperplasia
      (6) Corpus luteum cysts
2. Polycystic ovary syndrome (Stein-Leventhal syndrome)
   a. Triad of **secondary amenorrhea, obesity, and hirsutism**
   b. Increased LH and testosterone
   c. Stromal fibrosis and small follicular cysts in the ovary
3. Endometriosis
   a. Non-neoplastic endometrial tissue located outside the uterus
   b. Responds to hormonal variations of menstrual cycle
   c. Most commonly occurs in the ovary (bilateral)
   d. Presents as pain and excessive bleeding during menstruation
   e. Large blood-filled sacs (**chocolate cysts**) seen
   f. May result in infertility

III. Menopause
A. Last physiological menstrual cycle usually occurs in the **mid 40s or early 50s**
B. Estrogen levels fall (due to reduced ovarian function) and FSH levels increase
C. Early signs
   1. Anxiety
   2. Mood swings
   3. Irritability
   4. Depression
   5. **Hot flashes:** bouts of sweating and flushing
D. Late signs
   1. Vaginal dryness
   2. Painful intercourse
   3. Urinary tract infections
   4. Atrophy of breast tissue due to lack of estrogen stimulation
   5. **Osteoporosis**
   6. **Decreased high-density lipoproteins (HDL)** leading to an increased risk of **coronary artery disease**
E. Does not result in a decreased sex drive

PREGNANCY AND ITS ASSOCIATED COMPLICATIONS

I. Normal pregnancy
A. For clinical purposes, assume that a **woman of childbearing age is pregnant** unless proven otherwise
B. Normal gestation is **40 weeks**
C. Clinical signs include missed periods, swollen breasts, fatigue, nausea, and **elevated β-hCG**
D. Hormonal regulation
   1. Fertilization: **β-hCG** produced by the placenta **prevents corpus luteum regression**
   2. First trimester: **corpus luteum** produces estrogen and progesterone
   3. Second and third trimester
      a. Progesterone is produced by the **placenta**
      b. Estrogen production is regulated by the interplay among fetal adrenal gland, fetal liver, and placenta
   4. Parturition (delivery of baby): initiating event is unknown
   5. Lactation
      a. Estrogen and progesterone block the effect of prolactin on the breast
      b. Prolactin levels rise throughout pregnancy and suppress ovulation
      c. Estrogen/progesterone levels fall after delivery
E. Prenatal diagnostic procedures
   1. **Amniocentesis** is an aspiration of fluid from the amniotic sac at 10–14 weeks after fertilization
      a. Alpha fetoprotein (**AFP**) assay for neural tube defects
      b. **Spectrophotometry** to determine hemolytic disease of the newborn (see System 9 "Hematopoietic and Lymphoreticular System")
      c. Sex chromatin studies for X-linked disease
      d. **Cell culture** studies for chromosomal abnormalities
      e. Enzyme and DNA analysis
   2. Maternal serum AFP
      a. Elevated in neural tube defects
      b. Reduced in Down's syndrome

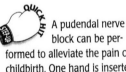
A pudendal nerve block can be performed to alleviate the pain of childbirth. One hand is inserted into the vagina to locate the ischial spine, which is used as a landmark, while the other hand inserts a needle, which contains anesthetic for the skin lateral to the vaginal opening.

The narrowest diameter that the fetus must transverse during birth is the pelvic outlet, from ischial spine to ischial spine (interspinous distance).

3. Chorionic villus sampling (CVS)
   a. Can be performed at 10 weeks of pregnancy
   b. Cells are aspirated from the chorionic villi
   c. Cells are evaluated for genetic abnormalities
4. **Ultrasound**
   a. Can be performed at 12 weeks of pregnancy
   b. Measures fetal size, determines sex, and diagnoses fetal malformations
E. Apgar score
   1. Used for physical assessment of child 1 minute and 5 minutes after birth
   2. Five categories are scored 0, 1, or 2, with 2 being indicative of better performance.
      a. Color (blue=0, trunk pink=1, all pink=2)
      b. Heart rate (0=0, <100=1, 100+=2)
      c. Reflexes (none=0, grimace=1, grimace and irritable=2)
      d. Muscle tone (none=0, some=1, active=2)
      e. Respiration (none=0, irregular=1, regular=2)

II. Abnormal placental attachment
A. **Abruptio placentae**
   1. Placenta separates from the uterine wall prior to parturition
   2. Usually leads to fetal **death**
   3. May result in disseminated intravascular coagulation (**DIC**) in mother
B. **Placenta accreta**
   1. Direct connection of uterus wall to placenta
   2. Due to prior surgery or trauma during pregnancy
   3. Improper separation results in massive **hemorrhage**
C. **Placenta previa**
   1. Placenta attaches to lower uterus and blocks the cervical os
   2. Associated with **bleeding**

III. Ectopic pregnancy
A. Risk factors
   1. **Pelvic inflammatory disease (PID)** (e.g., chronic salpingitis)
   2. Previous surgery
   3. Endometriosis
   4. Previous ectopic pregnancy
B. Clinical features
   1. Amenorrhea
   2. Pelvic pain and cervical tenderness
   3. Tissue mass (usually in the fallopian tubes)
   4. Elevated β-hCG

IV. Preeclampsia
A. Triad of **hypertension, albuminuria,** and **edema**
B. Most common in the last trimester of first pregnancy
C. May result in eclampsia if untreated
   1. Eclampsia has similar manifestations to preeclampsia, but also includes seizures and possibly DIC
   2. Eclampsia can be characterized by Hypertension, Elevated Liver enzymes, and Low Platelets (**HELLP** syndrome)

V. Hydatidiform mole
A. Placental villi that enlarge abnormally early in pregnancy
B. **"Cluster of grapes"** with marked increase in β-hCG
C. Manifests as vaginal bleeding and an increase in uterine size
D. Two types:

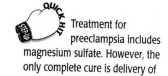

Treatment for preeclampsia includes magnesium sulfate. However, the only complete cure is delivery of the fetus.

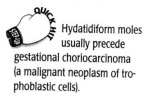

Hydatidiform moles usually precede gestational choriocarcinoma (a malignant neoplasm of trophoblastic cells).

THE REPRODUCTIVE SYSTEM

1. **Complete mole**
   a. Diploid XX karyotype
   b. No embryo present
   c. Completely paternal in origin
2. **Partial mole**
   a. Triploid (XXX or XXY) karyotype
   b. Embryo present

VI. Gestational diabetes
A. Insulin resistance occurs in normal pregnancy
B. Mother may be unable to meet the increased metabolic demands of pregnancy
C. Two or more of the following venous glucose values must be reached after a 100 g oral glucose load
   1. Fasting > 105 mg/dL
   2. 1 hour > 190 mg/dL
   3. 2 hour > 165 mg/dL
   4. 3 hour > 145 mg/dL
D. High blood glucose leads to hypoglycemia in the infant, macrosomia (enlarged body), increased risk of trauma, and increased likelihood of cesarean section due to large size of fetus

VII. Infections causing birth defects (TORCHES)
A. The **TORCHES** are **t**oxoplasmosis, **o**ther infections, **r**ubella, **c**ytomegalovirus infection, and **her**pes simplex and **s**yphilils
B. This group of infectious organisms can cause birth defects if the mother is infecting during pregnancy, especially in the first trimester.

GYNECOLOGIC DIAGNOSTIC TESTS

I. Wet mount
A. Vaginal epithelial scrapings placed on a glass slide with a drop of saline
B. Microbes detected:
   1. Trichomonas appears as pear-shaped organisms with sporadic movement
   2. Bacterial vaginosis appears as vaginal epithelium with roughened edges (**clue cells**)

II. Potassium hydroxide (KOH) preparation
A. KOH is added to a microscope slide prepared with vaginal epithelial scrapings
B. Epithelium is dissolved with KOH
C. Microbes detected:
   1. Candida, which is resistant to KOH, remains on the slide and is identified by its **budding cells with short hyphae**
   2. KOH reacts with bacterial amines producing a "**fishy odor**" characteristic of bacterial vaginosis

III. Papanicolaou (Pap) smear
A. Cells from the cervix are scraped onto a glass slide.
B. Microbes detected:
   1. Human papilloma virus (HPV) is characterized by **koilocytes** (large epithelial cells with perinuclear clearing)
   2. Cytomegalovirus (CMV) appears as intranuclear inclusions with a halo around them (**owl's eye** cells)

3. Herpes simplex virus (HSV) appears as multi-nucleated giant cells
C. Precancerous lesions detected: Cervical intraepithelial neoplasia (**CIN**) 1, 2, 3
D. Cancers detected
   1. Invasive **squamous cell carcinoma** (most common)
   2. Endometrial adenocarcinoma

SEXUALLY TRANSMITTED DISEASES (STDs) (Table 7-4)

Between 20%–50% of those patients with one sexually transmitted disease (STD) will have a coexisting infection with another. The sexual partners of those diagnosed with an STD should be treated. However, the physician cannot inform the partner, except when the physician feels that the patient is unreliable and the partner will go untreated.

TABLE 7-4	Sexually Transmitted Diseases (STDs)
Microbe	**Disease**
Calymmatobacterium granulomatis	Granuloma inguinale; biopsy shows **Donovan bodies**
Chlamydia trachomatis	Urethritis and **acute PID** from serotypes D–K; ulcerative lesions of the genitalia as a result of the L1–L3 serotypes
Gardnerella vaginalis	Vulvovaginitis
Haemophilus ducreyi	Chancroid; ulcerative lesions of the genitalia
Herpes simplex virus-2	Genital herpes; urethritis; **painful** ulcerative lesions of the genitalia
HIV type 1 and 2	**AIDS**
Human papilloma virus types 6 and 11	**Condyloma acuminatum** of vulva
Human papilloma virus (especially types 16, 18, 31, 45)	Genital or anal **warts; squamous cell carcinoma** of cervix, vagina, anus, or penis
Neisseria gonorrhoeae	Urethritis; **acute PID;** pharyngitis; monoarticular **arthritis**
Treponema pallidum	Syphilis; **painless** ulcerative lesions of the genitalia —Primary syphilis—hard chancres —Secondary syphilis—gray wartlike lesions on the genitalia (condyloma lata) —Tertiary syphilis—neurologic manifestations such as tabes dorsalis and ascending aortic aneurysm
Trichomonas vaginalis	Vulvovaginitis; male urethritis

AIDS=acquired immunodeficiency syndrome; *HIV*=human immunodeficiency virus; *PID*=pelvic inflammatory disease

 Chlamydia is the most common STD in the world in part due to the fact that it goes undetected when the patient is co-infected with gonorrhea. Treatment for gonorrhea should also be supplemented with chlamydia therapy for both the patient and their partner.

PID can be diagnosed via bimanual pelvic examination eliciting "**the chandelier sign**" (cervical motion tenderness).

Salpingitis, often associated with PID, can lead to infertility if left untreated.

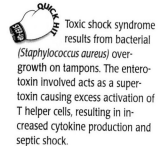 Some non-sexually transmitted infections of the GU tract include: *Candida albicans* which causes vulvovaginitis, *Staphylococcus aureus* that can result in toxic shock syndrome, and *Escherichia coli* and *Staphylococcus saprophyticus,* which can both cause UTI's.

Toxic shock syndrome results from bacterial (*Staphylococcus aureus*) overgrowth on tampons. The enterotoxin involved acts as a supertoxin causing excess activation of T helper cells, resulting in increased cytokine production and septic shock.

FEMALE GYNECOLOGIC NEOPLASMS

Tumors of the gynecologic organs may manifest themselves as dysfunctional uterine bleeding (DUB), and as such, a heightened level of suspicion must be maintained with this presentation. Many of these neoplasms can be detected and even prevented (as is the case with cervical cancer) by routine gynecologic exams.

(text continued on page 170)

● Ovarian Neoplasms of Epithelial Origin (Table 7-5)

QUICK HIT

CA125 (cancer antigen 125) is elevated in over 80% of ovarian carcinomas.

QUICK HIT

75% of ovarian neoplasms are epithelial in origin. These tumors are usually seen in middle-aged to elderly women.

TABLE 7-5 Ovarian Neoplasms of Epithelial Cell Origin

Neoplasm	Morphology	Clinical Presentation
Serous cystadenoma	Cystic	Benign; frequently bilateral
Serous cystadenocarcinoma	Cystic	Malignant; frequently bilateral; most common (50% of ovarian neoplasms)
Mucinous cystadenoma	Mucin-filled cysts	Benign
Mucinous cystadenocarcinoma	Mucin-filled cysts	Malignant; **pseudomyxoma peritonei** (diffuse peritoneal metastasis secreting mucin)
Endometrioid tumor	Resembles endometrium	Malignant
Brenner tumor	Resembles **transitional epithelium**	Benign; rare tumor
Clear cell tumor	Abundant **clear cytoplasm**	Usually unilateral; rare

[handwritten annotations: "psomma bodies", "Jelly Belly", "warthin nests", "Bilateral", "malignant", "young"]

● Ovarian Neoplasms of Germ Cell Origin (Table 7-6)

QUICK HIT

Germ cell tumors account for only 25% of ovarian neoplasms, but are the most common ovarian tumors found in women under 20 years of age.

TABLE 7-6 Ovarian Neoplasms of Germ Cell Origin

Neoplasm	Morphology	Clinical Features
Dysgerminoma	Large cells with clear cytoplasm	Malignant; **equivalent of seminoma;** occurs in children
Endodermal sinus (yolk sac)	Resembles yolk sac	Malignant; produces alpha-fetoprotein **(AFP)**
Immature teratoma	Elements from multiple embryonic layers; poorly differentiated; resembles fetal or embryonic tissue	Malignant
Mature teratoma (dermoid cyst)	Elements from multiple embryonic layers; including: hair, bone, tooth, and nervous tissue; duplication of maternal genetics; resembles adult tissue	**Most common germ cell neoplasm** (90%); **benign** (vs. malignant in males)
Monodermal teratoma	Elements from multiple embryonic layers; one tissue type develops, most commonly thyroid tissue **(struma ovarii)**	Benign; hyperthyroidism
Choriocarcinoma	Usually seen in combination with other germ cell tumors	Malignant; produces β-human chorionic gonadotropin **(β-hCG)**
Granulosa-theca	Lipid-laden cells; fibroblast proliferation; cuboidal cells in cords; eosinophilic follicles **(Call-Exner bodies)**	Benign; may secrete estrogen leading to precocious puberty or endometrial hyperplasia or carcinoma
Thecoma-fibroma	Fibroblast proliferation	Benign; rare; in combination with ascites and hydrothorax referred to as **Meigs' syndrome**
Sertoli-Leydig cell	Tubules containing testicular cells	Produces testosterone; virilization
Metastasis	Most commonly from GI, breast, or ovary; **Krukenberg tumor:** primary in stomach with signet-ring cells bilaterally	Only 5% of ovarian neoplasms

[handwritten annotations: "Durod bodies", "+ α1 Trypsin", "adults.", "Kids"]

THE REPRODUCTIVE SYSTEM

● Tumors of the Uterus (Cervix and Body) (Table 7-7)

TABLE 7-7 Tumors of the Uterus (Cervix and Body)

Neoplasm	Clinical Features
Cervical intraepithelial neoplasia (CIN)	• May be classified as CIN I, CIN II, or CIN III • Neoplastic changes in the endometrium beginning at the **squamocolumnar junction** • CIN I: mild dysplasia extending less than 1/3 of the thickness of the epithelium • CIN II: cells appear more malignant with increased mitotic figures and variation in nuclear size; approximately 2/3 of the epithelium involved • CIN III: also called carcinoma in-situ (CIS); involves the full thickness of the cervical epithelium • Associated with human papilloma virus 16, 18, 31, 33, 45 infection (HPV)
Squamous cell carcinoma of the cervix	• Evolves from a progression of CIN • Increased incidence is associated with **early sexual activity** and **multiple sex partners**
Leiomyoma	• Benign tumor of the uterine body • The **most common tumor of women** (the most common malignancy in women is breast cancer) • Often multiple • Size increases with pregnancy and decreases with menopause
Leiomyosarcoma	• Uncommon • Does not arise from a preexisting dysplastic or neoplastic condition
Endometrial carcinoma	• The **most common malignancy** of the female genital tract • Associated with nulliparity • More often found in older women • Exogenous **estrogen** administration or estrogen-producing tumors may be predisposing factors • Also predisposed by diabetes, tamoxifen, hypertension, and obesity • Usually presents as vaginal bleeding

insitu (handwritten annotation)

adenocarcinoma (handwritten annotation)

QUICK HIT Estrogens can be synthesized by adipose tissue. This may be partially responsible for predisposing obese women to endometrial carcinoma.

● Tumors of the Vulva and Vagina (Table 7-8)

TABLE 7-8 Tumors of the Vulva and Vagina

Tumor	Description
Papillary hidradenoma	• **Most common** benign tumor of the vulva • Often presents as an ulcerated and bleeding nodule • Originates from apocrine sweat glands • Can easily be surgically removed
Squamous cell carcinoma of the vulva	• Similar to squamous cell carcinoma of the cervix • Highest occurrence in **older women** • Vulvar dystrophy precedes carcinoma • Associated with infection of HPV 16, 18, 31, 33, 45
Paget's disease of the vulva	• Histologically similar to Paget's disease of the breast • Is not always associated with underlying adenocarcinoma (vs. Paget's disease of the breast)

hydradenoma (handwritten annotation)

(continued)

TABLE 7-8 **Tumors of the Vulva and Vagina** *(Continued)*

Tumor	Description
Malignant melanoma	• Similar to malignant melanoma of the skin • 10% of malignant tumors of the vulva
Squamous cell carcinoma of the vagina	• The vagina is rarely a primary site of cancer formation • Usually an extension of squamous cell carcinoma of the cervix
Clear cell adenocarcinoma	• A rare malignant tumor • Occurs in the daughters of women given **diethylstilbestrol (DES)** during pregnancy
Sarcoma botryoides	• A type of rhabdomyosarcoma • Usually occurs in **girls under 5** years of age • **"Bunch of grapes"** that protrude from the vagina

BREAST PATHOLOGY (Table 7-9)

Risk factors for breast cancer include: over 45 years of age, nulliparity, early menarche, late menopause, high fat diet, HER-2/neu oncogene activation, first degree relative with positive history, and a history of breast cancer in the contralateral breast.

QUICK HIT Breast cancer is the **most common cancer** of women, but the second leading cause of cancer death after lung cancer. The most common location is the **upper, outer quadrant**.

QUICK HIT The presence of estrogen and/or progesterone receptors on breast cancer reflects a good prognosis due to the ability to employ hormonal (anti-estrogen) therapy.

QUICK HIT Gynecomastia (enlargement of the breast tissue in males) can be caused by alcoholism, cimetidine, ketoconazole, spironolactone, and digitalis.

QUICK HIT Male breast cancer represents 1% of all breast cancer.

TABLE 7-9 **Breast Pathology**

Condition	Pathology	Clinical Features
Acute mastitis	Entry of ***Staphylococcus aureus*** through nipple; abscess	Most often occurs during **nursing**; may be due to eczema
Fibrocystic changes	Breast mass; tender during menstruation; usually **bilateral; "blue-domed"** cysts	**Most common breast disorder;** non-neoplastic; predisposition to cancer only with evidence of cellular atypia
Fibroadenoma	Painless; rubbery mass	Benign; **most common tumor in patients under 25 years of age**
Intraductal papilloma	Tumor of the lactiferous ducts	Benign; may present as serous or bloody discharge
Phyllodes	Large mass; cysts; ulceration of skin	Malignant potential; may recur
Invasive ductal carcinoma	Firm mass; cells form glands; fibrous stroma	Malignant; **most common carcinoma** of the breast
Lobular carcinoma	Cancer cells fill ducts; **bloody discharge;** may be bilateral; cells line up **"Indian file"**	Malignant; may be progression of lobular carcinoma in situ
Paget's disease	Superficial lesion of nipple or areola; **Paget cells** in epidermis (large cell with marginal clearing seen)	Malignant; indicative of **underlying ductal carcinoma**
Medullary carcinoma	Soft, fleshy tumor; characterized by lymphocytic infiltrate	Malignant

THE PROSTATE (Figure 7-9)

FIGURE
7-9 **The Prostate**

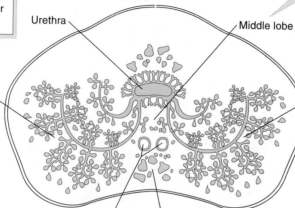

Prostatic carcinoma
- Most common male cancer
- Enlarged, firm, nodular prostate on DRE
- Elevated serum PSA and alkaline phosphatase
- Frequent metastasis is to bone (especially the spine)
- Affects the lateral lobe (posterior lobe in older nomenclature)

Benign prostatic hyperplasia
- Most common cause of male urinary tract obstruction
- Bladder distention or hypertrophy
- UTI's
- Increased residual volume and frequency
- Nocturia, difficulty initiating stream
- Caused by age-related increase in testosterone and estrogen
- Common after 40 years of age
- Affects middle lobe (lateral and middle lobe in older nomenclature)

Urethra — Middle lobe

Lateral lobe — Lateral lobe

Ejaculatory ducts   Posterior lobe

DRE=digital rectal examination; *PSA*=prostate-specific antigen; *UTI*=urinary tract infection

TESTICULAR PATHOLOGY

Anatomic disorders of the testis occur more often in young children, whereas the infection and neoplastic diseases are more likely to occur in the young-adult, sexually active population. Routine testicular examinations can often prevent and detect serious complications. When detected early, testicular neoplasms are one of the most curable cancers.

● **Testicular Disorders (Table 7-10)**

TABLE 7-10	**Testicular Disorders**
Disorder	**Clinical Features**
Hydrocele	• **Serous fluid** collects in the tunica vaginalis • Caused by **patency** between the peritoneal cavity and the tunica vaginalis
Hematocele	• **Blood** collects in the tunica vaginalis • Usually caused by **trauma**
Varicocele	• **Engorgement of the veins** of the spermatic cord • Most noticeable when patient is standing
Spermatocele	• Epididymal cyst containing **sperm**

(continued)

QUICK HIT **Benign prostatic hyperplasia (BPH) is not a pre-cancerous disorder** and it cannot be accurately diagnosed by measuring prostate specific antigen (PSA).

QUICK HIT Prostate cancer is the second most common cause of cancer death in males. The leading cause is lung cancer.

QUICK HIT The digital rectal exam (DRE) is essential, since many of the male pelvic organs can be assessed. When the examining finger is introduced into the rectum, anal tone (S2-S4 innervation) can be evaluated. Anteriorly, from inferior to superior, lie the lower border of the prostate, the posterior aspect of the prostate, and the bladder if distended.

THE REPRODUCTIVE SYSTEM

(text continued on page 174)

TABLE 7-10	Testicular Disorders *(Continued)*
Disorder	**Clinical Features**
Cryptorchidism	• **Failure** of one or both of the testes to **descend** • Increased incidence of **germ cell testicular cancer,** such as seminoma and embryonal carcinoma (see Table 7-11 on testicular neoplasms) • Failure of descent leads to testicular **atrophy** and **sterility**
Testicular torsion	• **Twisting** of the spermatic cord • If untreated, will result in **testicular necrosis**
Orchitis	• Testicular infection and inflammation • May be viral or bacterial in origin • Can lead to **sterility if bilateral**
Epididymitis	• **Inflammation and infection** of the epididymis • Most often caused by ***Neisseria gonorrhoeae, Chlamydia trachomatis,*** *Escherichia coli, Mycobacterium tuberculosis*

● **Testicular Neoplasms (Table 7-11)**

TABLE 7-11	Testicular Neoplasms	
Neoplasm	**Site of Origin; Morphology**	**Clinical Features**
Seminoma	Germ cell; arranged in lobules or nests	Malignant; incidence highest in 35–40 year-olds; painless enlargement of testis; **most common germ cell tumor;** similar to dysgerminoma of the ovary; radiosensitive and curable
Embryonal carcinoma	Germ cell; variable morphology with papillary convolutions	Malignant; highest incidence in 20's; more aggressive than seminomas; very common in mixed tumors
Yolk sac tumor (endodermal sinus tumor)	Germ cell; anastomosing cords	Malignant; presents with pain or metastasis; similar to ovarian tumor; peak incidence in childhood (infants to 3 years of age); **increased AFP**
Teratoma	Two or more embryonic layers; **multiple tissue types** such as cartilage, epithelium, liver, and muscle	Malignant; occurs at any age, but more common in children; mature: heterogeneous tissue in organoid fashion; immature: incompletely differentiated
Mixed germ cell tumor	Variable; variable	Malignant; aggressive; more than one neoplastic pattern; **most common**
Leydig cell tumor (interstitial)	Testicular stroma; intracytoplasmic **Reinke crystals**	Benign; produces androgens, estrogens, and/or corticosteroids; often seen with **precocious puberty** or gynecomastia; similar to ovarian Sertoli-Leydig cell tumor
Sertoli cell tumor (androblastoma)	Testicular stroma; form cord-like structures	Benign; minor endocrine abnormalities; similar to ovarian Sertoli-Leydig cell tumor
Choriocarcinoma	Trophoblastic cells; villous structures resembling placenta	Malignant; hemorrhagic; **β-hCG elevated;** peaks in early adulthood

AFP=alpha fetoprotein

Human Immunodeficiency Virus (HIV) (Figure 7-10)

FIGURE
7-10 Replication of the Human Immunodeficiency Virus and Its Effect

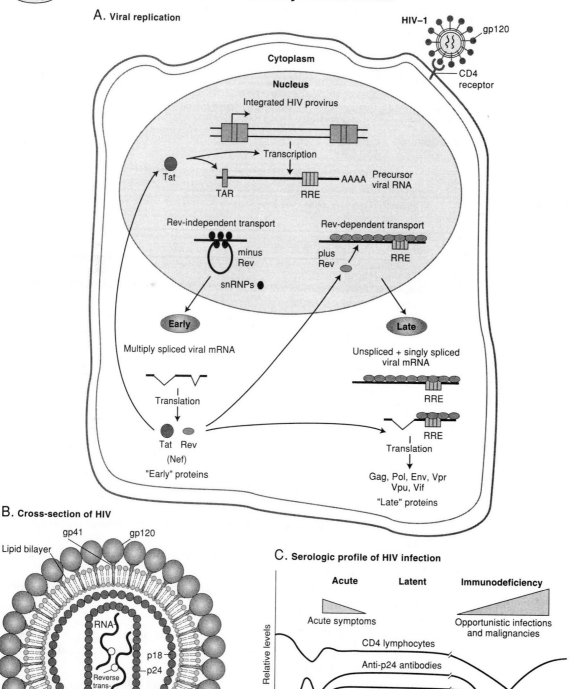

A. Viral replication

B. Cross-section of HIV

C. Serologic profile of HIV infection

gp=glycoprotein; *HIV*=human immunodeficiency virus; *mRNA*=messenger ribonucleic acid; *RNA*=ribonucleic acid; *snRNP*=small nuclear ribonucleoprotein particle

I. Etiology
   A. HIV-1 (more common) or HIV-2 **retrovirus**
   B. Transmitted by:
      1. Sexual contact
      2. **Intravenous (IV) drug** abusers sharing needles
      3. Contact with bodily fluids (blood, semen, breast milk)
      4. Mother to fetus (transplacentally)
   C. Not transmitted through:
      1. Casual contact
      2. Toilet seats
      3. Kissing
      4. Mosquitoes
   D. Occupational risk to health care worker is low. A needle stick with an HIV patient's blood carries a **0.3% chance of transmission**

II. Pathology
   A. Primary infection
      1. Transmitted virus infects **T-helper lymphocytes** (CD4) via the interaction of viral proteins **gp120** and **gp41** with each other and the CD4 marker (see Figure 7-10 and Table 7-12)

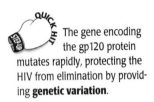

The gene encoding the gp120 protein mutates rapidly, protecting the HIV from elimination by providing **genetic variation**.

TABLE 7-12	HIV proteins and function
Gene	**Product and Function**
GAG	Viral core proteins p17, p24
POL	Protease, integrase, reverse transcriptase, RNAse H
ENV	gp 120, gp41
TAT	Transcriptional transactivator (increases gene expression); essential for replication
REV	Transition from early to late gene expression; protein transport from nucleus to cytoplasm; essential for replication
NEF	Transcriptional silencer; may produce latent infection
VIF	Viral infectivity gene; cell to cell transmission
VPU	Viral protein U; viral particle export
VPR	Viral protein R; activates viral and cellular promoters

      2. The virus also infects macrophages and monocytes (proposed portal of entry into CNS)
      3. Viremia is accompanied by the **"acute retroviral syndrome"** (a flu-like illness)
      4. 1st month is the **window period,** as p24 antigen is not yet detectable in the blood (patient is contagious)
   B. Chronic Infection
      1. Immune response lowers viral blood counts but active replication persists
      2. **No clinical symptoms** for approximately **10 years (latent period)**
      3. CD4 count steadily declines
      4. Near end of latent period, develop constitutional symptoms
         a. Weight loss
         b. Fever
         c. Night sweats
         d. Adenopathy
   C. Acquired Immunodeficiency Syndrome (AIDS)
      1. Defined as a **CD4 count of 200 cells/microliter** or less coupled with the presence of certain **opportunistic** infections

2. Infections typically seen with AIDS:
   a. **Pneumocystis carinii pneumonia** (80%)
   b. **Kaposi's sarcoma**
   c. B-cell lymphoma (brain and bone marrow)
   d. Toxoplasma gondii (brain tissue infection)
   e. CMV (leads to retinitis)
   f. Cryptococcus neoformans (meningeal infection)
   g. Mycobacterium avium-intracellulare (MAI)
   h. Tuberculosis (TB)
   i. Candida albicans (thrush, esophagitis)
   j. Cryptosporidium (chronic diarrhea)

D. Epidemiology
   1. In the U.S., during the 1980s, the infection first spread among **male homosexuals.**
   2. **IV drug abusers** and **hemophiliacs** (before tests were developed to screen blood) were the next populations affected.
   3. **Heterosexual** transmission is rising in the U.S. and is now the leading cause of infection in Africa.

E. Laboratory diagnosis
   1. **The enzyme-linked immunosorbent assay (ELISA) test** for antibodies lends a presumptive diagnosis
   2. This must be confirmed by the **Western blot** test which demonstrates antibodies to gp41 or p24 (see Figure 7-10)

F. Treatment (see therapeutics list)
   1. Nucleoside analogues and protease inhibitors
   2. **Combination therapy** has drastically improved HIV treatment by forestalling the development of resistance to medication

THERAPEUTICS

Antimicrobials

Aminoglycosides	Doxycycline	Penicillin
Carbenicillin	Erythromycin	Trimethoprim-
Cephalosporin	Metronidazole	sulfamethoxazole
Clarithromycin		

Antineoplastics

5-Fluorouracil	Dactinomycin	Methotrexate
Aminoglutethimide	Doxorubicin	Paclitaxel
Bleomycin	Estrogens	Tamoxifen
Cisplatin	Flutamide	Vinblastine
Cyclophosphamide		

HIV therapeutics

Dideoxyinisine (ddI)	Ritonavir	Zidovudine (AZT)
Lamivudine (3TC)	Saquinavir	

Sex hormones

Antiprogesterone (RU-486)	Finasteride	Norgestrel
Clomiphene	Flutamide	Oxandrolone
Estradiol	Medroxyprogesterone	Premarin
	Norethindrone	Tamoxifen

Urinary tract antiseptics

Ciprofloxacin   Nalidixic acid   Nitrofurantoin

Uterine-Modifying Agents Used During Pregnancy

Carboprost   Magnesium sulfate   Ritodrine
Prostaglandin E$_2$ Naproxen   Terbutaline
Ergonovine   Oxytocin

SPECIAL SECTION

TIMELINE OF THE DEVELOPMENTAL STAGES OF LIFE (Figure 7-11)

FIGURE 7-11 **Stages of Development**

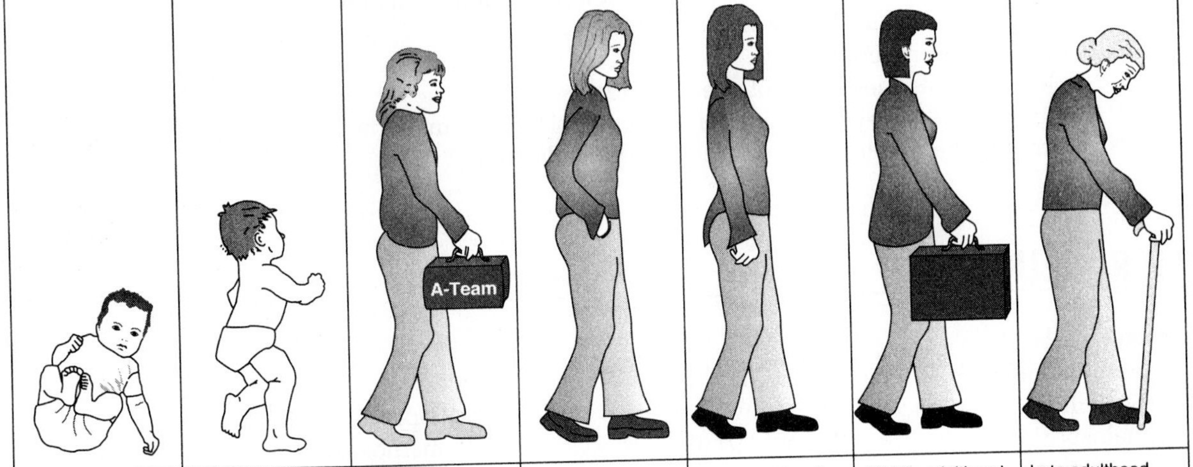

	Infancy (0–1y)	Toddler (1–3y)	School age (3–11y)	Adolescence (11–20y)	Early adulthood (20–40y)	Middle adulthood (40–60y)	Late adulthood (60–80y)
Freud	Oral	Anal	Phallic-oedipal (3–6y); latency (6–11y)	Genital			
Erikson	Trust vs Mistrust	Autonomy vs shame and doubt	Initiative vs guilt (3–6y); industry vs inferiority	Identity vs role confusion	Intimacy vs isolation	Generativity vs stagnation	Ego integrity vs despair
Piaget	Sensorimotor (0–2y)	Preoperational (2–7y)	Concrete operations (7–11y)	Formal operations			
Characteristics	Reflexes: • Palmer grasp (0–2m) • Rooting (0–3m) • Babinski (0–12m) Milestones: • Turn over (5m) • Sit (6m) • Walk (12m)	Terrible two's ("no"); band-aid (2–4y); parallel play (2–4y); balance on one foot (2y); climb stairs (3y)	Cooperative play (4–7y); conservation of mass (7–11y); button clothes (4y); throw a ball (4y);	First menstruation (11y); first ejaculation (13y); peer pressure	New family; children; role in society solidified; period of reassessment	Height of career; mid-life crises; menopause (45–55y)	Depression (ECT); women outlive men by 6–8 years; Kübler-Ross (stages of grief and dying) • Denial • Anger • Bargaining • Depression • Acceptance

y = years of age; m = months old

THE FAMILY UNIT AND RELATED CONCEPTS

I. The Family Cycle
A. Phase 1: **Marriage**
   1. Married couples are mentally and physically healthier than unmarried couples.
   2. Nearly half of all marriages end in divorce.
B. Phase 2: **Child-rearing**
   1. Children raised in single-parent families have higher rates of depression, drug abuse, suicide, and criminal activity.
   2. Children from divorced families are more likely to become divorced themselves later in life.
C. Phase 3: **Children leave home**
D. Phase 4: **Physical decline** and final distribution of goods

 The death of a child or the suicide of a spouse is the most severe psychological stressor.

II. Postpartum depression
A. Up to 50% of all women develop a short-lived depression after giving birth (postpartum blues)
B. Etiology
   1. Change in hormone levels
   2. Increased responsibility
   3. Fatigue
C. Major depression seen in 5%–10% of all women after childbirth

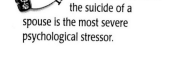 Depression is defined as a 2-week course marked by 4 of the following 8 criteria: 1) anhedonia, 2) increased or decreased sleep, 3) feelings of guilt, 4) decreased energy level, 5) inability to concentrate 6) changes in appetite, 7) psychomotor retardation, 8) suicidal ideation

III. Attachment of child to mother
A. **Anaclitic depression:** sustained absence of mother between 6–12 months of age leads to a withdrawn and unresponsive infant
B. **Harlow** showed that monkeys raised in isolation did not develop normally.
   1. Males were more affected than females.
   2. Recovery was not possible if isolation lasted longer than 6 months.
C. **Bowlby** showed that physical contact between mother and child was crucial to development.
D. **Spitz** observed that children without proper mothering were slow to develop and had a greater number of medical problems.
E. **Mahler** documented development as a process where the infant separates from the mother.
   1. Normal autistic phase (0–1 month): infant has little interaction
   2. Symbiotic phase (1–5 months): infant is close to mother
   3. Separation-individuation phase (5–16 months): child realizes individuality and begins to explore environment

IV. Child Abuse
A. Includes physical abuse, sexual abuse, and emotional neglect
B. Risk factors
   1. Substance abuse by parents
   2. Poverty
   3. Marital problems or single-parent home
D. Physical abuse is marked by numerous fractures, bruises, subdural hematomas, or burns (at various stages of healing)
E. Sexual abuse of children is marked by trauma to the genitalia, sexually transmitted diseases, or urinary tract infections.
F. Abuse predisposes the child to post-traumatic stress disorder (PTSD), dissociative disorders, depression, anorexia, phobias, and personality disorders.
G. Physician intervention is necessary.

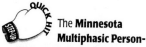 The **Minnesota Multiphasic Personality Inventory** (MMPI) is the most commonly used objective personality test, while the **Rorschach** test is the major projective test of personality. Intelligence is measured by the **Stanford-Binet** scale as an intelligence quotient (IQ) and is relatively stable throughout life.

VI. Family therapy
A. Involves all members of a family even though only one person might have a problem
B. Identifies dysfunctional behavior and encourages communication and problem-solving
C. Based on the concept that the family system is composed of subsystems where boundaries are established and mutual accommodation occurs

SEXUALITY

I. Gender
A. **Gender identity** is an individual's sense of being male or female, while **gender role** is the expression of one's gender.
B. Sexual orientation is a physical preference for one or both genders (heterosexual, homosexual, bisexual).
C. Psychological factors play a role in gender identity and sexual orientation.
  1. **Transsexual:** a person who has the sense of being in the wrong-sex body and has a strong desire to correct it.
  2. **Homosexual:** a person who has a sexual preference for same-sex individuals.
  3. **Transvestite:** a man who dresses in women's clothing for pleasure

II. Sexual dysfunction

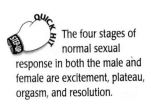

The four stages of normal sexual response in both the male and female are excitement, plateau, orgasm, and resolution.

A. Premature ejaculation (early climax without reaching plateau phase) is the **most common** male sexual disorder.
B. The most common sexual dysfunction in women is **sexual arousal disorder** where lubrication cannot be maintained throughout the sexual act.
C. Impotence
  1. Failure to achieve erection and/or ejaculation
  2. Usually has an organic component but may be psychogenic (e.g., caused by stress or anxiety)
    a. Often due to alcohol abuse
    b. Psychogenic cause can be confirmed by observing erections during REM sleep.
C. Vaginismus
  1. Spasm in the outer third of the vagina
  2. Difficulty during intercourse or pelvic examination
  3. Often results from rape, incest, or abuse
D. Paraphilias (Table 7-13)

TABLE 7-13 **Paraphilias**

Category	Description (How sexual pleasure is derived)
Exhibitionism	Exposing one's genitalia
Fetishism	Inanimate objects (e.g., women's high-heeled shoes or undergarments)
Frotteurism	Furtively rubbing genitalia against a woman (e.g., pushing up against a woman in a crowded subway)
Necrophilia	Corpses
Pedophilia	Children

(continued)

TABLE 7-13 Paraphilias *(Continued)*	
Category	**Description (How sexual pleasure is derived)**
Masochism	Receiving physical or psychological pain and humiliation
Sadism	Inducing physical or psychological pain and humiliation in others
Transvestic fetishism	Wearing women's clothing (such men are still attracted to women)
Voyeurism	Furtively watching individuals engage in intercourse or seductive activities
Zoophilia	Animals

1. Involves unusual objects of sexual desire
2. Are found almost exclusively in men

RAPE

I. An act of sexual aggression in which the penis penetrates the outer vulva.

II. Rapists tend to be male and tend to rape women of own race
   A. Roughly, half of the assailants are black and half are white
   B. Use of weapons and alcohol is common
   C. Rapists are usually young (under 25 years of age)
   D. Rapes are underreported (usually only 15% of total)
      1. Victims are generally 15–30 years of age
      2. Rape usually occurs inside the woman's home by an individual whom she knows
   E. Rape usually results in rape trauma syndrome, which involves emotional lability for over one year
      1. Group therapy and support are important treatment modalities
      2. Post-traumatic stress disorder (PTSD) may occur even after treatment
         a. PTSD occurs in a subgroup of individuals exposed to trauma
         b. Usually develops in adolescents or young adults

SUICIDE

I. Second-leading cause of death in persons 15–24 years of age and 8th leading cause of death in the United States.

II. Women attempt suicide 4 times more often than men, but men are 3 times more successful due to the lethality of method used

III. Marriage reduces the risk of suicide

IV. Professional women may be at an increased risk for suicide

V. Suicide risk should be assessed during the mental status exam.
   A. Patients with a **plan** are at higher risk.
   B. Indications for hospitalization include impulsiveness, lack of social support, and a plan.

QUICK HIT
Pedophilia is the **most common** paraphilia and needs to be reported to the authorities upon discovery by the physician.

QUICK HIT
The core set of symptoms in PTSD is re-experiencing the traumatic event, avoidance, numbing, and arousal or hypervigilance.

QUICK HIT
Divorced white males over 65 years of age, who have a plan, and are taking 3 or more medications have the highest risk of suicide.

THE REPRODUCTIVE SYSTEM

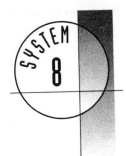

The Musculoskeletal System

DEVELOPMENT

I. Bone Formation
A. **Endochondral bone**
1. Forms over a cartilage frame
2. Becomes the **long bones** of the skeleton **(e.g., femur)**
B. **Membranous bone**
1. Forms without a cartilage frame
2. Becomes the **flat bones** of the skeleton, (e.g., bones of the cranium)

II. Skeletal Muscle
A. Derives from **somites**
B. Each somite produces its own **myotome**

III. Pharyngeal Arches
A. **Arch 1**
1. Innervated by the mandibular branch of the trigeminal nerve [cranial nerve V **(CN V)**]
2. Gives rise to the following muscles:
   a. Muscles of mastication (temporalis, masseter, lateral pterygoid, medial pterygoid)
   b. Two tensor muscles (tensor veli palatini, tensor tympani)
   c. Two other muscles (mylohyoid, anterior belly of the digastric)
B. **Arch 2**
1. Innervated by the facial nerve **(CN VII)**
2. Gives rise to the following muscles:
   a. Muscles of facial expression (obicularis oculi, obicularis oris, buccinator)
   b. Three other muscles (stylohyoid, stapedius, and the posterior belly of the digastric)
C. **Arch 3**
1. Innervated by the glossopharyngeal nerve **(CN IX)**
2. Gives rise to the stylopharyngeus muscle
D. **Arch 4**
1. Innervated by the vagus nerve (pharyngeal and superior laryngeal branches of **CN X**)
2. Gives rise to the following muscles:
   a. Cricothyroid muscle
   b. All the muscles of the soft palate and pharynx except the stylopharyngeus muscle and tensor veli palatini
E. **Arch 6**
1. Innervated by the vagus nerve (recurrent laryngeal branch of **CN X**)
2. Gives rise to the intrinsic muscles of the larynx except the cricothyroid

*Of all the intrinsic muscles of the larynx (posterior cricoarytenoid, lateral cricoarytenoid, arytenoid, thyroarytenoid, cricothyroid, transverse arytenoid, oblique arytenoid, and vocal muscle), the posterior cricoarytenoid muscle is the only muscle that **abducts** the vocal cords.*

IV. Skin (Figure 8-1)

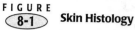

Skin Histology

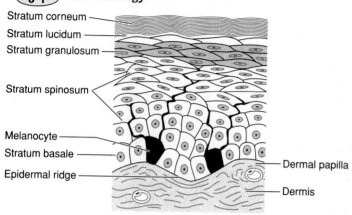

Stratum corneum
Stratum lucidum
Stratum granulosum

Stratum spinosum

Melanocyte
Stratum basale
Epidermal ridge

Dermal papilla

Dermis

Stratum basale is actively mitotic, and gives rise to the other four layers.

A. Epidermis forms from **ectoderm** and dermis forms from mesoderm.
B. Melanocytes contain melanin pigment and are derived form neural crest.
C. Renews every 2–3 weeks
D. Function
    1. Barrier to infection
    2. Thermoregulation
    3. Protection from desiccation
D. Two types of skin
    1. Thick skin (e.g., palms and soles of feet)
       a. Stratum basale (deepest layer)
       b. Stratum spinosum
       c. Stratum lucidum
       d. Stratum granulosum
       e. Stratum corneum (most superficial layer)
    2. Thin skin (e.g., face, genitalia, and back of hands)- stratum lucidum is absent in thin skin (though it has all the other layers).

BONE FUNCTION AND METABOLISM (Figure 8-2)

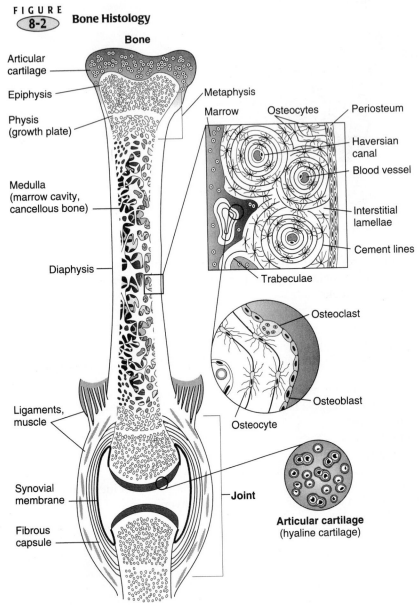

FIGURE 8-2 Bone Histology

(Adapted from Damjanov: *Histopathology: A Color Atlas and Textbook.* Baltimore, Williams & Wilkins, 1996. p 422)

I. Osteoblasts

A. Synthesize collagen to form cartilage

B. Calcium and phosphate are deposited on the cartilaginous matrix to form mineralized bone.

C. Blood supply goes to osteoblasts via vessels within the **haversian canals**

D. When osteoblasts become surrounded by bone matrix they become osteocytes

II. Osteocytes

A. Are influenced by parathyroid hormone **(PTH)** to stimulate osteoclastic bone resorption

B. Resorption allows Ca^{2+} to be transferred rapidly into the blood

III. Osteoclasts
   A. Multi-nucleated cells formed from **monocytes**
   B. Contain acid phosphatase
   C. Resorb bone under influence of **PTH**

IV. Hormonal control
   A. **Parathyroid hormone**
   1. Stimulates osteoclastic activity causing osteolysis and release of Ca^{2+} from bone
   2. Promotes the reabsorption of Ca^{2+} in the kidney
   3. Inhibits phosphate (PO_4^{3-}) reabsorption in the kidney
   4. Converts vitamin D to its active form, 1,25-dihydroxycholecalciferol
   5. Raises blood calcium and lowers phosphate
   B. **Calcitonin**
   1. Inhibits osteoclasts which inhibits bone reabsorption
   2. Lowers blood calcium
   C. **Vitamin D**
   1. Assists PTH in the reabsorption of bone
   2. Increases Ca^{2+} absorption from the intestine
   3. Increases Ca^{2+} reabsorption from the kidney
   4. Increases PO_4^{3-} reabsorption from the kidney
   5. Raises blood calcium and phosphate

> **QUICK HIT**
> Exogenous estrogen administration slows the rate of bone loss that occurs after menopause, by stimulating osteoblasts via estrogen receptors.

BONE, CARTILAGE, AND JOINT DISEASE

In the healthy adult, bone mass peaks between 20 and 25 years of age. Bone diseases can adversely affect the mass and strength of the skeleton, predisposing the patient to fractures.

● **Diseases That Affect Bone Formation (Table 8-1)**

TABLE 8-1   Diseases that Affect Bone Formation

Disease	Etiology	Clinical Features
Osteitis fibrosa cystica (von Recklinghausen's disease of bone)	Caused by increased levels of **PTH**; primary or secondary hyperparathyroidism	Cystic spaces in the bone that are lined with osteoclasts; often colored brown due to hemorrhage, hence the name "brown tumor of bone"
Achondroplasia	Caused by failure of long bones to elongate due to narrow epiphyseal plates and sealing of these plates with the metaphysis; **autosomal dominant** disease; **most common cause of dwarfism**	Short limbs; normal-sized head and trunk
Osteogenesis imperfecta	Group of gene mutations that cause **defective collagen synthesis**; most common type of mutation is autosomal dominant; often called "brittle bone disease"	Multiple fractures occur with only minor trauma; **blue sclera**; deformities of teeth and skin

(continued)

TABLE 8-1 Diseases that Affect Bone Formation *(Continued)*

Disease	Etiology	Clinical Features
Osteopetrosis	**Increased density of bone** due to failure of reabsorption by osteoclasts; "marble bone" disease; the most severe form is autosomal recessive	Multiple **fractures** despite increased density; narrowing of marrow spaces causes anemia; narrowing of other cavities causes blindness, deafness, and cranial nerve compression
Paget's disease of bone	Increased osteoblastic and osteoclastic activity by an unknown cause; occurs most commonly in the elderly; may involve one or more bones	**Skeletal deformities;** complications include bone pain due to **fracture,** multiple **AV shunts** in bone causing high output cardiac failure, hearing loss due to thickening of bony structures in ear; may lead to osteosarcoma; 3 phases of disease: • Osteolytic phase—resorption due to osteoclasts • Mixed phase—osteoclastic and osteoblastic activity leads to a **mosaic pattern** in the bone • Late phase—increase in bone density due to osteoblastic activity

AV=arteriovenous; *PTH*=parathyroid hormone

● **Metabolic and Infectious Bone Disease (Table 8-2)**

TABLE 8-2 Metabolic and Infectious Bone Disease

Disease	Etiology	Clinical Features
Osteoporosis	Decreased synthesis or increased reabsorption of bone due to physical inactivity, increased thyroid levels, postmenopausal state, increased cortisol level, decreased calcium levels	**Decrease in bone mass** leads to fractures (especially of the weight-bearing bones of the spine) and radiolucent bone on radiograph
Scurvy	Lack of Vitamin C intake; defective **proline and lysine hydroxylation** in collagen synthesis	Impaired bone formation and lesions result; painful subperiosteal hemorrhage; osteoporosis; bleeding gums
Rickets (children) Osteomalacia (adults)	Impaired calcification of bone due to deficiency of vitamin D; if caused by renal disease, termed "renal osteodystrophy"	Skeletal malformations, craniotabes (thinned and softened bones of the skull), late fontanelle closure, decreased height, rachitic rosary (costochondral junction thickening resembling string of beads), pigeon breast due to a protruding sternum in children; radiolucency in adults
Avascular necrosis	Death of osteocytes and fat necrosis via the following mechanisms: vascular compression, vascular interruption (fracture), thrombosis (sickle cell disease, caisson disease), vessel injury	Joint pain; osteoarthritis; sites include head of the femur (**Legg-Calvé-Perthes** disease), tibial tubercle (**Osgood-Schlatter** disease)

(continued)

QUICK HIT The most common cause of avascular necrosis is steroid-induced vascular compression. Caisson disease, which leads to necrosis via thrombosis and embolism, is caused by gas emboli resulting from decompression syndrome (e.g., rapid ascension from deep levels while scuba diving).

THE MUSCULOSKELETAL SYSTEM

TABLE 8-2 Metabolic and Infectious Bone Disease *(Continued)*

Disease	Etiology	Clinical Features
Pyogenic osteomyelitis	Infection of bone most often caused by **Staphylococcus aureus;** routes of infection include: hematogenous, extension from adjacent infection, open fracture/surgery	Acute febrile illness; pain; tenderness; usually affects metaphysis of distal femur, proximal tibia, and proximal humerus; forms sequestrum and involucrum
Tuberculous osteomyelitis	Tuberculous infection spreads to bone from elsewhere in body	Seen in hips, long bones, hands, feet, and vertebrae **(Pott's disease)**

Quick Hit: Patients with sickle cell disease often contract pyogenic osteomyelitis as a result of salmonella infections, while intravenous drug users often become infected with pseudomonas.

● Tumors of Bone and Cartilage (Table 8-3)

Tumors of the bone and cartilage, while rare, occur most commonly in the lower extremities of young males. Metastases are more common than primary tumors of the bone. Tumors of the prostate, breast, and lung account for 80% of bone metastases.

TABLE 8-3 Tumors of Bone and Cartilage

Tumor	Morphology	Clinical Features
Osteochondroma	Benign bone tumor; **most common benign tumor;** originates in metaphysis of long bones	Most common in men younger than 25 years of age; usually occurs on the lower end of the femur or upper end of the tibia
Giant cell tumor	Benign bone tumor; spindle-shaped cells with multinuclear giant cells; occurs on epiphyseal end of long bones	Most common in women 20–55 years of age; has **"soap bubble"** appearance on radiograph; usually occurs on the lower end of the femur or upper end of the tibia
Osteoma	Benign bone tumor; mature bone (dense tissue)	Most common in men; affects skull or facial bones; protrudes from surface
Osteoid osteoma	Benign bone tumor; nidus rimmed by osteoblasts and surrounded by vascular, spindled stroma	Most common in men 20–30 years of age; occurs near the ends of the tibia and femur; painful; radiolucent **nidus** is seen on radiograph
Osteosarcoma	Malignant bone tumor; origin usually in metaphyseal long bones; destructive masses with hemorrhage and necrosis	Most common in boys in their teenage years; usually occurs in tibia or femur near the knee; local pain; tenderness; swelling; metastasizes to lung first; growth under bone results in **Codman's triangle** on radiograph
Chondrosarcoma	Malignant cartilage tumor; lobulated translucent tumors; necrosis; calcification	Most common in men in mid- to late life; central skeleton is affected; radiograph shows localized area of bone destruction
Ewing's sarcoma	Malignant cartilage tumor; similar to lymphoma; **t(11;22);** sheets of small round cells producing Homer-Wright pseudorosettes	Most common in boys from 10–15 years of age; occurs in long bones, ribs, pelvis, scapula; early metastasis; responds to chemotherapy; painful, warm, swollen mass

(continued)

Gardner syndrome.

Quick Hit: Osteochondromas generally do not undergo malignant transformation to chondrosarcoma, except in the familial variety which is characterized by multiple lesions.

Quick Hit: Predisposing factors for osteosarcoma include Paget's disease of the bone, mutations of the p53 gene on chromosome 17 (Li-Fraumeni syndrome), familial retinoblastoma, radiation, and bone infarcts.

Quick Hit: The most common bone sarcoma in children is an osteosarcoma, followed by Ewing's sarcoma.

THE MUSCULOSKELETAL SYSTEM

QUICK HIT

Café au lait spots are also seen in Peutz-Jeghers syndrome and neurofibromatosis type 1 (Von Recklinghausen's disease).

TABLE 8-3 Tumors of Bone and Cartilage (Continued)

Tumor	Morphology	Clinical Features
Fibrous dysplasia	Benign; bone replaced haphazardly by fibrous tissue	"Chinese figures" configuration on radiograph; 3 types: • single bone involvement • several bones involved • several bones involved, along with precocious puberty and café au lait spots
Metastasis	Malignant; usually lytic lesions unless arising from prostate or breast	Originate from prostate, breast, kidney, lung; ectopic hormone production **[parathyroid hormone related protein (PTHrP)]**

● Arthritic Joint Disease (Table 8-4)

The etiology of arthritic joint diseases is not well understood. For this reason, treatment is often palliative rather than curative.

Two factors to consider in the differential diagnosis of an acutely painful joint include infection and urate deposition. These two entities may be distinguished from each other, in part, by aspiration of the joint fluid with evaluation for white blood cells, bacteria on gram stain, or crystals.

QUICK HIT

Osteoarthritis may affect only one joint and can affect the distal interphalangeal (DIP) joints of the hands. Rheumatoid arthritis is bilaterally symmetric and does not affect the DIP joints. Also, rheumatoid arthritis is characterized by joint stiffness in the morning that is relieved as the day goes on, while osteoarthritis pain gets worse as the day goes on.

TABLE 8-4 Arthritic Joint Disease

Disease	Etiology	Clinical Features
Osteoarthritis	Degeneration of joint cartilage followed by growth of surrounding bone; the **most common type of arthritis**; primary type has no specific risk factor; secondary type related to trauma, metabolic disorder, or inflammatory arthropathy; **knee** is the most common site	Joint mice" form from pieces of torn and frayed joint cartilage and broken pieces of osteophytes; erosion of cartilage results in **eburnation** (polishing) of the underlying bone; cysts visible in bone on radiograph; Heberden's nodes are osteophytes at the distal interphalangeal (DIP) joint; Bouchard's nodes are osteophytes of the proximal interphalangeal (PIP) joints
Rheumatoid arthritis	Inflammation of joints and tendons most likely due to autoimmune reaction; **rheumatoid factor**—IgM antibody to IgG is characteristic; more common in women; associated with **HLA-DR4**	Acute inflammation of the synovium with edema and cellular infiltrate; synovial hypertrophy and hyperplasia; granulation tissue (**pannus**) over articular cartilage; subcutaneous rheumatoid nodules; **swan-neck** and **boutonniere** deformity develop due to inflammation, muscle atrophy, and contracture; DIP joints are spared
Ankylosing spondylitis	Unknown cause; high association with **HLA-B27**; negative rheumatoid factor; males are more commonly affected	Chronic low back pain and stiffness; improves with movement; calcification of spinal ligaments and fusion of the facet joints produces a **"bamboo spine"**; may produce extra-skeletal manifestations of **apical lung fibrosis, aortic insufficiency,** or **cauda equina syndrome**

(continued)

THE MUSCULOSKELETAL SYSTEM

TABLE 8-4 Arthritic Joint Disease *(Continued)*

Disease	Etiology	Clinical Features
Psoriatic arthritis	Unknown cause; may present similar to rheumatoid arthritis; HLA-B27 association; **no rheumatoid factor;** no male or female preponderance	**Asymmetric** involvement of **DIP joints,** PIP joints, feet, ankles, and knees; **"pencil in a cup"** deformity of the proximal phalanges
Reiter's syndrome	Caused by reaction to systemic illness that originated either enteropathically or urogenitally; HLA-B27 association; most common in males, usually 20–40 years of age	Classic triad of genitourinary inflammation **(urethritis),** ocular inflammation **(conjunctivitis),** and acute asymmetric **arthritis**

HLA=human leukocyte antigen; *Ig*=immunoglobulin

● **Infectious and Metabolic Joint Disease (Table 8-5)**

TABLE 8-5 Infectious and Metabolic Joint Disease

Disease	Etiology	Clinical Features
Gout	Inflammatory reaction in joints caused by **urate crystal** deposition; IgG opsonization of the crystals followed by phagocytosis stimulates inflammation; often precipitated by a large meal or by drinking excessive amounts of alcohol	Great toe involvement is called **podagra; tophi** (nodules of fibrous tissue and crystals) occur near the joints, on the ear, and on the Achilles' tendon; renal damage may occur when crystals deposit in collecting tubules; urate crystals have **strong negative birefringence** under polarized light
Non-gonococcal septic arthritis	Inflammation of joints; most commonly **Staphylococcus aureus** and streptococcus species	Monoarticular arthritis, usually affecting the knee; chills and fever; **positive Gram stain** and synovial fluid cultures
Gonococcal septic arthritis	Inflammation of joints and other systemic effects due to sexually acquired gonococcal infection; **most common form of arthritis in sexually active adults**	Monoarticular arthritis, usually affects the knee; chills and fever; rash (including papules and pustules); Gram stain and synovial fluid cultures often negative
Lyme disease	Infection with *Borrelia burgdorferi* which is transmitted by the tick, *Ixodes dammini;* arthritis occurs late in the disease	**Erythema chronicum migrans,** a characteristic expanding bull's eye rash; knees are most common site of arthritis; may cause myocardial, pericardial, and neurologic manifestations

Ig=immunoglobulin

 Hypertrophic osteoarthropathy, which manifests as clubbing of the digits and periostitis, is one of the sequelae of systemic disorders such as chronic lung disease, cirrhosis, inflammatory bowel disease, and congenital cyanotic heart disease.

Lesch-Nyhan syndrome is an **X-linked** deficiency of **hypoxanthine-guanine phosphoribosyl transferase** (HGRPT) that results in elevated levels of uric acid and manifests as mental retardation, gout, and self-mutilation. It can be treated with allopurinol which blocks xanthine oxidase, an important enzyme in the formation of uric acid.

 Pseudogout, caused by **calcium pyrophosphate** crystals, resembles gout in its presentation. However, calcium pyrophosphate crystals have weak positive birefringence under polarized light.

SYSTEMIC LUPUS ERYTHEMATOSUS (SLE)

I. Prototypical connective tissue disorder which more frequently affects women

II. Clinical Features
   A. Fever, lymphadenopathy, weight loss, and general malaise
   B. **Immune complex deposition** in the vessels of almost all organs

C. Pulmonary fibrosis characterized by interstitial fibrosis or diffuse alveolitis
D. **Libman-Sacks** endocarditis
   1. **Mitral valve** affected
   2. Verrucous lesions seen on both sides of the leaflets
E. Pericarditis and pleuritis
F. Glomerular disease
   1. May range from mild to diffuse proliferative change
   2. Subendothelial and mesangial immune complex deposits
   3. Endothelial proliferation (**wire-loops**) and thickened basement membranes (membranous glomerulonephritis)
G. Arthralgia and arthritis
H. Vasospasm of small vessels, especially of the fingers (**Raynaud's phenomenon)**
I. Cotton-spot lesions in fundus of eye
J. Skin rash
   1. Characteristic **butterfly rash** over the malar eminences of the face
   2. Rashes can also be prevalent elsewhere on the body
   3. Rashes associated with exposure to sunlight (photosensitivity)

III. Laboratory Findings

A. Anti-nuclear antibodies are seen in almost all cases.
   1. Presence of antibodies to **double-stranded DNA** is highly specific for SLE
   2. Antibodies to **Smith antigen** (Sm) are also specific for SLE
B. Decreased level of complement (C3 and C4) in the serum
C. Skin biopsies show immune complex deposition.
D. **False-positive test for syphilis**
E. **Hypercoagulable** state in vitro due to anti-cardiolipin antibodies

> **QUICK HIT**
> In vitro, the hypocoagulable state is due to antibodies that react with the cardiolipin test substrate. However, this reaction does not occur in vivo as the SLE patient is prone to excessive clotting, not excessive bleeding.

● **Other Connective Tissue Disorders (Table 8-6)**

Inherited disorders of the bone, skin, cartilage, and blood vessels are some of the most common genetic conditions in humans. These diseases are characterized by widespread manifestations.

TABLE 8-6 | **Other Connective Tissue Disorders**

Disorder	Etiology	Clinical Features
Marfan's syndrome	Deficiency of **fibrillin** (a glycoprotein in microfibrils) results in skeletal, visual, and cardiovascular defects; **autosomal dominant** inheritance	Abnormally long fingers (**arachnodactyly),** arms, and legs; hyperextensible joints; tall and thin body habitus; high palate; ocular lens dislocation (**ectopia lentis);** cardiovascular defects including mitral valve prolapse, proximal aorta aneurysm, aortic valve insufficiency, and **aortic dissection**
Ehlers-Danlos syndrome	Genetic defect in collagen and **elastin** formation	Frequent hemorrhage; **hyperextensibility of joints** and skin; fragility of tissue
Progressive systemic sclerosis (scleroderma)	Diffuse fibrosis and degeneration of almost every organ due to autoimmune reaction; **anti-scl-70** (anti-nuclear antibody); anti-centromere antibody present in **CREST** (**C**alcinosis, **R**aynaud's phenomenon, **Es**ophageal dysfunction, **S**clerodactyly, **T**elangiectasia); occurs more frequently in women	Hypertrophy of subcutaneous collagen leads to thickened skin, fixed facial expression, claw-like hand (sclerodactyly); Raynaud's phenomenon; fibrosis of esophagus, GI tract, lungs, heart, and kidney

(continued)

TABLE 8-6   **Other Connective Tissue Disorders** *(Continued)*

Disorder	Etiology	Clinical Features
Sjögren's syndrome	Auto-immune reaction; **anti-SS-A (Ro)** and **anti-SS-B (La)** antibodies; anti-SS-B antibody is highly specific; occurs more often in women	Classic triad: • Dry eyes (**xerophthalmia**) • Dry mouth (**xerostomia**) • Presence of **other connective tissue or autoimmune disease** (often rheumatoid arthritis) Enlarged parotid glands due to lymphocytic infiltration; hypergammaglobulinemia
Polymyositis	Autoimmune inflammatory disorder; occurs more frequently in women; often **associated with malignancy**	Weakness in the proximal muscles of the extremities; high level of creatine kinase in serum; termed **dermatomyositis** when skin is involved
Mixed connective tissue disease (MCTD)	Autoimmune disorder; occurs more frequently in women; renal involvement is rare (as opposed to other connective tissue diseases); anti-nuclear ribonucleoprotein **(anti-nRNP)** is a highly specific ANA	Raynaud's phenomenon; arthralgia; muscle inflammation; esophageal dysmotility

ANA=antinuclear antibody

QUICK HIT Xerostomia and xerophthalmia alone are characteristic of **sicca syndrome**, which is also autoimmune in nature.

● Nerve Damage and Regeneration (Figure 8-3)

FIGURE

8-3   **Nerve Damage and Regeneration**

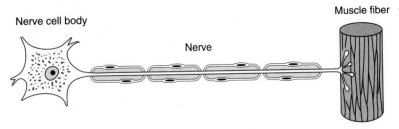

Nerve cell body   Muscle fiber

Nerve

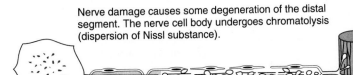

Nerve damage causes some degeneration of the distal
segment. The nerve cell body undergoes chromatolysis
(dispersion of Nissl substance).

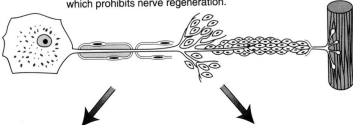

The muscle continues to atrophy for 3 weeks. In the PNS,
Schwann cells proliferate and help direct the regenerating
neuron. In the CNS, astrocyte proliferation forms a scar
which prohibits nerve regeneration.

If the nerve fibers don't find the degenerating
segment, a neuroma is formed

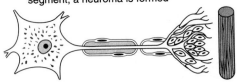

Successful nerve regeneration allows the muscle
fiber to return to its original size

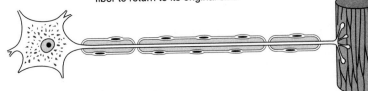

CNS=central nervous system; *PNS*=peripheral nervous system

BRACHIAL PLEXUS (Figure 8-4)

FIGURE
8-4
Brachial Plexus

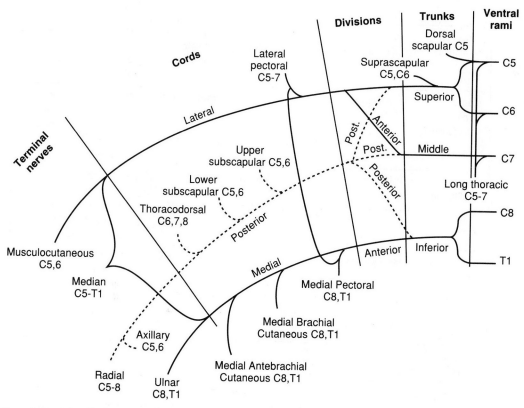

C=cervical vertebra; *T*=thoracic vertebra

● **Lesions of the Brachial Plexus and its Branches (Table 8-7)**

TABLE 8-7	Lesions of the Brachial Plexus and its Branches		
Disorder	**Lesion**	**Cause**	**Clinical Features**
Erb-Duchenne palsy	Upper brachial plexus (C5 and C6)	**Hyper-adduction** of the arm	**"Waiter's tip"** position (arm extended and adducted, forearm pronated)
Klumpke's palsy	Lower brachial plexus (C7-T1)	**Hyper-abduction** of the arm	Claw hand from ulnar nerve involvement; wrist and hand dysfunction; associated with **Horner's syndrome**
Claw hand	Ulnar nerve	Occurs in children with **epiphyseal separation** of the medial epicondyle of the humerus	Weak finger adduction; medial hand numbness; dysfunction of 4th and 5th digit flexion
Radial nerve palsy	Radial nerve	**Fracture of mid-humerus**	**Wristdrop;** inability to extend wrist or fingers; *(continued)*

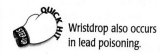

Horner's syndrome is the combination of unilateral miosis, ptosis, and anhidrosis due to a lesion of the cervical sympathetic chain. This condition is often seen with a Pancoast's tumor.

Wristdrop also occurs in lead poisoning.

THE MUSCULOSKELETAL SYSTEM

The radial nerve is also involved in lateral epicondylitis (tennis elbow).

The median nerve can also be damaged in fractures of the distal third of the humerus and elbow (causing total loss of thumb opposition) or slashing of the wrist.

Lateral winging is caused by accessory nerve lesions leading to trapezius paralysis.

TABLE 8-7	Lesions of the Brachial Plexus and its Branches *(Continued)*		
Disorder	**Lesion**	**Cause**	**Clinical Features**
			loss of sensation from dorsum of hand
Carpal tunnel syndrome	Median nerve	**Repetitive wrist motion** (tendons in the flexor retinaculum compress nerve)	Wrist flexion elicits pain; wrist extension relieves pain; symptoms worse at night
Medial winging of the scapula	Long thoracic nerve	Surgery (e.g., **mastectomy**)	Limited arm abduction and flexion; serratus anterior paralysis; medial scapula protrudes if patient pushes wall
Shoulder dislocation	Axillary nerve	**Anterior dislocation** (due to forced abduction and extension)	Loss of innervation to deltoid; compromised shoulder flexion and extension; palpable depression under acromion
Surgical neck fracture of the humerus	Axillary nerve	A fall landing on the elbow	Loss of innervation to deltoid; compromised shoulder flexion and extension; palpable depression under acromion

● Other Traumatic Injuries (Table 8-8)

Musuloskeletal dysfunction can be due to derangement of bone, nerve, musculature, or any combination of these elements. Insult to the body can result in problems that are acute (e.g., a torn anterior cruciate ligament) or chronic (e.g., tennis elbow).

The anatomical snuffbox is bounded dorsally by the extensor pollicis longus and on the palmar side by extensor pollicis brevis and the abductor pollicus longus, with the scaphoid and the trapezium bones creating the base.

TABLE 8-8	Other Traumatic Injuries
Injury	**Description**
Anterior cruciate ligament (ACL) tear	Positive **anterior drawer sign** (lower leg pulled forward with knee flexed); often manifests as **"terrible triad"** (i.e., torn medial collateral ligament, medial meniscus damage, and torn ACL)
Clavicle fracture	**Middle one third** of clavicle; upward displacement of proximal fragment; downward displacement of distal fragment; severe pain
Compartment syndrome	Fascial sheets separate the limbs into anterior and posterior compartments; hemorrhage into these compartments, due to crush injury or fracture, results in **compression of neurovascular structures** and further complications
Inversion sprain of ankle	Most common ankle injury; results from forced inversion; stretches or tears lateral ligaments (especially the **anterior talofibular**)
Scaphoid fracture	Tenderness in the anatomical snuffbox; may lead to **avascular necrosis** if left untreated; easily missed on radiographs
Scoliosis	Complex lateral deviation and torsion of the spine; may be idiopathic or congenital or may result from a short leg, hip displacement, or polio
Shoulder separation	Downward displacement of the clavicle due to laxity of the acromioclavicular and coracoclavicular ligaments

(continued)

TABLE 8-8	Other Traumatic Injuries (Continued)	
Injury	**Description**	
Subacromial bursitis	Inflammation of the subacromial bursa; **most common bursitis** in the body	
Tennis elbow	Sprain of radial collateral ligament (lateral epicondyle); pain on wrist extension and forearm supination	
Waddling gait	Limp due to superior gluteal nerve injury affecting gluteus medias and minimus; inability to abduct thigh; results in **Trendelenburg's sign**	

Golf elbow has manifestations similar to those of tennis elbow, except that it involves the medial epicondyle.

Trendelenburg's sign results in tilting of the pelvis to the side opposite that of injury when standing on the foot of the injured side. It can also be seen in a hip dislocation or a fracture of the neck of the femur.

MUSCLE FUNCTION AND DYSFUNCTION (Figure 8-5)

FIGURE
8-5 **Myocyte Contraction** (continued)

A.. **The cross-bridge cycle of skeletal muscle**

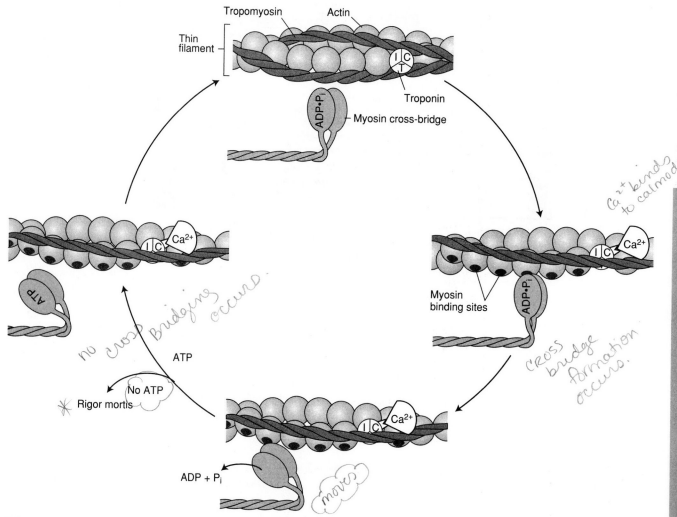

ADP=adenosine diphosphate; ATP=adenosine triphosphate; Ca=calcium; P=phosphate; T=troponin

FIGURE
8-5 *(Continued)*

B. **Gross, histologic, microscopic anatomy of skeletal muscle**

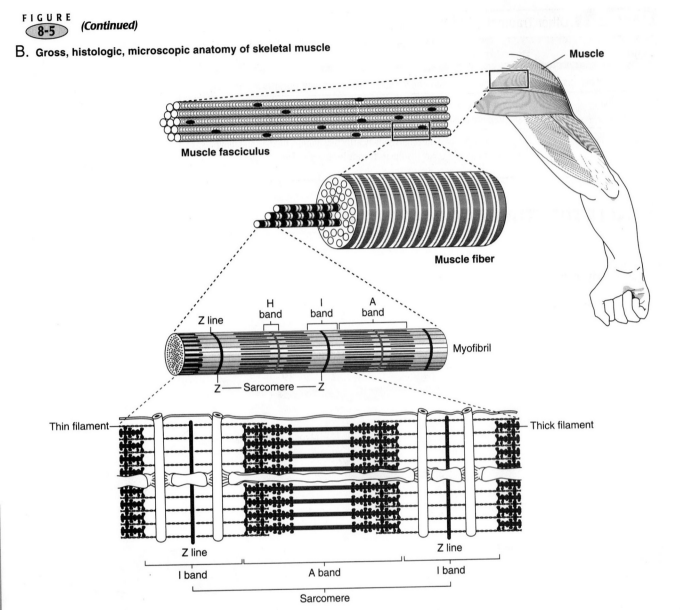

● Comparison of Muscle Fibers (Table 8-9)

Smooth muscle plays a significant role in the maintenance of the lumens of the respiratory and gastrointestinal tracts, and blood vessels. **Cardiac muscle** contracts the heart and propels blood through the vasculature.

TABLE 8-9	**Comparison of Muscle Fibers**		
Category	**Smooth Muscle Fiber**	**Cardiac Muscle Fiber**	**Skeletal Muscle Fiber**
Nuclei	Centrally located single nucleus	Centrally located single nucleus	Peripherally located multiple nuclei
Banding	No distinct bands	Distinct bands	Distinct bands
Z line (convergence actin filaments)	None; dense bodies present	Present	Present
Transverse (T) tubules (membrane invaginations)	None	At Z line; diads	At A-I junction; triads
Junctional communication	Gap junctions	Intercalated disks	None
Neuromuscular junction	None	None	Present
Regeneration	High	None	Some
Calcium source	Sarcoplasmic reticulum; extracellular	Sarcoplasmic reticulum; extracellular	Sarcoplasmic reticulum
Mechanism of calcium release	IP_3	Calcium-induced	Depolarization of T-tubule
Calcium binding protein	Calmodulin	Troponin	Troponin

IP_3 = inositol-1,4,5-triphosphate

● Skeletal Muscle Fiber Types (Table 8-10)

Skeletal muscle maintains posture and produces movement. Muscle can be divided into **two subtypes** with differing physiologic roles.

TABLE 8-10	**Types of Skeletal Muscle Fiber**	
Category	**Type 1**	**Type 2**
Action	Sustained force; weight-bearing muscles	Sudden movement; directed action
Lipid stores	Abundant	Few
Glycogen stores	Few	Abundant
Energy utilization	Aerobic; many mitochondria	Anaerobic; few mitochondria; easily fatigued
Twitch	Slow	Fast
Color	Red (due to blood supply)	White

● **Muscle Tumors (Table 8-11)**

Pathology of muscles can take many forms. Metabolic dyscrasias, which can be induced or inherited, are far more common than neoplasms.

TABLE 8-11 Muscle Tumors

Category	Leiomyoma	Leiomyosarcoma	Rhabdomyosarcoma
Morphology	Benign; elongated nuclei; whorled bundles of smooth muscle cells; no larger than 2 cm	Malignant; "cigar-shaped" nuclei; dense bodies	Malignant; embryonal, alveolar, and pleomorphic types; rhabdomyoblast is diagnostic cell
Location	Smooth muscle; **uterus**	Smooth muscle; skin; deep soft tissues	Skeletal muscle; head and neck; GU tract; retroperitoneum
Immunohisto-chemistry	Antibodies to actin and desmin	Antibodies to vimentin, actin, and desmin	Antibodies to vimentin, actin, desmin, and myoglobin
Prognosis	Indolent course; easily cured	Variable; prognosis worse with increased size	Aggressive; treat with surgery, radiation, chemotherapy
Notes	Afflicts women more often than men; **most common tumor in women**	Uncommon	**Most common soft tissue sarcoma of childhood** and adolescence

The embryonal type of rhabdomyosarcoma is related to sarcoma botryoides resulting in a "bunch of grapes" appearance (see System 7 "Reproductive System").

● **Other Neuromuscular Disorders (Table 8-12)**

TABLE 8-12 Other Neuromuscular Disorders

Disorder	Etiology	Clinical Features	Notes
Lactic acidosis	Shock; sepsis; methanol poisoning; metformin toxicity; liver failure	Increased serum lactate; **metabolic acidosis;** increased anion gap	May lead to coma or death
Myasthenia gravis	Acetylcholine receptor **autoantibodies at the neuromuscular junction;** linked to HLA-DR3; associated with thymus disorders	Muscle weakness with use; ptosis; manifests itself in facial, ocular, and limb muscles; proximal muscles affected first	Four times more common in women; anticholinesterase (e.g., edrophonium) improves condition
Duchenne's muscular dystrophy	**X-linked recessive;** deficiency in **dystrophin** leading to lack of actin stabilization	Progressive; proximal muscle weakens; **pseudohypertrophy** of muscles (e.g., calf); positive Gower's maneuver; leads to death via respiratory and/or cardiac failure	Increased creatine kinase and lactate dehydrogenase
Mitochondrial myopathy	Transmitted via mitochondrial DNA (mtDNA); non-Mendelian inheritance	**Ragged red fibers** seen on muscle biopsy; proximal muscle weakness	**Maternal** mode of transmission

DNA=deoxyribonucleic acid; HLA=human leukocyte antigen

Increased anion gap metabolic acidosis may also be due to salicylate poisoning, alcohol intoxication, acute renal failure, diabetic ketoacidosis, and aspirin ingestion. Normal anion gap metabolic acidosis is due to diarrhea and renal tubular acidosis.

Becker's muscular dystrophy is similar to Duchenne's, but is much less severe.

FIGURE
8-6 **Muscle Glycogen Storage Disorders**

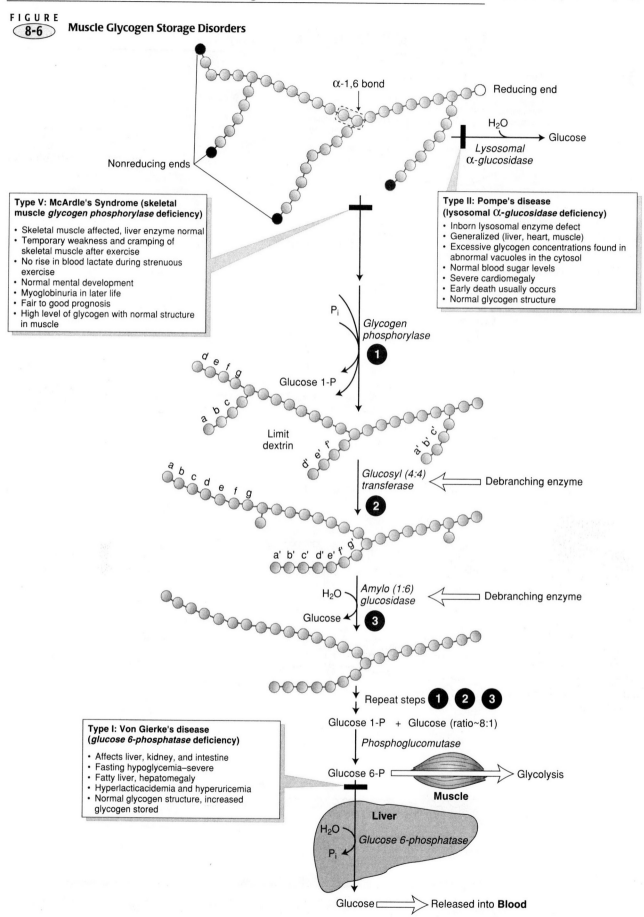

α-1,6 bond

Reducing end

H_2O → Glucose

Lysosomal
α-glucosidase

Nonreducing ends

Type V: McArdle's Syndrome (skeletal muscle *glycogen phosphorylase* deficiency)

- Skeletal muscle affected, liver enzyme normal
- Temporary weakness and cramping of skeletal muscle after exercise
- No rise in blood lactate during strenuous exercise
- Normal mental development
- Myoglobinuria in later life
- Fair to good prognosis
- High level of glycogen with normal structure in muscle

Type II: Pompe's disease (lysosomal *α-glucosidase* deficiency)

- Inborn lysosomal enzyme defect
- Generalized (liver, heart, muscle)
- Excessive glycogen concentrations found in abnormal vacuoles in the cytosol
- Normal blood sugar levels
- Severe cardiomegaly
- Early death usually occurs
- Normal glycogen structure

P_i

Glycogen phosphorylase ❶

Glucose 1-P

Limit dextrin

Glucosyl (4:4) transferase ❷ ← Debranching enzyme

H_2O

Amylo (1:6) glucosidase ❸ ← Debranching enzyme

Glucose

Repeat steps ❶ ❷ ❸

Glucose 1-P + Glucose (ratio~8:1)

Phosphoglucomutase

Type I: Von Gierke's disease (*glucose 6-phosphatase* deficiency)

- Affects liver, kidney, and intestine
- Fasting hypoglycemia–severe
- Fatty liver, hepatomegaly
- Hyperlacticacidemia and hyperuricemia
- Normal glycogen structure, increased glycogen stored

Glucose 6-P ⇒ Glycolysis

Muscle

Liver

H_2O

Glucose 6-phosphatase

P_i

Glucose ⇒ Released into **Blood**

THE MUSCULOSKELETAL SYSTEM

(Adapted from Champe PC and Harvey RA: *Lippincott's Illustrated Reviews: Biochemistry, 2nd edition.* Philadelphia, Lippincott-Raven Publishers, 1994. p. 140. Used by permission of Lippincott Williams & Wilkins.)

COLLAGEN SYNTHESIS (Figure 8-7)

FIGURE
8-7   **Collagen Synthesis**

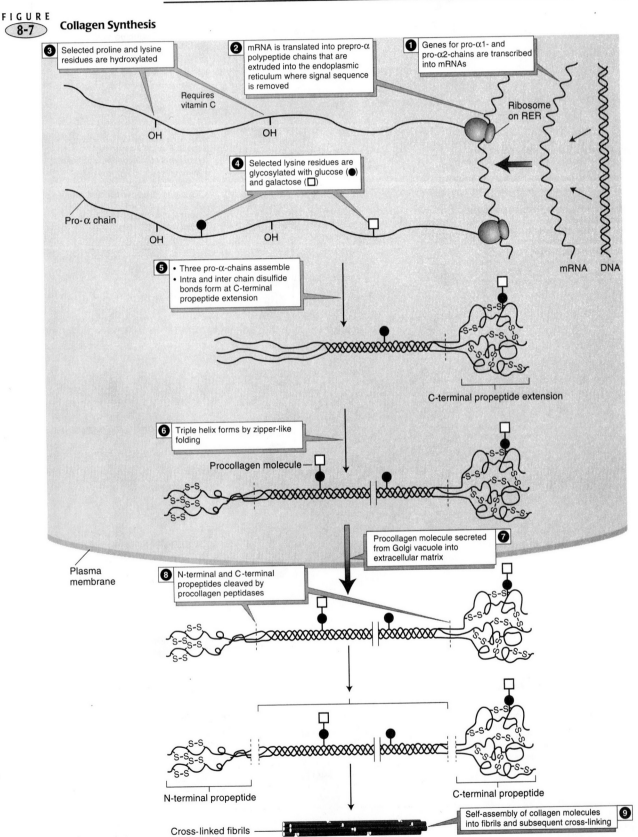

❸ Selected proline and lysine residues are hydroxylated

❷ mRNA is translated into prepro-α polypeptide chains that are extruded into the endoplasmic reticulum where signal sequence is removed

❶ Genes for pro-α1- and pro-α2-chains are transcribed into mRNAs

Requires vitamin C

OH   OH

Ribosome on RER

❹ Selected lysine residues are glycosylated with glucose (●) and galactose (□)

Pro-α chain

OH   OH

mRNA   DNA

❺ • Three pro-α-chains assemble
• Intra and inter chain disulfide bonds form at C-terminal propeptide extension

C-terminal propeptide extension

❻ Triple helix forms by zipper-like folding

Procollagen molecule

❼ Procollagen molecule secreted from Golgi vacuole into extracellular matrix

Plasma membrane

❽ N-terminal and C-terminal propeptides cleaved by procollagen peptidases

N-terminal propeptide   C-terminal propeptide

❾ Self-assembly of collagen molecules into fibrils and subsequent cross-linking

Cross-linked fibrils

THE MUSCULOSKELETAL SYSTEM

(Adapted from Champe PC and Harvey RA: *Lippincott's Illustrated Reviews: Biochemistry, 2nd edition. Philadelphia, Lippincott-Raven Publishers, 1994. p. 41. Used by permission of Lippincott Williams & Wilkins.*)
DNA=deoxyribonucleic acid; *mRNA*=messenger ribonucleic acid; *RER*=rough endoplasmic reticulum

THE INGUINAL CANAL (Figure 8-8) (see Tables 8-13 and 8-14)

FIGURE
8-8   The Inguinal Canal

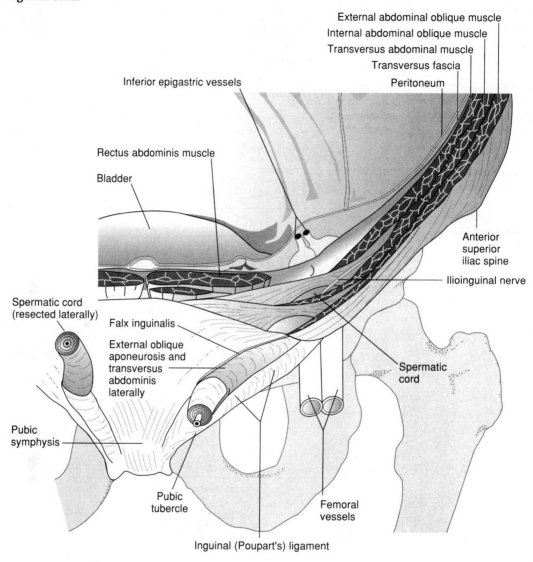

The Inguinal Canal

● The Inguinal Canal (Table 8-13)

TABLE 8-13   The Inguinal Canal

Border	Anatomic composition
Superior	**Falx inguinalis:** internal abdominal oblique (IAO) and transversus abdominis muscles
Inferior	Inguinal ligament
Anterior	External abdominal oblique (EAO) aponeurosis; IAO and transversus abdominis muscles laterally
Posterior	Transversalis fascia; falx inguinalis medially

QUICK HIT — The inguinal canal contains the ilioinguinal nerve (sensory to the anterior aspect of labia or scrotum), spermatic cord in males (ductus deferens, testicular artery, pampiniform plexus), and the round ligament of the uterus in females.

THE MUSCULOSKELETAL SYSTEM

● **Hernias (Table 8-14)**

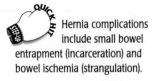

Hernias may cause small bowel obstruction. However, small bowel obstructions are most commonly caused by adhesions.

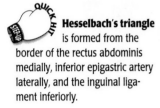

Hernia complications include small bowel entrapment (incarceration) and bowel ischemia (strangulation).

Hesselbach's triangle is formed from the border of the rectus abdominis medially, inferior epigastric artery laterally, and the inguinal ligament inferiorly.

TABLE 8-14 **Hernias**			
Hernia	**Pathology**	**Clinical Features**	**Diagnosis**
Direct inguinal hernia	Parietal peritoneum passes directly through abdominal wall (**Hesselbach's** triangle)	More common in older males	Medial to inferior epigastric artery; located above pubic tubercle
Indirect inguinal hernia	Parietal peritoneum passes through internal inguinal ring and follows the inguinal canal	**Most common** type; occurs in young adult males more frequently than in females	Lateral to inferior epigastric artery; located above pubic tubercle
Femoral hernia	Parietal peritoneum passes through the femoral canal	More common in females	Located below the pubic tubercle

SKIN DISORDERS (Table 8-15)

TABLE 8-15 **Skin Disorders**	
Disorder	**Description**
Keloid scarring	• **Excessive scarring** that occurs after minor trauma • Results in raised, firm lesions on the skin • Occurs more frequently in African-Americans • Genetic predisposition is a factor
Xanthomas	• Accumulation of foam-filled histiocytes within the dermis • Often associated with **hyperlipidemia** or lymphoproliferative disorders • Often found on the Achilles tendon and the extensor tendons of the fingers
Seborrheic keratosis	• Common **benign neoplasm** in the elderly • Raised papules and plaques that appear to be "pasted on"
Albinism	• **Lack of melanin pigment** production • Ocular type limited to eyes; X-linked • Oculocutaneous type involves the skin, eyes, and hair; autosomal recessive; lack of tyrosinase enzyme which converts tyrosine to DOPA
Hemangiomas	• Large-vessel malformation composed of masses of blood-filled channels • **Port-wine stain** birthmarks are the most common manifestation • Cavernous hemangiomas are a subset with large cavernous vascular spaces that can occur in von Hippel-Lindau disease
DOPA=3,4-dihydroxyphenylalanine	

A lack of pigment, such as in albinism, predisposes one to a variety of skin disorders including actinic keratosis, basal cell carcinoma, squamous cell carcinoma, and malignant melanoma.

● Skin Cancers and Premalignant Conditions (Table 8-16)

Skin disorders are often characterized by pruritus, inflammation, and irritability. Skin lesions that are suggestive of malignancy demonstrate asymmetry, irregular borders, variations in color, and increasing size.

TABLE 8-16 Skin Cancers and Premalignant Conditions

Disorder	Description
Acanthosis nigricans	• A thickening and **hyperpigmentation** of the axilla, neck, and groin region • Benign type—several causes • Malignant type—is an important marker of an underlying **adenocarcinoma**
Actinic keratosis	• A series of dysplastic changes that occur before the onset of **squamous cell carcinoma** • A buildup of keratin due to excessive exposure to sunlight leads to a **"warty"** appearance
Squamous cell carcinoma	• Malignant tumor of the skin caused by excessive exposure to sunlight • Rarely metastasizes • Characterized by ulcerated, scaling nodules • Appears microscopically as islands of neoplastic cells with **whorls of keratin** ("pearls")
Basal cell carcinoma	• **Most common** skin tumor • Appears grossly as a pearl-like papule on sun-exposed areas • Appears histologically as a dark cluster with **palisading peripheral cells** • Almost never metastasizes

Malignant melanoma	• Aggressive tumor that arises from melanocytes
	• Associated with excess exposure to sunlight
	• Two growth patterns:
	  • **Benign radial manner** (growth within skin layer)
	  • **Aggressive vertical manner** (growth through deeper layers)
	• Associated with the S-100 tumor marker

THERAPEUTICS

Anti-cancer therapeutics
5-Fluorouracil   Methotrexate
Dactinomycin   Vincristine

Anticholinesterase inhibitors
Edrophonium   Neostigmine   Physostigmine

Antigout therapeutics
Allopurinol   Colchicine   Sulfinpyrazone

Antipyretics and Analgesics
Acetaminophen   Aspirin

Antimicrobials
Ampicillin   Penicillin   Tetracycline
Cephalosporins (first generation)   Sulfamethoxazole plus trimethoprim (SMX-TMP)   Thiabendazole

Muscle Relaxants

Baclofen   Benzodiazepine   Dantrolene

Nonsteroidal Anti-inflammatory Drugs

Aspirin   Indomethacin   Piroxicam
Ibuprofen   Naproxen

Rheumatoid arthritis therapeutics

Aurothioglucose   Cyclophosphamide

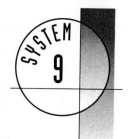

Hematopoietic–Lymphoreticular System

HEMATOPOIESIS TIMETABLE

I. **Week 3:** Embryonic visceral mesoderm gives rise to angioblasts.

II. **1st Trimester:** Yolk sac produces red blood cells (RBCs).

III. **2nd Trimester:** Liver and spleen produce RBCs.

IV. **3rd Trimester:** Central and peripheral skeleton produces RBCs.

V. **Adulthood:** Axial skeleton (vertebral bodies, sternum, ribs, pelvis) produces RBCs.

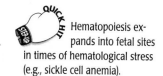

Hematopoiesis expands into fetal sites in times of hematological stress (e.g., sickle cell anemia).

THE CELLS (Table 9-1)

The hematopoietic-lymphoreticular system is composed of a multitude of cells. Most of these cells can be found circulating in the bloodstream, while a few are found within peripheral tissues.

TABLE 9-1 The Cells of the Hematopoietic-Lymphoreticular System

Cell	Relative Amounts	Life Span	Morphology	Functions	Secretion	Notes
Neutrophils (PMNs)	40%–75% of WBCs	Less than 7 days	Multilobed nucleus, azurophilic granules (lysosomes), **myeloperoxidase**	Phagocytic, acute inflammatory response	Lysosomal contents released upon cell death	Lysosomes contain lysozyme which is **bactericidal**
Basophils	<1% of WBCs	Years	Bilobate, basophilic	Allergies	Heparin, histamine, SRS-A	**Bind IgE** antibody to their membrane
Eosinophils	0.5%–5% of WBCs	Less than 2 weeks in connective tissues	Bilobed, azurophilic granules	Phagocytic for Ag-Ab complexes, **antiparasitic,** inactivated histamine and SRS-A	Histaminase arylsulfatase	Large numbers found in lamina propria of GI tract
Mast cells	Found in connective tissue	9–18 months	Basophil-like, round nucleus	Bind IgE; mediate **Type I hypersensitivity** reaction	ECF, histamine, leukotrienes, heparin	**Cromolyn sodium** prevents degranulation by stabilizing membrane
Macrophages	Found **only in tissues,** not in the blood	Extended life in tissues	Ameboid	Phagocytize bacteria, RBCs, and damaged cells	IL-1, **IL-2,** TNFα	Activated by LPS and INF-γ

QUICK HIT Neutrophils are hypersegmented in megaloblastic anemia.

QUICK HIT Slow-reacting substance of anaphylaxis (SRS-A) is comprised of leukotriene C_4 and leukotriene D_4 which bronchoconstrict, vasoconstrict, and increase vascular permeability.

QUICK HIT Eosinophilia occurs in response to trematodes (also called flukes) including Schistosomas, Chlonorchis sinensis, and Paragonimus westermani; or cestodes (also called tapeworms) including Taenia solium, T. saginata, Diphyllobothrium latum, and Echinococcus granulosus. Eosinophilia can also result from neoplasms, allergy, asthma, and connective tissue disorders.

QUICK HIT An acute allergic reaction is a type I hypersensitivity reaction.

Cell	Count	Lifespan	Morphology		Function	Mediators	Notes
Monocytes	3×9% of WBC's	Less than 3 days in the blood	Large kidney-shaped nucleus	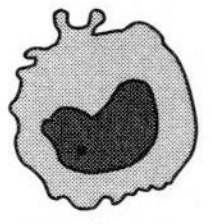 Monocyte	Differentiate into macrophages and osteoclasts	IL-1, IL-6	Chemotactically **attracted to sites of inflammation**
T-lymphocytes	15%–18% of WBCs, 75% of lymphocytes	Years	Basophilic, large nucleus, scant cytoplasm	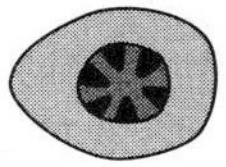 Large T-lymphocyte	**Cell-mediated immune response**	IL-2, IL-3, IL-4, IL-5, IL-6, INFγ, TNFα, TNFβ	Several types (see Figure 9–5)
B-Lymphocyte	5%–7% of WBCs, 25% of lymphocytes	Months	Basophilic, large nucleus, scant cytoplasm	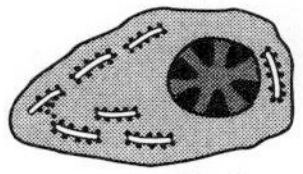 Plasma cell	**Humoral immune response**	INFα	Differentiate into plasma cells and long-lived memory cells
Erythrocytes	5×10^6/cc in men, 4.55×10^6/cc in females	120 days	**Anucleate, biconcave disc**	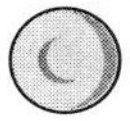 Erythrocyte	Gas exchange	See Figure 9-3 "RBC physiology"	Anaerobic metabolism exclusively
Platelets	250,000 to 400,000/cc	6–8 days	Irregularly shaped, membrane bound	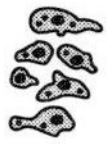 Platelets	Prevention of bleeding by **clot formation**	Histamine, PDGF, serotonin, TxA_2	Disorders of number or function can result in bleeding

Ag-Ab=antigen-antibody; *ECF*=eosinophilic chemotactic factor; *GI*=gastrointestinal; *Ig*=immunoglobulin; *IL*=interleukin; *INF-γ*= gamma interferon; *LPS*=lipopolysaccharide; *RBC*=red blood cell; *SRS-A*=slow-reacting substance of anaphylaxis; *TxA₂*=thromboxane A₂; *TNF*=tumor necrosis factor; *WBC*=white blood cell

QUICK HIT
STEP-UP
Monocyte-derived osteoclasts have calcitonin receptors but not parathyroid receptors.

QUICK HIT
STEP-UP
Gamma interferon (INF-γ) is used to treat chronic granulomatous disease (CGD).

THE ORGANS OF THE LYMPHORETICULAR SYSTEM

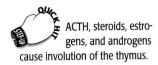

ACTH, steroids, estrogens, and androgens cause involution of the thymus.

I. Thymus
A. Derived from the **third pharyngeal pouch**
B. The cortex contains thymocytes (immature T-lymphocytes).
C. The medulla contains mature T-lymphocytes and **Hassall's corpuscles** (whorl-like bodies which contain keratin). As T-lymphocytes mature, they express T-cell receptors and CD receptors. T-lymphocytes that recognize "self" undergo apoptosis, while those that recognize "non-self" undergo clonal expansion.

Virchow's (sentinel) nodes are supraclavicular nodes often enlarged by metastasis from gastric carcinoma.

II. Lymph Nodes (Figure 9-1)
A. Derived from mesenchymal cells
B. Outer cortex contains B-lymphocytes
C. Inner cortex (also called the paracortex) contains T-lymphocytes and is thymic-dependent
D. Medulla contains B-lymphocytes, plasma cells, and macrophages

FIGURE
9-1   **The Lymph Node**

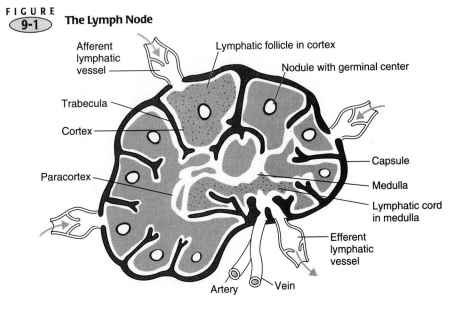

III. Lymph
A. Fluid that returns lipids, proteins, and water-soluble substances to the circulation via the lymphatic vessels.
B. The left side of the head, the left thorax, the left upper limb, and everything below the diaphragm drain into the thoracic duct. This duct terminates at the junction of the left subclavian and left internal jugular veins.
C. The **right upper quadrant of body** (right side of head, right upper limb, and right thorax) empties into the **great vessels of the right side.**

IV. Spleen (Figure 9-2)
A. Derived from mesenchyme beginning in the 5th week
B. White pulp: B-lymphocytes surround the central artery, and T-lymphocytes are arranged into periarteriolar lymphatic sheaths (PALS)
C. Marginal zone: where blood meets spleen parenchyma; antigen-presenting cells (APCs) and macrophages are present.

HEMATOPOIETIC SYSTEM

D. Red pulp: contains splenic (Billroth) cords separated by sinusoids; also has plasma cells, macrophages, lymphocytes, and RBCs

FIGURE
9-2   The Spleen

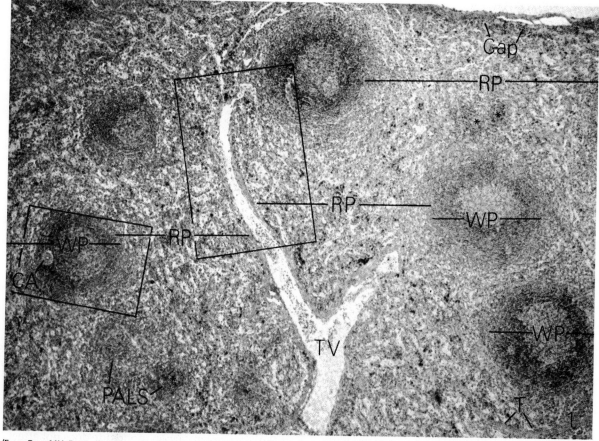

(From Ross MH, Romrell LJ, Kaye GI: *Histology: A Text and Atlas,* 3rd edition. Baltimore: Williams & Wilkins, 1995. p. 365. Used by permission of Lippincott Williams & Wilkins.)

V. Liver
A. Endoderm of foregut (hepatic diverticulum) grows into surrounding mesoderm (septum transversum)
B. Hepatic cords from diverticulum, arranged around umbilical and vitelline veins, form hepatic sinusoids.
C. Produces **fetal hemoglobin (HbF) during second trimester**
D. Produces **clotting factors** of coagulation cascade
E. Can function to sequester and break down RBCs if spleen is removed

VI. Gut-Associated Lymphatic Tissue
A. Found in tonsils, Peyer's patches of the jejunum, appendix, and cecum
B. M-cells: present antigens to lymphocytes and secrete IgA

RED BLOOD CELL PHYSIOLOGY (Figure 9-3)

FIGURE
9-3   RBC physiology

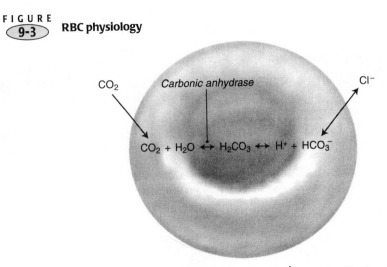

CO_2=carbon dioxide; H_2O=water; H_2CO_3=carbonic acid; H^+=hydrogen ion; HCO_3^-=bicarbonate; Cl^-=chloride

● Hemoglobin-Oxygen Dissociation Curve (Figure 9-4)

Red blood cells deliver oxygen to tissues and carry carbon dioxide (CO_2) to the lungs. In the tissues, CO_2 diffuses into the RBC, combines with water via **carbonic anhydrase** (CA), and produces carbonic acid. This dissociates into hydrogen ions and bicarbonate. The **bicarbonate leaves** the RBC in exchange for chloride **(chloride shift)**. In the lungs, this process is reversed. Thus, **bicarbonate in the plasma** is the **major route** for CO_2 transport to the lungs.

Deoxyhemoglobin exists in the **tense state** which resists oxygen binding. Binding of the first oxygen molecule requires considerable energy and precipitates a conformational change from the tense state to the relaxed state. Binding of further oxygen molecules requires less energy **(positive cooperativity).** Certain factors affect hemoglobin affinity for oxygen (see Figure 9-4). However, carbon monoxide does not affect hemoglobin affinity for oxygen, and therefore does not shift the hemoglobin-oxygen dissociation curve. Instead, due to its 200-fold greater affinity for the oxygen binding sites on hemoglobin, carbon monoxide causes hypoxia.

> **QUICK HIT**
>
> Carbon monoxide poisoning causes hypoxic injury to the basal ganglia and results in a cherry-red color of the skin and viscera. The treatment is 100% oxygen.

FIGURE
9-4   **Hemoglobin-Oxygen Dissociation Curve**

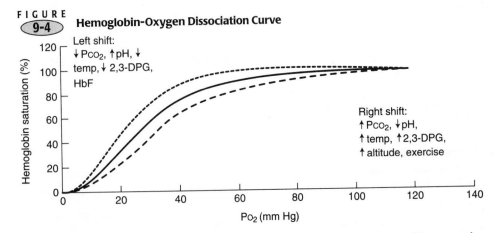

$2,3$-DPG=2,3-diphosphoglycerate; HbF=hemoglobin F; $mmHg$=millimeters of mercury; PCO_2=partial pressure of carbon dioxide; pH=hydrogen ion concentration; PO_2=partial pressure of oxygen

LYMPHOCYTE DIFFERENTIATION

The CD4: CD8 ratio is normally 2:1. In AIDS, this ratio is **reversed.**

T-helper (Th) lymphocytes express **MHC class II** and **CD4 proteins** on their membranes. They participate in the cellular response to **extracellular** antigens (e.g., bacteria). Cytotoxic T-lymphocytes (T-cyt) **express MHC class I and CD8 proteins** on their membranes. T-cyt cells are involved in the immune response to **intracellular** antigens (e.g., viruses and obligate intracellular organisms such as *Chlamydiae* or Rickettsiae). Natural killer (NK) cells are a form of T lymphocytes that do not pass through the thymus for maturation. As one of the body's innate defenses, NK cells kill **tumor cells and viral infected cells** by secreting cytotoxins (perforins). They do not require antibodies to kill, but their potency is increased when antibody is present [i.e., antibody-dependent cellular cytotoxicity (ADCC)].

ADCC is one of the mechanisms by which type II hypersensitivity reactions can occur. Other mechanisms are complement fixing antibodies (e.g., Goodpasture's syndrome) and anti-cell surface receptor antibodies (e.g., Graves' disease).

● **T-cell Differentiation (Figure 9-5)**

FIGURE 9-5 **T-cell Differentiation**

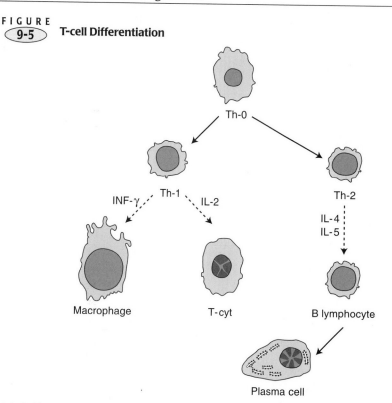

IL=interleukin; *INF-γ*=gamma interferon; *T-cyt*=cytotoxic T-lymphocytes; *Th*=T-helper lymphocytes

IMMUNOGLOBULINS

I. Characteristics

A. Glycoproteins

B. Consist of **light (L) chain** and **heavy (H) chain**

C. Two identical H chains and two identical L chains linked by **disulfide bonds** in a "Y" shape

D. **Variable region** exists on both L and H chains

E. H chain composes **Fc** and **Fab** fragment

F. L chain composes Fab fragment only

G. Types (Table 9-2)

TABLE 9-2 Immunoglobulin (Ig) Properties					
	IgM	**IgG**	**IgE**	**IgA**	**IgD**
Percentage of Total Ig	9%	75%	0.004%	15%	0.2%
Structure	Monomer/ pentamer -Pentamer held together by J chain	Monomer	Monomer	Monomer/ dimer -Dimer held together by J chain	Monomer
Function	-Fixes complement -Antigen receptor on B cell surface -**Primary response**	-Fixes complement -Opsonizes -**Crosses the placenta** -Neutralizes bacterial toxins -**Secondary response**	-Allergic response **(type I hypersensitivity)** -Binds to basophils and mast cells -Antihelminthic	-Found in **secretions** -Prevents bacterial and viral attachment	-Unknown -May be antigen receptor on B cell surface

COMPLEMENT SYSTEM (Figure 9-6)

FIGURE 9-6 Complement Pathway

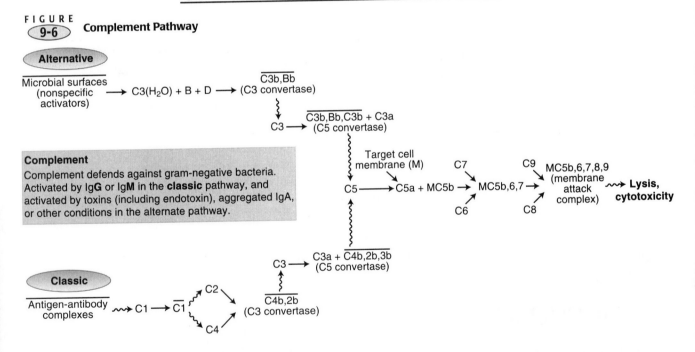

Complement
Complement defends against gram-negative bacteria. Activated by IgG or IgM in the **classic** pathway, and activated by toxins (including endotoxin), aggregated IgA, or other conditions in the alternate pathway.

(Adapted from Bhushan V, Le T, Amin C. *First Aid for the USMLE Step 1*. Stamford, Connecticut, Appleton & Lange, 1999. p. 207.)

I. Function of complement
    A. Causes **lysis** of target cell
    B. Defends against **gram-negative bacteria**

II. Activation of Pathways

A. IgG and IgM activate the **classic pathway**
1. The activation is initiated by antigen-antibody complexes.
2. The first step of activation involves formation of complex by C1, C2, and C4.

B. Antigens activate the **alternative pathway**
1. The activation is initiated by microbial surfaces and aggregated IgA.
2. The first step of activation involves C3.

III. Properties of complement cascade components

A. **C1:** only component not made in liver [made in gastrointestinal (GI) epithelium]
B. **C1-C4:** involved in viral neutralization
C. **C3b:** involved in opsonization
D. C3a: produces anaphylatoxin I
E. **C5a:** produces anaphylatoxin II, neutrophil and macrophage chemotaxis
F. **C5b-C9:** also known as the membrane attack complex (MAC)
G. **C1-Inhibitor:** deficiency of this component leads to hereditary angioedema
H. Alteration in the complement cascade—complement deficiencies—are discussed in Table 9-3.

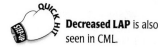

QUICK HIT
The membrane attack complex has only one component each of C5b, C6, C7, and C8, but has numerous C9's.

QUICK HIT
Decreased LAP is also seen in CML.

TABLE 9-3	Complement Deficiencies	
Disease	**Defect**	**Significant Features**
Hereditary angioedema	Decreased C1 inhibitor	Increased capillary permeability, edema
Paroxysmal nocturnal hemoglobinuria (PNH)	Deficiency of decay accelerating factor (DAF); increased complement activation	Complement-mediated hemolysis; brown urine in morning; **decreased leukocyte alkaline phosphatase (LAP)**

C1 = first component of complement.

Deficiencies of C1, C3, C5, C6, C7, and C8 lead to increased bacterial infections. C3 defect causes increased susceptibility to *Staphylococcus aureus.* **C6, C7, C8 deficiencies lead to *Neisseria gonorrheae* infection and meningitis. C2 and C4 deficiencies have manifestations resembling autoimmune diseases such as systemic lupus erythematosus (SLE).** C2 deficiency is the most common complement deficiency.

● Cytokines (Table 9-4)

Cytokines are hormones which have a low molecular weight and are involved in cell-to-cell communication.

TABLE 9-4	Cytokines		
Cytokine	**Secreted by**	**Function**	
IL-1	Macrophages	Endogenous **pyrogen;** stimulates T cells	
IL-2	T helper cells	Activates T helper and cytotoxic cells	
IL-4	T helper cells	Stimulates growth of B cells; increases IgE and IgG	
IL-5	T helper cells	Differentiation of B cells; increases IgA	
IL-10	T helper cells	Inhibits development of Th-1 cells; inhibits INF-γ production	
IL-12	Macrophages	Promotes Th-1 cell development; stimulates gamma interferon production	
INF-γ	T helper cells	Stimulates macrophages and NK cells; increases MHC expression; stimulates phagocytosis and killing	

(continued)

HEMATOPOIETIC SYSTEM

TABLE 9-4 Cytokines *(Continued)*		
Cytokine	**Secreted by**	**Function**
Tissue necrosis factor	Macrophages	At low concentrations, activates neutrophils and increases IL-2 receptor synthesis; at high concentrations, mediates septic shock and results in tumor necrosis
Transforming growth factor	T cells, B cells, macrophages	Inhibits growth and activities of T cells; enhances collagen synthesis; dampens the immune response

Ig=immunoglobulin; *IL*=interleukin; *INF-γ*=gamma interferon; *MHC*=major histocompatibility complex; *NK*=natural killer

HYPERSENSITIVITY REACTIONS

There are four types of hypersensitivity reactions. They vary in onset of symptoms, severity, and mechanism.(Table 9-5)

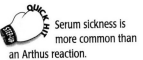

Radioimmunosorbent test (RIST) is a radioimmunoassay (RIA) which measures total IgE. A radioallergosorbent test (RAST) is an RIA that determines specific IgE concentration. Both the RIST and RAST can be used to measure IgE concentration to predict anaphylactic response.

Serum sickness is more common than an Arthus reaction.

TABLE 9-5 Hypersensitivity Reactions	
Reaction Type	**Description**
Type I **(anaphylaxis)**	Mediated by **IgE** antibody bound to mast cells or basophils Antigens crosslink antibody Release **histamine,** SRS-A, eosinophilic chemotactic factor, and platelet-activating factor Results in asthma, **wheal,** and **flare**
Type II (cytotoxic)	Antibody-dependent cellular cytotoxicity Antibody produced to specific cell-surface antigens IgM and IgG mediated lysis via complement Examples: **Rh incompatibility, Goodpasture's syndrome,** myasthenia gravis, hemolytic anemia
Type III (immune-complex)	**Antigen-antibody complexes** induce inflammatory response Deposition of complexes in tissue Examples: **Arthus reaction, serum sickness,** glomerulonephritis, rheumatoid arthritis
Type IV (delayed or cell-mediated)	**Helper (CD4) T lymphocyte mediated** Response is delayed (from hours to days) Predominantly mononuclear cell infiltration Examples: **tuberculin (PPD) test, chronic transplant rejection,** contact hypersensitivity

Ig=immunoglobulin; *PPD*=purified protein derivative; *Rh*=rhesus (factor)

● Transplant Rejection Timeline (Figure 9-7)

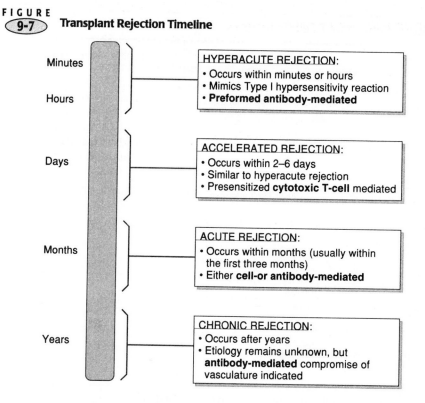

FIGURE
9-7 Transplant Rejection Timeline

Minutes

Hours

HYPERACUTE REJECTION:
• Occurs within minutes or hours
• Mimics Type I hypersensitivity reaction
• **Preformed antibody-mediated**

Days

ACCELERATED REJECTION:
• Occurs within 2–6 days
• Similar to hyperacute rejection
• Presensitized **cytotoxic T-cell** mediated

Months

ACUTE REJECTION:
• Occurs within months (usually within the first three months)
• Either **cell-or antibody-mediated**

Years

CHRONIC REJECTION:
• Occurs after years
• Etiology remains unknown, but **antibody-mediated** compromise of vasculature indicated

> **QUICK HIT** Graft versus host disease (GVHD) is caused by donor lymphocytes attacking recipient cells. It is characterized by elevated IgE, elevated bilirubin and liver enzymes, and skin lesions. It is seen commonly in bone marrow transplants.

IMMUNODEFICIENCIES

Diseases affecting the immune system leave the individual prone to infection. The immune system can be affected on any level or at any time, from its development to its most distal signaling mechanisms.

● Congenital B Cell Deficiencies (Table 9-6)

TABLE 9-6 Congenital B Cell Deficiencies		
Disease	**Defect**	**Significant Features**
X-linked agammaglobulinemia (of Bruton)	Lack of maturation of B cells	Absence of plasma cells, serum IgG; recurrent **pyogenic infections** beginning after 6 months; one of most common congenital B cell diseases; lymphoid tissue has **poorly defined germinal centers**
Selective IgA deficiency	Lack of maturation of B cells; failure of gene switching in heavy chain	**Most common congenital B cell defect 1/700; pulmonary tract infections**
Common variable immunodeficiency	Failure of terminal B cell differentiation	See Table 9-8
Ig = immunoglobulin		

● Congenital T Cell Deficiencies (Table 9-7)

TABLE 9-7 Congenital T Cell Deficiencies		
Disease	**Defect**	**Significant Features**
Thymic aplasia (DiGeorge's syndrome)	Deficiency of development of 3rd and 4th branchial pouches; T-cell defect	Defective development of the thymus, parathyroid glands, ear, mandible, aortic arch; leads to recurrent infections by **viral and fungal organisms; hypocalcemia** from low PTH leads to tetany
Chronic mucocutaneous candidiasis	Lack of T-cell response to Candida	Recurrent candidal skin and mucous membrane infections
Hyper IgM syndrome	Mutation in CD4+ helper T-cell interaction with CD40 on B-cell prevents class switching	Increased IgM; decreased IgG, IgA, IgE; normal numbers of T and B cells

Ig=immunoglobulin; *PTH*=parathyroid hormone

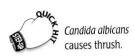

Candida albicans causes thrush.

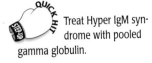

Treat Hyper IgM syndrome with pooled gamma globulin.

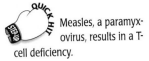

Measles, a paramyxovirus, results in a T-cell deficiency.

● Congenital Combined T and B Cell Deficiencies (Table 9-8)

TABLE 9-8 Congenital Combined T and B Cell Deficiencies		
Disease	**Defect**	**Significant Features**
Severe combined immunodeficiency (SCID)	**Autosomal recessive** (defect in tyrosine kinase ZAP-70, or adenosine deaminase deficiency) and X-linked forms (IL-2 receptor defect)	Susceptible to recurrent bacterial, viral, fungal, and protozoal infections
Wiskott-Aldrich syndrome	IgM response to capsule polysaccharide (e.g., pneumococcus) is weak	**Eczema, thrombocytopenia, recurrent infections;** becomes notable in first year of life
Ataxia-telangiectasia	IgA deficiency and lymphopenia	Autosomal recessive; becomes noticeable in first 2 years of life; ataxia (cerebellar dysfunction), telangiectasia, recurrent infections, thymic aplasia

IL=interleukin; *ZAP*=zeta-associated protein

SCID caused by adenosine deaminase (ADA) deficiency was one of the first diseases successfully treated with gene therapy.

● Plasma Cell Abnormalities (Table 9-9)

TABLE 9-9	Plasma Cell Abnormalities		
Disease	**Etiology**	**Clinical Features**	**Notes**
Multiple myeloma	Clonal plasma cell tumor	**Lytic, punched-out bone lesions** especially in the skull; hyperglobulinemia; **Bence Jones proteinuria**	**Rouleaux formation** ("stack of coins" appearance)
Waldenström's macroglobu-linemia	Excessive production of IgM by lymphoid cells	Slowly progressive course; usually in men over 50 years of age; platelet function abnormal; hyper-viscosity syndrome	No bone lesions (which differentiates this from multiple myeloma)
Benign monoclonal gammopathy	Increased production of monoclonal antibodies from an unknown origin	Asymptomatic; occurring in older individuals	Monoclonal spike without Bence Jones proteinuria (versus multiple myeloma)

Ig=immunoglobulin

● Phagocyte Deficiencies (Table 9-10)

TABLE 9-10	Phagocyte Deficiencies	
Disease	**Defect**	**Significant Features**
Chronic granulo-matous disease (CGD)	Neutrophils **lack NADPH oxidase**	**X-linked** (some autosomal recessive); no oxidative burst; B and T cells normal; opportunistic infections (e.g., *Staphylococcus aureus, Aspergillus,* enteric gram-negative rods)
Chédiak-Higashi syndrome	Failure of neutrophils to empty lysosomes	Autosomal recessive; recurrent pyogenic infections (e.g., *Staphylococcus, Streptococcus*)
Job's syndrome	T helper lymphocytes fail to produce INF-γ	Eczema; increase in Th-2 (see Figure 9-5) leads to increase in IgE, causing increased histamine release
Leukocyte adhe-sion deficiency	Defect in adhesion protein LAF-1	Pyogenic infections early in life; poor phagocytosis

INF-γ=gamma interferon; *LAF-1*=leukocyte-activating factor; *NADPH*=reduced nicotinamide adenine dinucleotide

● Acquired Immunodeficiencies (Table 9-11)

TABLE 9-11	Acquired Immunodeficiencies	
Disease	**Defect**	**Significant Features**
Common variable hypogamma-globulinemia	Acquired or congenital (unknown) B-cell defects	Recurrent pyogenic bacterial infections (e.g., pneumococcus, *H. influenzae*); decreased IgG production
AIDS	**HIV virus infects CD4 cells**	Opportunistic infections (e.g., **mycobacterium-avium intracellular**, C. neoformans, **P. carinii**, C. albicans); increased tumors (e.g., **Kaposi's**)

AIDS=acquired immunodeficiency syndrome; *HIV*=human immunodeficiency virus

THROMBOSIS AND THE CLOTTING CASCADE

(Figure 9-8)

Aspirin functions as an anti-thrombotic by permanently **acetylating cyclooxygenase** (COX), thereby inhibiting TxA_2 production. TxA_2 triggers the aggregation of platelets. Aspirin also inhibits prostaglandin formation, but unlike platelets, endothelium can synthesize new COX.

FIGURE 9-8 Thrombosis and the Clotting Cascade

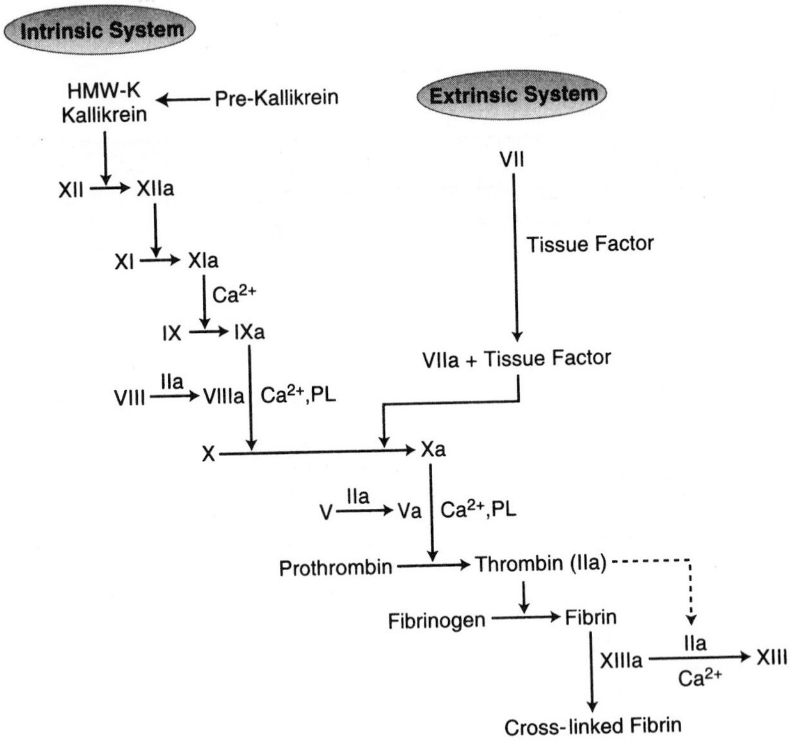

Ca^{2+}=calcium; *HMW-K*=high-molecular-weight kininogen; *PL*=phospholipid

Factors II, VII, IX, X require vitamin K for synthesis and are produced in the liver.

Thrombosis is the intravascular coagulation of blood and involves the interaction of platelets, coagulation proteins, and endothelial cells. With intact endothelium, a balance exists between prothrombotic [platelet-derived thromboxane A_2 (TxA_2)] and anti-thrombotic [endothelium-derived prostaglandin I_2 (PGI_2)] mediators. With damaged endothelium, exposed collagen causes adhesion of platelets through glycoprotein receptors and von Willebrand's factor (vWf). This adhesion triggers platelet release of adenosine diphosphate (ADP), serotonin, histamine, and platelet-derived growth factor (PDGF), resulting in primary plug formation and cessation of bleeding. Stabilization of the primary plug (formation of secondary plug) is mediated by fibrin and factor XIIIa, a result of activation of the clotting cascade.

Factor XIa in the presence of Ca^{2+} activates factor IX. Factor IXa requires Ca^{2+} and a phospholipid to activate factor X. Activated factor X requires Ca^{2+}, phospholipid, and factor Va to activate prothrombin to thrombin. Thrombin and Ca^{2+} inactivate factor XIII, which promotes the cross-linking of fibrin.

● Key Players in Inhibition of Coagulation

α-1-Antitrypsin	Inhibits factor XIa
α-2-Macroglobulin	Inhibits serine proteases
Antithrombin III	Inhibits factor Xa and thrombin
Inhibitor of first component of complement (C1 INH)	Inhibits factor XII and kallikrein
Heparin cofactor II	Inhibits thrombin
Protein C	Inactivates Va, VIIIa
Protein S	Is cofactor for Protein C

● Coagulation Disorders (Table 9-12)

Abnormalities of the coagulation cascade, endothelial cells, or platelets can lead to inappropriate bleeding or clot formation. These coagulopathies can be manifested as symptomatology involving skin, joints, vasculature, or internal organs.

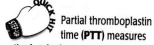

Partial thromboplastin time (PTT) measures the **intrinsic system.** Therapeutic drug monitoring of heparin is measured using PTT. Heparin overdose is treated with intravenous protamine sulfate.

Prothrombin time (PT) measures the **extrinsic system.** Therapeutic drug monitoring of warfarin is measured using PT. Warfarin overdose is treated with administration of vitamin K.

Factor VIII is the only clotting factor increased in liver disease.

Factor XIII is the only clotting factor that is not a serine protease.

TABLE 9-12	Coagulation Disorders		
Disease	**Etiology**	**Clinical Features**	**Notes**
Disseminated intravascular coagulation (DIC)	Multifactorial, causes include sepsis, trauma, and neoplasms	**Thrombocytopenia; diffuse hemorrhage;** microthrombus formation	Activation of factors V, VIII, and protein C
von-Willebrand factor (vWf) deficiency disease	**Autosomal dominant** disorder	Impaired platelet adhesion; **decreased factor VIII** (vWf binds factor VIII in the blood); **increased bleeding time**	Most common hereditary bleeding disorder; similar diseases include Bernard-Soulier disease and Glanzmann's thrombasthenia
Hemophilia A	**X-linked** factor VIII deficiency	Bleeding into muscle, subcutaneous tissues, and joints	**Most common type of hemophilia;** variable penetrance
Hemophilia B (Christmas disease)	X-linked factor IX deficiency	Bleeding into muscle, subcutaneous tissues, and joints	Presentation is identical to hemophilia A
Idiopathic thrombocytopenic purpura (ITP)	**Antiplatelet antibodies**	Thrombocytopenia	Follows URI in children and is self-limiting; chronic in adults
Thrombotic thrombocytopenic purpura (TTP)	Idiopathic systemic disease	Hyaline occlusions and microangiopathic hemolytic anemia leading to schistocytes and helmet cells	May cause neurologic abnormalities
URI=upper respiratory tract infection			

HEMATOPOIETIC SYSTEM

● vWf Deficiency versus Hemophilia A (Table 9-13)

TABLE 9-13 vWf Deficiency versus Hemophilia A

	vWf Deficiency	Hemophilia A
Factor VIII: coagulant activity	↓	↓
vWf level	↓	Normal
Ristocetin cofactor activity	↓	Normal
Ristocetin aggregation	↓	Normal
Bleeding time	↑	Normal
Inheritance	**Autosomal dominant**	**X-linked**

Ristocetin, an antibiotic not used for clinical disease, has platelet aggregation properties. vWf=von Willebrand factor

● Clotting Time Algorithm (Table 9-14)

TABLE 9-14 Clotting Time Algorithm

	PT normal	PT prolonged
PTT normal	Factor XIII deficiency	Factor VII deficiency
PTT prolonged	Factor VIII, IX, XI deficiencies in patients with bleeding; factor XII, prekallikrein, HMWK deficiencies in patients without bleeding	Common pathway deficiency: factor V, X, II, I; severe hepatic diseases; DIC

DIC=disseminated intravascular coagulation; HMWK=high-molecular-weight kininogen; PT=prothrombin time; PTT=partial thromboplastin time

LYMPHOMA

I. Tumors of the lymphoid system

II. Present as enlarged, firm, fixed, painless nodes

III. Are classified as Hodgkin's and Non-Hodgkin's disease

QUICK HIT

Staging of lymphoma (Ann Arbor System): (1) One node or organ affected; (2) Two nodes or organs on same side of diaphragm affected; (3) Both sides of diaphragm, spleen or other organ affected; (4) Disseminated foci

• Comparison of Hodgkin's and Non-Hodgkin's Disease (Table 9-15)

TABLE 9-15 Hodgkin's versus Non-Hodgkin's Disease

Hodgkin's Disease	Non-Hodgkin's Disease
Number of **Reed-Sternberg cells** [binucleated giant cells] proportional to severity	Malignant neoplasm of lymphocytes (90% B cell, 10% T cell) within lymph nodes (especially periaortic)
Causes inflammation, fever, diaphoresis **(night sweats), leukocytosis,** hepatosplenomegaly, pruritus	Causes painless peripheral lymphadenopathy
Usually affects **young men** (peak incidence in adolescents)	
Often curable More reactive lymphocytes signal better prognosis	Classification criteria -Nodular type has better prognosis than diffuse -Small cell type has better prognosis than large cell
Rye classifications (low-grade to high-grade): -Lymphocytic predominance (least common, best prognosis) -Mixed cellularity (most frequent) **-Nodular sclerosis** (predominantly in **women;** fibrous bands in lymph nodes; lacunar cells; often found in the mediastinum) -Lymphocytic depletion (worst prognosis; rare necrosis and fibrosis of lymphocytic tissue)	Working classification (low-grade to high-grade): -Small lymphocytic cell (B-cell; elderly; indolent course; CLL related) -Follicular small cell (cleaved B-cell; elderly; **most common non-Hodgkin's lymphoma t(14;18),** expression of bcl-2 oncogene) -Large cell (elderly and children; usually B-cell) -Lymphoblastic (T-cell; children; **mediastinal mass** progressing to ALL) -Small non-cleaved [**(Burkitt's)** B-cell, EBV infection; **"starry-sky"** appearance; related to B-cell **ALL; t(8;14),** expression of c-myc oncogene] -Cutaneous T-cell (*Mycosis fungoides,* Pautrier's microabscesses, Sezary's syndrome, skin lesions)

ALL=acute lymphocytic leukemia; *CLL*=chronic lymphocytic leukemia; *EBV*=Epstein-Barr virus

LEUKEMIA (Table 9-16)

The symptoms of leukemia include fatigue, dyspnea on exertion, bleeding, pallor, and hepatosplenomegaly.

TABLE 9-16 Classification of Leukemia

Acute Myeloblastic	Acute Lymphoblastic	Chronic Myeloid	Chronic Lymphocytic
Myeloblasts; defect in maturation beyond myeloblast or promyelocyte stage; **Auer rods;** predominantly affects **adults;** poor prognosis	Small lymphoblasts; decreased cytoplasm; predominantly affects **children;** responsive to therapy	t(9;22) results in **Philadelphia chromosome** (BCR-ABL); leukocytosis; **decreased LAP;** splenomegaly; onset at **35–55** years of age; ends in blastic crisis	Usually B cells; "smudge cells" in smear; warm autoimmune hemolytic anemia; hypogammaglobulinemia; lymphadenopathy; hepatosplenomegaly; more common in **men over 60** years of age

BCR=B-cell reactivity; *LAP*=leukocyte alkaline phosphatase

QUICK HIT: ALL is the **most common malignancy** in children.

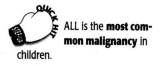

ANEMIA (Table 9-17)

Anemia, a decrease in circulating red blood cell mass, is usually defined as hemoglobin less than 12 g/dL in female patients and less than 14 g/dL in male patients.

QUICK HIT
Heme regulates its own production by inhibiting synthesis (transcription and translation) of ALA synthetase.

QUICK HIT
Heme keeps the translational initiation complex active on the ribosome, which increases the production of globin.

QUICK HIT
In sickle cell disease, the 6th amino acid of the β chain of hemoglobin is changed from glutamate to valine in HbS. Sickling only occurs when the RBCs are **deoxygenated.** Oxygenated HbS RBCs function normally.

TABLE 9-17	Classification of Anemia	
Microcytic (MCV <80)	**Normocytic (MCV 80–100)**	**Macrocytic (MCV >100)**
Iron deficiency	Aplastic anemia	Liver disease
Lead poisoning	Acute blood loss	B12 deficiency
Sickle cell	Hemolytic anemia	Folate deficiency
Chronic disease		
Sideroblastic		
Thalassemia		

MCV = mean cell volume

I. Microcytic Anemia

A. Iron deficiency
1. **Most common anemia**
2. **TIBC is increased, serum iron,** and **bone marrow stores are low**
3. Occurs in menstruating or pregnant women, infants, and preadolescents
4. Caused by dietary deficiency or bleeding (menorrhagia, GI bleeding, GI cancers, and inflammatory bowel disease)
5. Pale, easy fatigability, dyspneic, may be associated with Plummer-Vinson syndrome (characterized by glossitis, esophageal web)

B. Lead poisoning
1. Inhibits heme synthesis (delta-ala dehydratase and ferrochetalase)
2. **Basophilic stippling** of RBCs is seen microscopically.
3. Finger, wrist, and foot drop occur from neurotoxicity.
4. Renal lesions, GI colic, and gingival lead lines occur.
5. Treatment is with ethylenediamine tetraacetic acid (EDTA).

C. Sickle cell disease [sickle cell hemoglobin or hemoglobin S(HbS)]
1. Primarily seen in **African Americans**
2. The homozygous form is most severe.
3. Severe hemolytic anemia is seen.
4. Leads to painful crises; organ infarction **(autosplenectomy);** strokes
5. Aplastic crises occur, usually provoked by viral infection (usually Parvovirus B19).
6. Patients are especially susceptible to infection by **encapsulated bacteria** (*Streptococcus pneumoniae* and *Haemophilus influenzae*) and osteomyelitis caused by salmonella.
7. Sickle cells are seen in peripheral blood smear.
8. Treatment is with hydroxyurea to increase HbF.

D. Chronic disease
1. Second most common anemia
2. **Total iron-binding capacity (TIBC) is reduced (ferritin is increased)**
3. Low serum iron, but high iron stores in the bone marrow

E. Sideroblastic anemia
   1. Iron stain reveals ringed sideroblasts.
   2. TIBC is reduced, and serum iron is increased.
   3. RBC count is reduced.
F. Thalassemia
   1. This is a group of genetic disorders, all in some way deficient in α or β globin chain synthesis.
   2. **β-Thalassemia is more common** (especially in people of Mediterranean origin).
   3. The homozygous form, called thalassemia major (also known as Mediterranean or Cooley's anemia), causes splenomegaly, bone distortions, hemosiderosis, increased HbF, and is fatal in childhood.
   4. The heterozygous form of β-thalassemia (thalassemia minor) causes a minor anemia, but has no effect on life span.
   5. α-Thalassemia is caused by a deletion in one or more of the four alpha globin genes; loss of all four genes is not compatible with life.

II. Normocytic Anemias

A. Aplastic anemia
   1. Dysfunctional or deficient multipotent myeloid stem cells leads to pancytopenia.
   2. Caused by viruses, chemicals, radiation, renal failure (via decreased erythropoietin) or may be idiopathic
   3. Drugs causing aplastic anemia include nonsteroidal anti-inflammatory drugs **(NSAIDs), benzene,** and **chloramphenicol.**
   4. Symptoms include fatigue, pallor, mucosal bleeding, and petechia due to thrombocytopenia.
   5. Neutropenia occurs, leading to frequent infections.
   6. **Fat infiltration** into hypocellular marrow occurs.
B. Anemia due to acute blood loss
   1. Leads to a **transient normocytic** anemia
   2. May appear macrocytic due to increased reticulocyte release from bone marrow 7–10 days later
C. Hemolytic anemias
   1. Increased red cell destruction leads to an increase in unconjugated bilirubin, hemoglobinemia, hemoglobinuria, hemosiderosis, and decreased serum haptoglobin.
   2. Increase in reticulocytes occurs due to additional erythropoiesis.
   3. Extracorpuscular (acquired) hemolytic anemias
     a. Warm autoimmune hemolytic immunoglobulin (AIHI) (IgG): associated with lymphoma, spherocytosis, **positive direct Coombs' test**
     b. Cold AIHI (IgM): associated with lymphoid neoplasm, anti-I antibodies, ABO incompatibility, **Raynaud's phenomenon**
     c. Erythroblastosis fetalis (hemolytic diseases of the newborn): usually due to Rh blood group incompatibility; can result in kernicterus and death
     d. Caused by infections including bartonellosis, clostridia, malaria
   4. Intracorpuscular (genetic) hemolytic anemias
     a. Hereditary ovalocytosis (elliptocytosis): autosomal dominant
     b. Hereditary spherocytosis: autosomal dominant, **spectrin** deficiency
     c. Paroxysmal nocturnal hemoglobinuria: deficiency of decay accelerating factor (DAF), decreased leukocyte alkaline phosphatase (LAP)
     d. Glucose-6-phosphate dehydrogenase deficiency (G-6-PD): **X-linked;** more common in Mediterraneans and African Americans; precipitated by oxidative stress (primaquine therapy); **Heinz bodies** are seen.
     e. Pyruvate kinase deficiency: autosomal recessive, chronic

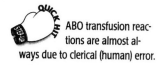
ABO transfusion reactions are almost always due to clerical (human) error.

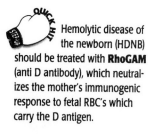
Hemolytic disease of the newborn (HDNB) should be treated with **RhoGAM** (anti D antibody), which neutralizes the mother's immunogenic response to fetal RBC's which carry the D antigen.

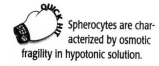
Spherocytes are characterized by osmotic fragility in hypotonic solution.

III. Macrocytic Anemias

    A. Liver disease—usually cirrhosis.

        1. Excess lipid is added to RBC membrane in diseased liver.

        2. Hypersplenism occurs.

        3. Spur cells are present.

    B. Vitamin B_{12} (cobalamin) deficiency

        1. **Megaloblastic anemia,** characterized by **hypersegmented neutrophils,** pancytopenia, achlorhydria

        2. Decreased DNA synthesis

        3. Most common form is **pernicious anemia** (caused by a deficiency of intrinsic factor); associated with increased incidence of gastric carcinoma.

        4. Other etiologies for vitamin B_{12} deficiency anemia include strict vegetarian diet, distal ileum pathology, bacterial overgrowth, D. latum infection; type A gastritis

        5. **Neurologic symptoms** due to demyelination of posterior and lateral columns, ataxia, and paresthesia in distal extremities

    C. Folate deficiency

        1. Megaloblastic anemia

        2. Hematological findings are identical to vitamin B_{12} deficiency.

        3. **No neurologic** deficits are present.

        4. Folate deficiency can mask vitamin B_{12} deficiency.

        5. Etiologies include dietary deficiency, sprue, *Giardia lamblia* infection, oral contraceptives, anti-neoplastics (methotrexate), and pregnancy.

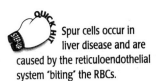

Spur cells occur in liver disease and are caused by the reticuloendothelial system "biting" the RBCs.

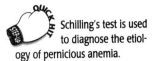

Schilling's test is used to diagnose the etiology of pernicious anemia.

MYELOPROLIFERATIVE DISORDERS

I. Polycythemia vera

    A. Chronic increase in the number of red cells due to bone marrow hyperplasia of unknown etiology

    B. Clinical manifestations

        1. Presents in middle age

        2. Symptoms are headache, vertigo, splenomegaly, pruritus.

    C. Differential diagnosis

        1. Absolute polycythemia vera

            a. Primary polycythemia—**Low or absent erythropoietin levels**

            b. Secondary polycythemia

                (1) Elevated erythropoietin levels

                (2) Appropriate: response to hypoxia

                (3) Inappropriate: secondary to an inappropriate secretion of erythropoietin due to a cyst or tumor

            c. Relative polycythemia vera (e.g., dehydration) is often due to a decrease in extracorpuscular volume, thus causing a relative increase in the hematocrit level.

    D. Diagnosis

        1. Major diagnostic criteria

            a. Increased red cell mass (hematocrit)

            b. Normal arterial oxygen saturation (>92%)

            c. Splenomegaly

         2. Minor diagnostic criteria

            a. Thrombocytosis

            b. Leukocytosis

            c. Elevated LAP

            d. Elevated serum B_{12}

3. Diagnosis requires all 3 major criteria or increased red cell mass, normal arterial oxygen saturation, and at least 2 minor criteria including leukocytosis and thrombocytosis.

II. Myelofibrosis

A. Generalized fibrosis of bone marrow characterized by pancytopenia in the face of increased megakaryocytes in the marrow

B. Clinical manifestations
   1. Presents in the late 50's
   2. **Tear-drop deformity** of RBCs occcurs, along with splenomegaly and extramedullary hematopoiesis
   3. "Dry tap" seen on bone biopsy

C. Differential diagnosis
   1. Primary myelofibrosis
      a. Marrow fibrosis
      b. Extramedullary hematopoiesis
   2. Secondary myelofibrosis
      a. Infections: tuberculosis, osteomyelitis
      b. Metastatic carcinoma
      c. Paget's disease

III. Essential Thrombocythemia

A. A primary disorder of unknown etiology resulting in increased platelets

B. Clinical manifestations
   1. Thrombocytosis
   2. Megakaryocytic hyperplasia
   3. Splenomegaly
   4. Hemorrhage and thrombosis
   5. Increased bone marrow reticulin and absence of bcr/abl gene

QUICK HIT Myelodysplastic syndromes also exist: refractory anemia; refractory anemia with ringed sideroblasts; refractory anemia with excess blasts; refractory anemia with excess blasts in transformation; and chronic myelomonocytic leukemia.

THERAPEUTICS

Therapeutics for Prevention of Bleeding

Aprotinin	Tranexamic acid	Menadiol
Vitamin K	[aminomethylcyclo hexanecarboxylic acid (AMCHA)]	Menadione

Therapeutics for correction of anemia

Iron	Cyanocobalamin (Vitamin B$_{12}$)	Erythropoietin
	Folic acid (Vitamin M)	Hydroxyurea

Anticoagulants

Warfarin	Heparin

Anti-thrombotics

Aspirin	Ticlopidine

Thrombolytics

t-PA (alteplase)	Anistreplase
Streptokinase	[anisoylated
Urokinase	plasminogen streptokinase activator complex (APSAC)]

SYSTEM 10

Basic Concepts

DNA, RNA, AND PROTEIN

I. Chemical components of DNA and RNA

A. Deoxyribonucleic acid (DNA) and ribonucleic acid (RNA) are made up of **nucleotides,** which contain:

1. A **nitrogenous base**—either a purine or pyrimidine (Figure 10-1)

FIGURE 10-1 **Bases**

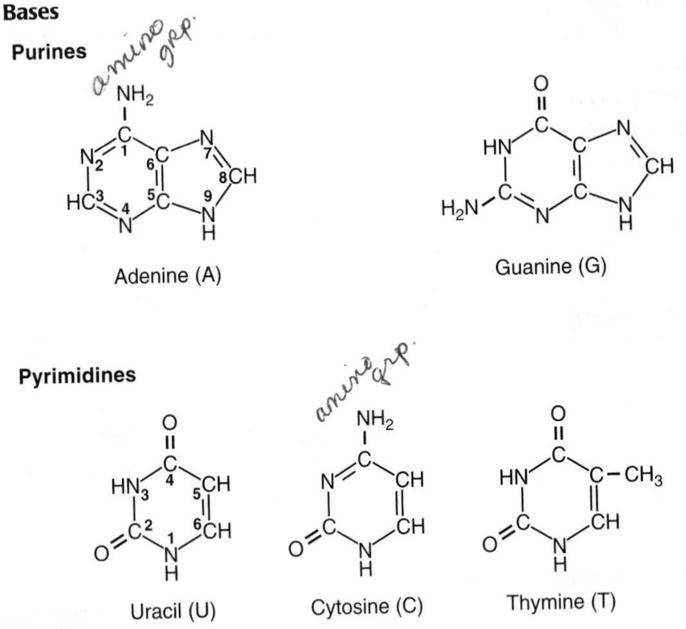

Purines
amino grp.
NH2
Adenine (A)
Guanine (G)
Pyrimidines
amino grp.
Uracil (U)
Cytosine (C)
Thymine (T)

C=carbon; *H*=hydrogen; *N*=nitrogen; *O*=oxygen

Pure As Gold (2) rings
CUT the PY (1) ring
G-C 3 H bonds
A-T 2 H bonds.

a. **Purines** are formed from:
   (1) Aspartate
   (2) CO_2
   (3) Glutamate
   (4) Glycine
   (4) N10-Formyl-tetrahydrofolate

b. **Pyrimidines** are formed from:
   (1) Aspartate
   (2) CO_2
   (3) Glutamine

2. A **pentose sugar**—either a **ribose** for RNA or a **2-deoxyribose** for DNA

3. One, two, or three phosphate groups: forming a -monophosphate, -diphosphate, or -triphosphate, respectively (Figure 10-2)

FIGURE
10-2 **Nucleotide structure**

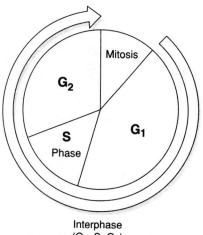

C=carbon; H=hydrogen; O=oxygen; P=phosphate

B. Nucleoside triphosphates (NTP) are linked together by a 3'–5' phosphodiester bond to form single stranded RNA or DNA.

C. **Adenine** (A) binds to **thymine** (T), while **guanine** (G) binds to **cytosine** (C) in DNA. **Uracil** (U) replaces thymine (T) in RNA.

II. DNA Replication

A. Is **semi-conservative**—when two DNA molecules are created from the original helix, one strand of parental DNA is incorporated with each new daughter strand

B. Takes place in the **S phase** of the cell cycle (Figure 10-3)

FIGURE
10-3 **The Cell Cycle**

M: mitosis: prophase–metaphase–anaphase–telophase

G₁: growth

S: synthesis of DNA

G₂: growth

G₀: quiescent G₁ phase

G_1 and G_0 are of variable duration. Mitosis is usually the shortest phase. Most cells are in G_0. Rapidly dividing cells have a shorter G_1.

(Adapted from Bhushan V, Le T, Amin C: *First Aid for the USMLE Step 1.* Stamford, Connecticut, Appleton & Lange, 1999. p. 165.)

C. DNA strand separation requires several proteins:

1. **DnaA**—20 to 50 of these proteins aggregate at the origin of replication and begin to separate the DNA strands

2. **Single strand binding (SSB) proteins** bind cooperatively to further separate the two strands of DNA.
3. **DNA helicase** unwinds the DNA.
D. Supercoiling is prevented by **DNA topoisomerase** type I and II
E. Replication process in prokaryotic cells (Figure 10-4)

F I G U R E
10-4   **DNA synthesis**

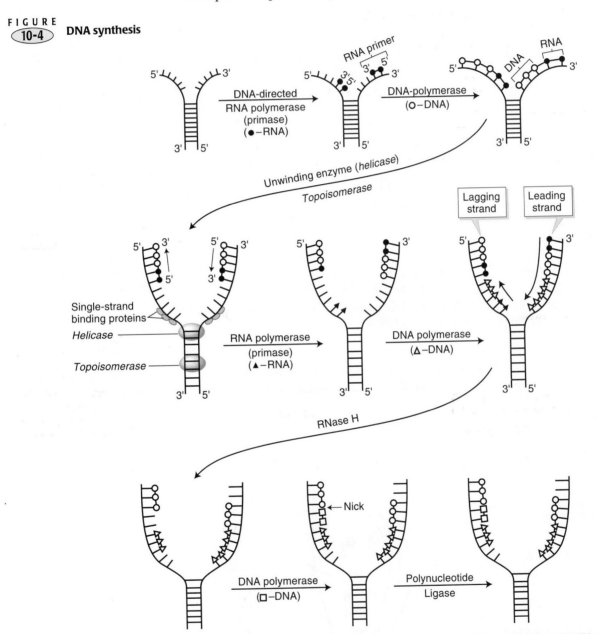

(Adapted from Marks DB: *BRS Biochemistry, 3rd edition.* Baltimore, Williams & Wilkins, 1999. Used by permission of Lippincott Williams & Wilkins.)

1. An RNA primer is placed on the separated DNA strands by RNA polymerase (also called **primase**) before replication can begin.
2. On the leading strand only one RNA primer is needed; on the lagging strand a new primer is required as the replication fork opens.
   a. Leading strand
      (1) The leading strand produces a continuously elongating strand of new DNA
      (2) The leading strand of DNA is copied continuously from 5′ to 3′ in the direction of the replication fork

b. Lagging strand
  (1) The lagging strand of DNA is copied piecewise in the direction opposite of the replication fork.
  (2) The lagging strand produces small pieces of new DNA with RNA interspersed, called Okazaki fragments.
3. The DNA chain is elongated by DNA polymerase III, which adds nucleotides with energy provided by breaking of the triphosphate bond.
4. When DNA strand synthesis is complete, it is proofread.
  a. The proofreading function of DNA polymerase III (3'–5' exonuclease) allows it to correct mismatched base pairs.
  b. The improperly placed base is hydrolytically removed and replaced with the appropriate one.
5. RNA primers are removed from the Okazaki fragments and leading strand.
  a. DNA polymerase I or III has **3'–5' exonuclease** activity which allows it to remove the RNA primer.
  b. Once the primer is removed, the space is filled with DNA.
6. The break in the strand backbone is sealed by **DNA ligase.**

F. Repair
  1. Damage due to ultraviolet light
    a. Ultraviolet light exposure results in **pyrimidine dimers** (especially thymine-thymine dimers).
  ✳ b. Dimers inhibit the replication process.
    c. Specialized **endonucleases** recognize a dimer and cleave it at its 5' end.
    d. An **exonuclease** then excises the dimer and leaves a gap in the DNA strand.
    e. The gap is filled with the appropriate nucleotides by DNA polymerase I.
    f. The strand is resealed by DNA ligase.
  2. Base alterations
    a. Bases may be changed spontaneously or slowly over time due to
    ✳ **alkylating agents** (cyclophosphamide and nitrosoureas). ✳
    b. Specialized **glycosylases** remove the improper base and leave an empty (apyrimidinic or apurinic) space.
    c. The empty space is filled by specific endonucleases or polymerases in the same manner that dimers are repaired.

III. DNA Packaging

A. Due to the incredible length of DNA, it must be properly coiled inside the cell.
B. **Histones** are a group of proteins designed to coil DNA.
  1. The high content of arginine and lysine gives histones a positive charge which attracts them to negatively charged DNA.
  2. Histones organize themselves into a group of eight to make a **nucleosome** core; each core contains 2 each of type H2A, H2B, H3, and H4 histones.
  3. DNA twists approximately twice around each core.
  4. Between cores a histone of type H1 is attached to the DNA.
  5. The arrangement of histones and DNA is called a nucleosome and produces a characteristic "beads on a string" appearance.
  6. The nucleosomes coil around themselves to produce a nucleofilament.
  7. Nucleofilaments are further packaged and coiled into more compact structures when DNA is not being replicated.

IV. RNA Synthesis

A. Initiation of transcription is influenced by a variety of factors:
  1. **RNA polymerase** binds to the promoter region of the DNA.
  2. The **TATAAT** nucleotide sequence is a section of the promoter located

QUICK HIT
DNA synthesis can be prevented by nucleoside analogs such as cytosine arabinoside, zidovudine, and acyclovir. These types of drugs are useful in antiviral and anticancer therapy.

*α & δ rep of lag + lead str DNA

QUICK HIT
In eukaryotic cells, replication is accomplished by POL enzymes similar to those in prokaryotic cells. POL α performs primase activity like prokaryotic primase, POL δ synthesizes the leading DNA strand, POL ε synthesizes the lagging strand, and POL β repairs and excises primers similarly to DNA polymerase I.

β & ε repair nuclear DNA.

*γ rep mito DNA

QUICK HIT
Xeroderma pigmentosum is a genetic disease in which cells cannot repair damaged DNA. People suffering from this disease cannot repair skin damage caused by sunlight and are predisposed to skin cancer.

(AR)
(thymidine dimers)

initiate synthesis of new chains.
no PRimer needed!

genes have a promoter region
to which RNA p'ase binds to. upstream from the start of transcription; it is contained in the Hogness box of eukaryotes and the Pribnow box of prokaryotes.

  3. The **CAAT box**, found in eukaryotes, and the −35 sequence, found in prokaryotes, are located further upstream from the TATAAT sequence and have promoter function.

B. After recognition of the promoter region by RNA polymerase, elongation begins.

  1. Elongation of RNA occurs in a manner similar to DNA replication, but does not require a primer for intiation.

  2. RNA polymerase does not have a proofreading function so it cannot correct mismatched base pairs that may occur.

C. In eukaryotic cells RNA undergoes **post-translational modification;** in prokaryotic cells transcription and translation occur simultaneously.

  1. RNA synthesized by eukaryotic **DNA polymerase II** is called **heterogeneous nuclear RNA (hnRNA)** and is found in the nucleus of the cell.

  2. This hnRNA is **capped at the 5′ end** by a 7-methyl-guanine molecule provided by S-adenosylmethionine (SAM).

  3. **A poly-A nucleotide tail is added to the 3′ end.**

  4. Introns are cleaved out.

  5. The molecule is now mature mRNA and is transported to the cytoplasm.

QUICK HIT

In eukaryotes, different RNA is synthesized by several different RNA polymerases. RNA polymerase I synthesizes ribosomal RNA, RNA polymerase II synthesizes messenger RNA, and RNA polymerase III synthesizes transfer RNA.

QUICK HIT

Point mutations include **silent mutations** (the same amino acid), **missense mutations** (a new amino acid), and **nonsense mutations** (stop codon). Insertions are the addition of extra amino acids, while deletions are the loss of amino acids.

RNA p'ase binds to promoter for DNA helix to occur.

Eukaryote
TATAAT
(Hogness)

Prokaryote
TATAAT
(Pribnow box)

V. Protein Synthesis (Figure 10-5)

FIGURE
10-5 Protein synthesis

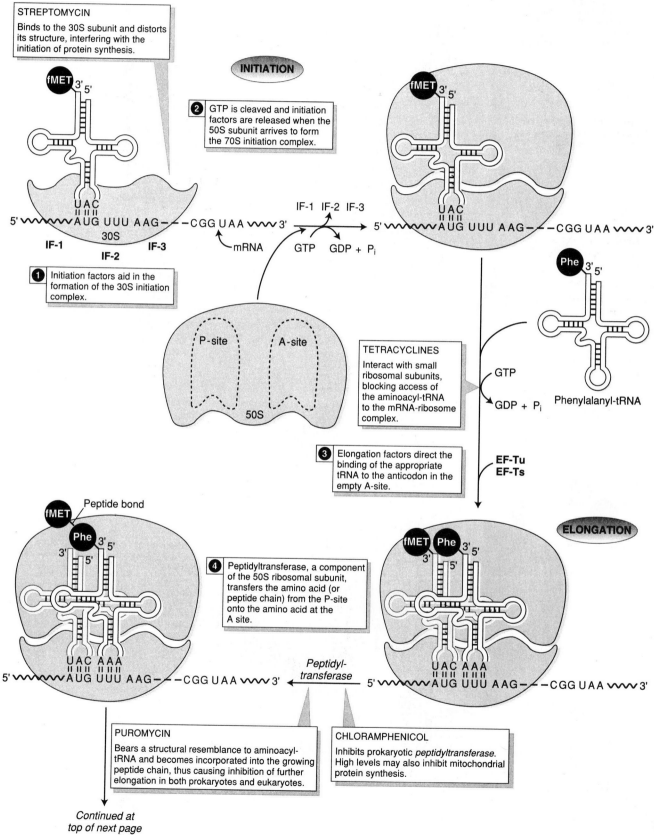

STREPTOMYCIN

Binds to the 30S subunit and distorts its structure, interfering with the initiation of protein synthesis.

INITIATION

2 GTP is cleaved and initiation factors are released when the 50S subunit arrives to form the 70S initiation complex.

fMET 3' 5'

IF-1 IF-2 IF-3

5' ∿∿∿UAC / AUG UUU AAG——CGG UAA ∿∿3'
30S
IF-1   **IF-3**
IF-2

mRNA   GTP   GDP + P_i

5' ∿∿∿AUG UUU AAG——CGG UAA ∿∿∿3'

1 Initiation factors aid in the formation of the 30S initiation complex.

Phe 3' 5'

P-site   A-site

50S

TETRACYCLINES

Interact with small ribosomal subunits, blocking access of the aminoacyl-tRNA to the mRNA-ribosome complex.

GTP
GDP + P_i   Phenylalanyl-tRNA

3 Elongation factors direct the binding of the appropriate tRNA to the anticodon in the empty A-site.

EF-Tu
EF-Ts

Peptide bond
fMET
Phe 3' 5'
3' 5'

4 Peptidyltransferase, a component of the 50S ribosomal subunit, transfers the amino acid (or peptide chain) from the P-site onto the amino acid at the A site.

ELONGATION

fMET Phe 3' 5'
3' 5'

UAC AAA
5' ∿∿∿AUG UUU AAG——CGG UAA ∿∿∿3'

Peptidyl-transferase

UAC AAA
5' ∿∿∿AUG UUU AAG——CGG UAA ∿∿∿3'

PUROMYCIN

Bears a structural resemblance to aminoacyl-tRNA and becomes incorporated into the growing peptide chain, thus causing inhibition of further elongation in both prokaryotes and eukaryotes.

CHLORAMPHENICOL

Inhibits prokaryotic *peptidyltransferase*. High levels may also inhibit mitochondrial protein synthesis.

Continued at top of next page

A=adenine; *Arg*=arginine; *C*=cytosine; *EF*=elongation factor; *fMET*=formyl methionine; *G*=guanine; *GDP*=guanine diphosphate; *GTP*=guanine triphosphate; *IF*=initiation factor; *P*=phosphate; *Phe*=phenylalanine; *RF*=release factor; *T*=thymine; *tRNA*=transfer ribonucleic acid; *U*=uracil (Adapted from Champe PC and Harvey RA: *Lippincott's Illustrated Reviews: Biochemistry, 2nd edition*. Philadelphia, Lippincott-Raven Publishers, 1994. pp. 396–7. Used by permission of Lippincott Williams & Wilkins.)

FIGURE
10-5 *(Continued)*

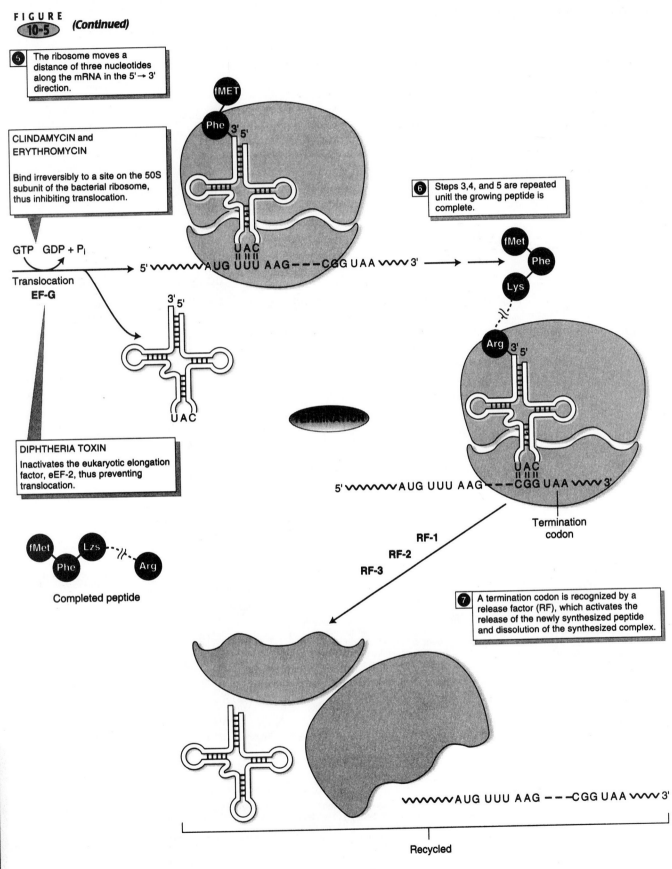

5 The ribosome moves a distance of three nucleotides along the mRNA in the 5'→ 3' direction.

CLINDAMYCIN and ERYTHROMYCIN

Bind irreversibly to a site on the 50S subunit of the bacterial ribosome, thus inhibiting translocation.

GTP GDP + P$_i$

Translocation
EF-G

DIPHTHERIA TOXIN

Inactivates the eukaryotic elongation factor, eEF-2, thus preventing translocation.

Completed peptide

6 Steps 3,4, and 5 are repeated unitl the growing peptide is complete.

TERMINATION

Termination codon

RF-1
RF-2
RF-3

7 A termination codon is recognized by a release factor (RF), which activates the release of the newly synthesized peptide and dissolution of the synthesized complex.

Recycled

A. Initiation is started with the binding of the ribosomal subunits to the messenger RNA (mRNA).

B. The start codon **AUG** is the first codon to be recognized and translated; initiation factor 2 (**IF-2** in prokaryotes, **eIF-2** in eukaryotes) and guanosine 5'-triphosphate (GTP) are required.

C. A methionine is added as the first amino acid.

D. Elongation requires a tRNA with the appropriate **anti-codon** to the codon on the mRNA, elongation factors, and GTP.

E. Termination requires a **UAA, UAG, or UGA** codon.

F. Regulation of RNA synthesis

    1. Eukaryotes

        a. Control is accomplished by gene **methylation, amplification,** and **rearrangement.**

        b. Histones play a role in gene suppression.

        c. Inducers activate gene expression.

        d. Some eukaryotic genes are regulated at transcription.

    2. Prokaryotes

        a. Protein synthesis is controlled at the level of transcription using operons.

        b. An **operon** is a set of adjacent genes that are activated or deactivated.

        c. Each operon has a **promoter** region upstream from the genes, an **operator** which activates or deactivates the genes, and a **repressor** protein which can bind to the operator and deactivate transcription. (Figure 10-6)

Operons

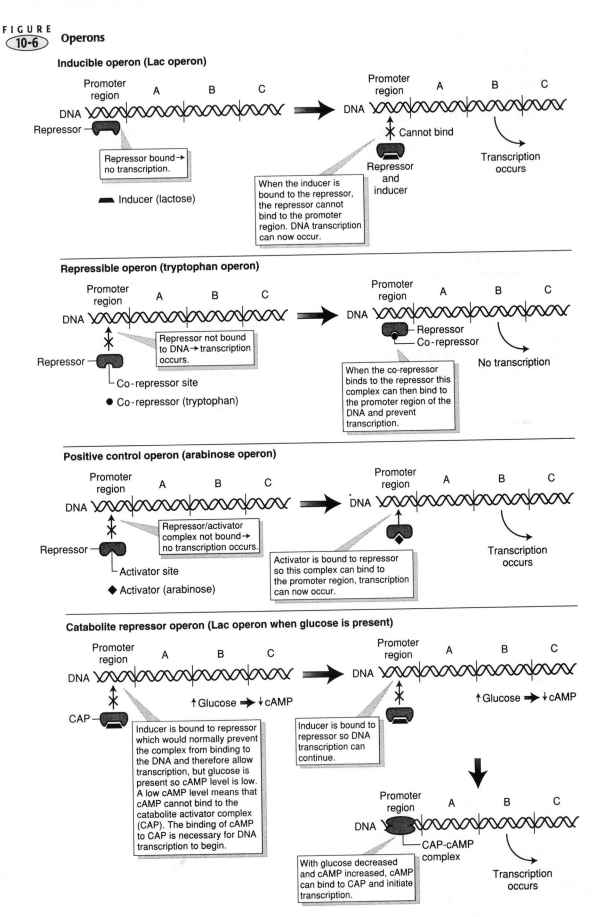

Inducible operon (Lac operon)

Promoter region · A · B · C — DNA — Repressor

Repressor bound→ no transcription.

Inducer (lactose)

When the inducer is bound to the repressor, the repressor cannot bind to the promoter region. DNA transcription can now occur.

Promoter region · A · B · C — DNA — Cannot bind — Repressor and inducer — Transcription occurs

Repressible operon (tryptophan operon)

Promoter region · A · B · C — DNA

Repressor not bound to DNA→ transcription occurs.

Repressor — Co-repressor site

Co-repressor (tryptophan)

When the co-repressor binds to the repressor this complex can then bind to the promoter region of the DNA and prevent transcription.

Promoter region · A · B · C — DNA — Repressor — Co-repressor — No transcription

Positive control operon (arabinose operon)

Promoter region · A · B · C — DNA

Repressor/activator complex not bound→ no transcription occurs.

Repressor — Activator site

Activator (arabinose)

Activator is bound to repressor so this complex can bind to the promoter region, transcription can now occur.

Promoter region · A · B · C — DNA — Transcription occurs

Catabolite repressor operon (Lac operon when glucose is present)

Promoter region · A · B · C — DNA

CAP

Inducer is bound to repressor which would normally prevent the complex from binding to the DNA and therefore allow transcription, but glucose is present so cAMP level is low. A low cAMP level means that cAMP cannot bind to the catabolite activator complex (CAP). The binding of cAMP to CAP is necessary for DNA transcription to begin.

↑Glucose ➡ ↓cAMP

Promoter region · A · B · C — DNA

Inducer is bound to repressor so DNA transcription can continue.

↑Glucose ➡ ↓cAMP

Promoter region · A · B · C — DNA — CAP-cAMP complex

With glucose decreased and cAMP increased, cAMP can bind to CAP and initiate transcription.

Transcription occurs

cAMP=cyclic adenosine monophosphate

VI. Post-Translational Folding of Proteins

A. Newly synthesized proteins have a linear structure **(primary structure).**

B. Based upon interactions between proteins, these linear structures can assume **secondary structures** such as an **α-helix** or **β-pleated sheet.**

C. The tertiary structure incorporates the secondary structures into a complete 3-dimensional configuration. This is the final conformation of many proteins.

D. A quaternary structure is formed when several tertiary structures are arranged together. This occurs in hemoglobin, for example, where two α and two β globular proteins form the complete hemoglobin molecule.

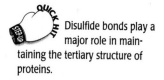 Disulfide bonds play a major role in maintaining the tertiary structure of proteins.

BACTERIAL MORPHOLOGY AND GENETICS

I. Cell Wall—the outermost component of all bacteria (except mycobacteria species, which only have a cell membrane).

A. Cell wall components

1. Peptidoglycan provides rigid support and protects against osmotic pressure changes, thick and multilayered in gram-positive organisms, thin and single layer in gram-negative organisms.

2. Gram-positive outer membrane is made up of teichoic acid.

3. Gram-negative outer membrane is made up of lipid-A (toxic component of endotoxin) and polysaccharide (major surface antigen).

4. Cytoplasmic membrane is a lipoprotein bi-layer without sterols, the site of oxidative and transport enzymes.

Peptidoglycan cross-linking is disrupted by penicillin and cephalosporins.

B. Gram stain

1. Separates most bacteria into two groups

   a. Gram-positive organisms stain blue.

   b. Gram-negative organisms stain red.

2. Procedure

   a. Crystal violet dye applied to the specimen stains all bacterial cells blue.

   b. Iodine, when added to the specimen, acts as a mordant and forms crystal violet-iodine complexes. Cells continue to appear blue.

   c. An organic solvent, such as ethanol, added to the specimen extracts the crystal violet-iodine complexes from gram-negative organisms. Gram-negative organisms now appear colorless, while gram-positive organisms remain blue.

   d. Safranin (red dye) is applied, staining the gram negatives red, while the gram positives maintain their blue color.

II. Bacterial Genome

A. Bacteria have a **haploid** genome as compared to the **diploid** human genome.

B. A typical bacterial cell has a **circular** DNA molecule with a molecular weight of approximately 2×10^9 with about 5×10^6 base pairs, which code for approximately 2000 proteins.

III. Mutation

A. Several types of mutations occur that can alter the bacterial genome.

B. Mutation is an important factor in bacterial survival as it allows the bacteria to adapt and change to their environment.

C. Mutations may be caused by a mistake committed by DNA polymerase, a chemical mutagen, ultraviolet light, a virus, or other cause.

D. Types of mutations

1. **Base substitution**

   a. One base replaces another

   b. Occurs at DNA replication

c. Can generate a missense mutation which causes the wrong amino acid to be placed in the protein, or it can generate a nonsense mutation, which is read as a stop codon.
d. Base substitution also occurs in eukaryotic cells, but can be repaired by the processes described above.

2. **Frameshift mutation**
a. One or more bases is added or removed (not a multiple of 3).
b. The reading frame is shifted on the mRNA molecule, causing massive errors in translation.
c. Often causes protein to end prematurely due to creation of a stop codon
d. Also occurs in eukaryotic cells

3. **Transposons** (Figure 10-7)

FIGURE 10-7 **Transposons**

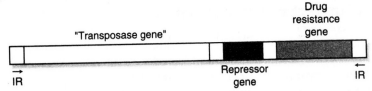

IR=inverted repeats

a. Called "jumping genes" because they transfer pieces of DNA from one bacterium to another
b. Transposons can integrate small pieces of DNA into the bacterial genome, plasmids, or bacteriophages.
c. Integration of transposon DNA into the host genome can occur within a pre-existing gene and render the host gene useless.
d. Each transposon has 4 domains:
   (1) **Inverted repeats**—appear at the ends and mediate integration of the transposon into a DNA molecule
   (2) **Transposase gene**—the enzyme that controls integration and removal of the transposon
   (3) **Repressor gene**—controls synthesis of transposase and whichever gene is in the fourth domain
   (4) **Drug resistance gene**—often appears in the fourth gene domain
e. Transposons replicate with the host DNA and are not capable of independent replication.
f. When transposons integrate and remove themselves from a DNA molecule, they can cause profound mutations.

IV. Genetic Transfer
A. Transfer within a cell
1. Transposons can transfer information between different areas of the same DNA molecule.
2. **Programmed rearrangements**
a. These are performed by certain bacteria including Neisseria, Borrelia, and Trypanosomes.
b. Programmed rearrangements cause a silent gene to be expressed.
c. Programmed rearrangements also allow the organism to evade the immune system.

● Transfer between cells (Table 10-1)

TABLE 10-1	Genetic Transfer Between Prokaryotic Cells	
Mode	**Mechanism**	**Notes**
Transduction	Transfer of DNA from one cell to another using a viral vector	**Generalized conduction** can transfer any gene and contains no viral DNA; **specialized conduction** can transfer only certain genes and contains viral DNA
Conjugation	Transfer of DNA from one bacterium to another via contact and exchange	Can transfer chromosomes or plasmids; utilizes a sex pilus

VIRAL GENETICS

● Comparison of Cells and Viruses (Table 10-2)

In contrast to infectious bacteria and fungi, viruses are not cells. They do not have a nucleus or organelles and are not capable of reproducing independently. Current antiviral agents such as acyclovir or foscarnet can only suppress viral replication. Viral elimination requires an intact host immune response.

TABLE 10-2	Comparison of Cells and Viruses		
	Eukaryotes	**Prokaryotes**	**Viruses**
Size (in micrometers)	7	2–6	0.01–0.2
Membrane-bound organelles	Present	Absent	Absent
Ribosomes	80S	70S	Absent
DNA	46 chromosomes	1 circular chromosome	DNA or RNA; circular, single strand, or multiple segments
Replication	Mitosis or meiosis	Binary fission	Production and assembly

I. Viral Structure (Figure 10-8)

A. Nucleic acid
  1. May be DNA or RNA, but never both
  2. May be single or double stranded
  3. May be linear, segmented, or circular
  4. Most are haploid, but retroviruses are diploid

QUICK HIT Conjugation is carried out by fertility plasmid (F plasmid). A bacterium containing the F plasmid (the male) has a sex pilus which can attach to an F plasmid-deficient bacterium (the female). Once attached, the female is reeled in and DNA is transferred.

QUICK HIT Prions lack most of the features associated with cells or viruses. Prions are thought to be abnormally folded proteins which are capable of catalyzing similar folding in the host's proteins. Accumulation of these abnormally folded proteins can cause spongiform diseases characterized by vacuolization of brain tissues, such as kuru or Creutzfeldt-Jakob disease.

QUICK HIT Viral structure is highly variable between viruses but constant for each particular virus.

FIGURE 10-8 Structure of Viruses

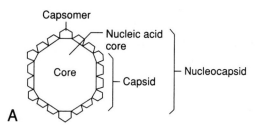

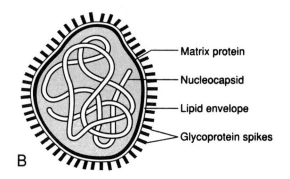

A

B

Matrix protein
Nucleocapsid
Lipid envelope
Glycoprotein spikes

Capsomer
Nucleic acid core
Core
Capsid
Nucleocapsid

B. Capsid
1. The protein coat around the nucleic acid core is composed of repeating units called **capsomeres.**
2. The capsid assumes one of two shapes:
   a. **Helical**—hollow rod shape
   b. **Icosahedral**—multiple triangles arranged into a small sphere
3. The capsid functions to protect the viral nucleic acid.
C. Envelope
1. Surrounds the capsid of some viruses
2. Causes the virus to be more susceptible to drying and lipid solvents
3. Composed of virus-specific lipids and proteins
4. Most **DNA viruses** derive their envelope from the host cell's **nuclear membrane,** while **most RNA viruses** derive their envelope from the host's **cellular membrane.**

II. Replication

A. Attachment
1. Viral surface proteins specifically attach to receptor proteins on the cell surface.
2. The non-covalent interaction of proteins determines host range.
B. Penetration
1. The virus may be engulfed by the host via a pinocytotic vesicle (**viropexis**).
2. Non-enveloped viruses may slip through the host membrane by direct **translocation.**
3. The viral **envelope may fuse with the host cell membrane.**
C. Uncoating
1. DNA viruses partially uncoat in the cytoplasm and undergo final uncoating in the nucleus (to protect the DNA from endonucleases in the cytoplasm).
2. RNA viruses uncoat in the cytoplasm.
D. Expression and replication
1. DNA viruses replicate in the nucleus (except poxvirus) using the host cell's RNA polymerase and other proteins.
2. **Positive single-stranded RNA viruses** contain an mRNA genome which **interacts directly with host ribosomes** for translation of a viral RNA polymerase which completes replication.
3. **Negative single-stranded and double-stranded RNA viruses** are packaged with a **viral RNA polymerase which produces positive RNA** for transcription.
4. Thousands of copies of viral proteins are produced.
5. For the retrovirus life cycle, see discussion of human immunodeficiency virus (HIV) (System 7 "Reproductive System").
E. Assembly
1. DNA viruses are assembled in the nucleus.
2. RNA viruses are assembled in the cytoplasm (except for the influenza virus, which is assembled in the nucleus).
F. Release
1. Non-enveloped viruses usually **rupture the host cell membrane** and release mature particles.
2. Enveloped viruses are released via **budding,** where each mature particle becomes surrounded by a portion of the host cell's membrane.

QUICK HIT The duration of a viral multiplication cycle ranges from 6 hours for poliovirus, to 48 hours for the papovavirus and adenovirus.

QUICK HIT The influenza and retroviruses are the only RNA viruses that replicate in the nucleus.

BASIC CONCEPTS

CONCEPTS IN PHARMACOLOGY

I. Absorption

A. There are many routes of administration (Figure 10-9).

FIGURE
10-9 **Routes of drug administration**

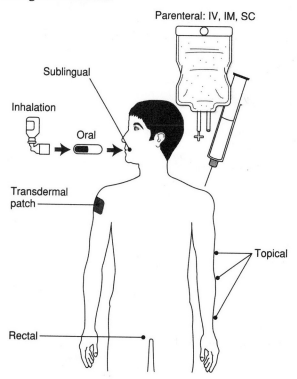

(Adapted from Mycek MJ, Harvey RA, and Champe PC: *Lippincott's Illustrated Reviews: Pharmacology, 2nd edition.*
Philadelphia, Lippincott-Raven Publishers, 1996. p. 2. Used by permission of Lippincott Williams and Wilkins.)
IM=intramuscular; *IV*=intravenous; *SC*=subcutaneous

B. **Oral** administration is the most common route.
C. Most drugs are absorbed in the **duodenum.**
   1. Drugs enter the portal circulation.
   2. They are subject to **first pass metabolism** by the liver.
D. Other factors affect absorption:
   1. pH
   2. Whether taken with food (slows transit allowing for further acid digestion)
   3. Whether the drug is a sustained-release preparation
   4. Whether gastrointestinal diseases or malabsorption syndromes are present

II. Distribution

A. Vd = TD/C

   Where: Vd = **V**olume of **d**istribution, TD = **T**otal **D**rug in body,
   C = plasma **C**oncentration

B. Distribution occurs more rapidly with high blood flow, high vessel
   permeability, and a **hydrophobic drug.**
C. Binding to **plasma proteins** (albumin and globulins) accelerates plasma
   absorption but slows diffusion into tissues.
D. Many disease states alter distribution.
   1. Edematous states (e.g., cirrhosis, heart failure, nephrotic syndrome)
     prolong distribution and delay clearance.

 If a drug is rapidly metabolized by the liver, the amount reaching the target tissues is significantly reduced. Such drugs include propranolol, lidocaine, verapamil, meperidine, and others.

Charged ions do not pass through the GI membrane as readily as uncharged ions. Therefore, the percent of drug in the uncharged state determines the rate of absorption.

$$pH = pK_a + log \frac{unprotonated}{protonated\ species}$$

 When infusing a drug, it takes 4.3 half lives to achieve 95% of the steady state concentration.

 Acidophilic drugs bind albumin while basophilic drugs bind globulins. The administration of a drug that binds to sites already occupied by a drug can displace the first drug. This leads to a surge in free drug, which in turn leads to increased activity and elimination.

2. Obesity allows for greater accumulation of lipophilic agents within fat cells, increasing distribution and prolonging half-life.
3. Pregnancy increases intravascular volume, thus increasing Vd.
4. Hypoalbuminemia allows drugs that are protein-bound to have increased availability due to lack of albumin for binding.

III. Pharmacokinetics

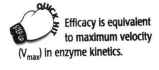

Efficacy is equivalent to maximum velocity (V_{max}) in enzyme kinetics.

A. The effect an agonist has on its receptors depends on concentration.
B. **Efficacy** is a measure of the maximum effect a drug can produce.
C. **Potency** is a measure of the amount of drug needed to produce a given effect (Figure 10-10).

FIGURE
10-10 **Dose response curve**

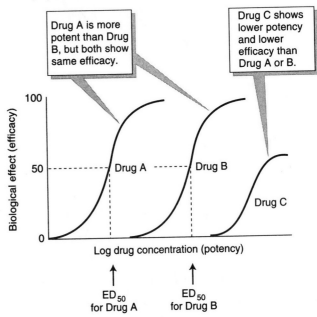

Drug A is more potent than Drug B, but both show same efficacy.

Drug C shows lower potency and lower efficacy than Drug A or B.

ED_{50} for Drug A

ED_{50} for Drug B

ED=effective dose; ED_{50}=dose effective in 50% of population

D. Effective Dose (ED) and Lethal Dose (LD)
1. ED is the dose of the drug which produces the desired effect.
2. ED_{50} is the dose of the drug which produces the desired effect in 50% of the population.
3. LD is the dose of the drug which produces death.
4. LD_{50} is the dose of the drug which produces death in 50% of the population.

5. Overlap of ED and LD determines therapeutic range (Figure 10-11)

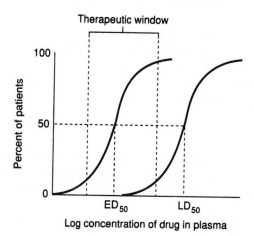

D. Antagonists (Figure 10-12)

Drug Antagonism

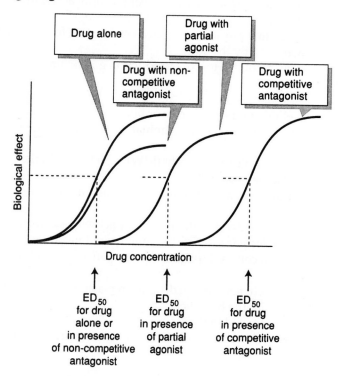

1. Competitive: antagonist competes for the same binding site as the agonist or drug
2. Non-competitive
   a. Antagonist prevents binding of the agonist or drug to the receptor or prevents activation of the receptor by the agonist
   b. Decreases the efficacy of the agonist
3. Partial: binds to the same receptor site as the agonist or drug, but has a lower potency

4. Complete: antagonist prevents all pharmacologic action(s) of the agonist or drug
E. A drug's **therapeutic index (TI)** is a measure of how safe it is to use: $TI = LD_{50}/ED_{50}$ LD=lethal dose for 50% of population, ED=effective dose for 50% of population
F. Pharmacokinetics are affected by disease states:
　1. Hyperthyroidism increases the heart's sensitivity to catecholamines
　2. Cirrhosis patients are more sensitive to sedative-hypnotics
　3. Patients with cirrhosis and congestive heart failure (CHF) will retain fluids if taking NSAIDs due to the role of prostaglandins in maintaining renal function.

IV. Metabolism

A. Drugs may be chemically altered to vary activity or aid excretion.
B. The enzymatic transformation of drugs usually follows one of two kinetics:
　1. **First order:** a constant **fraction** of drug is metabolized in a certain unit of time
　2. **Zero order:** a constant **amount** of drug is metabolized in a certain unit of time (e.g., ethanol)
C. The liver is the primary site of metabolism and employs two sets of reactions:
　1. **Phase 1:** drugs are modified or portions are removed (cytochrome p450 oxidation, enzymatic reduction, hydrolysis)
　2. **Phase 2:** conjugation reactions add elements to the drug (e.g., glucuronidation, sulfate or glutathione conjugation, acetylation, methylation)
D. **Prodrugs** are drugs that are administered in an inactive form and are metabolically activated by the body
E. Some drugs are metabolized to toxic products (e.g., acetaminophen)

V. Elimination

A. Most drugs are eliminated in the urine or bile
B. Volatile drugs (e.g., ethanol) can be eliminated through the lungs
C. **Renal excretion:**
　1. Substances with a molecular weight (MW) < 5000, free in the plasma, are filtered in the glomerulus.
　2. Higher concentrations of a substance within the tubules may favor some reabsorption.
　3. The proximal convoluted tubule (PCT) may actively secrete a drug.
　4. Urine pH, the molecular size, lipid solubility, and negative logarithm of the acid ionization constant (pK_a) of the drug affect renal excretion.
D. **Biliary excretion**
　1. Hepatocytes actively take up the drug from plasma, store it or metabolize it, and release it into the bile duct.
　2. Some drugs are excreted in feces.
　3. Some drugs are reabsorbed in the terminal ileum (**enterohepatic cycling**).

VI. Special circumstances

A. Older patients
　1. These patients often utilize multiple prescription and "over the counter" medications.
　2. Decreased body size, body water, and serum albumin, along with increased body fat alter drug distribution.
　3. **Decreased phase 1 reactions,** liver mass, and liver blood flow all slow metabolism.
　4. Decreased kidney mass, renal blood flow, and tubular function hamper drug excretion.

QUICK HIT Ethanol, barbiturates, and phenytoin induce p450 enzymes, while cimetidine and ketocoazole inhibit p450 enzymes, increasing and decreasing the metabolism of other drugs, respectively (e.g., warfarin). The macrolide antibiotics (e.g., erythromycin) inhibit p450 enzymes and increase the cardiac toxicity of cisapride.

QUICK HIT Filtration is dependent upon the amount of free drug in the blood, while active secretion is dependent upon the total plasma concentration (free and bound drug).

B. Pediatric patients
   1. **Most drugs cross the placenta** to some extent and their possible effects on the fetus are ranked as category A, B, C, D, and X (A=no risk, X=risk outweighs benefit).
   2. Absorption
      a. High gastric pH and delayed emptying affect enteral absorption in infancy.
      b. High surface area to volume ratio affects transdermal administration.
      c. Low muscle mass limits IM administration to the **vastus lateralis** in infancy.
   3. Albumin does not reach adult levels until one year of age.
   4. Both phases of metabolism are deficient to varying degrees until 1–2 years of age.
   5. Specific antibiotics avoided in childhood include **quinolones** (articular cartilage erosion) and **tetracycline** (depression of bone/teeth formation).
D. Pharmacogenetics
   1. Acetylation of isoniazid:
      a. **In patients who are slow acetylators,** there is increased incidence of neuropathy, bladder cancer, and familial Parkinson's disease.
      b. **Patients who are rapid acetylators** are the majority of the population.
      c. Also affects metabolism of hydralazine, dapsone, and phenytoin
   2. Succinylcholine sensitivity
      a. Atypical **pseudocholinesterase** does not hydrolyze scoline as effectively
      b. Leads to prolonged paralysis (scoline apnea)
      c. **Autosomal recessive**
   3. Ethanol metabolism
      a. **Aldehyde dehydrogenase** shows diminished activity in certain patients (50% of Chinese and Japanese)
      b. Acetaldehyde accumulation leads to facial flushing, headache, nausea, and vomiting.
C. Toxicology (Table 10-3)

TABLE 10-3 Toxicology	
Poison	**Therapy**
Acetaminophen	N-acetylcysteine
Aspirin	Alkalinization of urine
Benzodiazepine	Flumazenil
Carbon monoxide	100% oxygen
Cyanide	Sodium nitrite
Digitalis	Digitalis antibody or potassium (if serum potassium level is low)
Ethylene glycol, methanol, isopropyl alcohol	Ethanol
Heavy metals	Calcium EDTA (for lead); dimercaprol (for arsenic, mercury); penicillamine (for copper); deferoxamine (for iron)
Heparin	Protamine sulfate
Opioids	Naloxone
Propranolol	Glucagon
Tricyclic antidepressants	Gastric lavage, alkalinization of serum
Warfarin	Vitamin K
EDTA=ethylenediamine tetraacetic acid	

ENZYME KINETICS

I. Enzymes

A. An enzyme is a substance that **decreases the energy of activation for a reaction** (Figure 10-13)

FIGURE 10-13 **Enzyme effect on a chemical reaction**

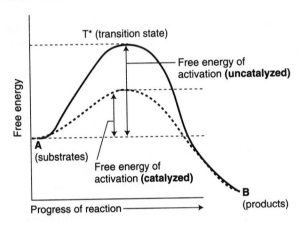

B. By lowering the energy of activation, enzymes increase the rate of reaction.

C. Enzymes **do not alter the equilibrium** of substrates and products, which is concentration-dependent.

II. Kinetics

A. **Velocity** (v) is the rate of reaction and is dependent upon enzyme concentration, substrate concentration, temperature, and pH.

1. Enzyme concentration: increased enzyme concentration leads to faster rate of reaction
2. Substrate concentration: increased concentration leads to increased rate of reaction, until a maximum is reached when all enzyme receptor sites are saturated
3. Temperature: increased temperature leads to increased rate of reaction up to a maximum, after which enzymes denature
4. pH: velocity of a reaction is maximum at its optimal pH. A pH that is either too high or too low leads to a slower reaction or may denature the enzyme

B. Michaelis-Menten equation

1. Enzymatically catalyzed reactions can be characterized by the Michaelis-Menten equation:

$$v = V_m \times [S] / (K_m + [S])$$

where: v is the velocity of the reaction.

V_m is the maximum velocity of the reaction.

[S] is the substrate concentration.

K_m is the Michaelis constant (the substrate concentration at which velocity is one-half of the maximum velocity of a given reaction; $v = 1/2V_m$).

2. Effect of substrate concentration on reaction velocity (Figure 10-14)

FIGURE
10-14 Effect of substrate concentration on reaction velocity

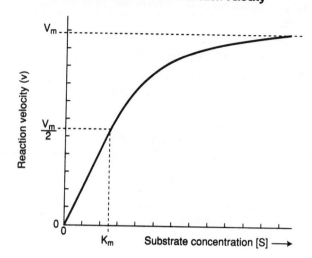

V_m = Maximum velocity
V = Velocity
K_m = Michaelis constant, where v = 1/2 V_m

C. Lineweaver-Burk plots (Figure 10-15)

FIGURE
10-15 Lineweaver-Burk plot

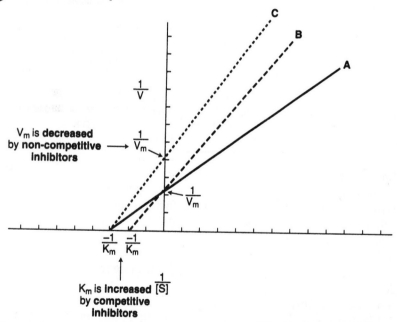

V_m is **decreased**
by **non-competitive** → $\frac{1}{V_m}$
inhibitors

$\frac{1}{V_m}$

$\frac{-1}{K_m}$ $\frac{-1}{K_m}$

K_m is **increased** $\frac{1}{[S]}$
by **competitive**
inhibitors

A = No inhibitor
B = Competitive inhibitor
C = Non-competitive inhibitor

[S] = Substrate concentration
v = Reaction velocity
V_m = Maximum velocity
K_m = Michaelis constant

$\frac{1}{V_m}$ is where the plot crosses the y axis

$\frac{-1}{K_m}$ is where the plot crosses the x axis

1. A Lineweaver-Burk plot is a linear representation of the Michaelis-Menten equation, which allows for easier interpretation of the maximum velocity of an equation
2. Lineweaver-Burk equation:

$$1/v = K_m / (V_m \times [S]) + 1/V_m$$

a. Competitive inhibitors increase the K_m
b. Non-competitive inhibitors decrease the V_m

BIOSTATISTICS AND EPIDEMIOLOGY

I. Sensitivity and Specificity (Table 10-4)

TABLE 10-4 Sensitivity and Specificity

Test Results		Disease States	
		Have disease	Do not have disease
	+	True Positive (TP)	False Positive (FP)
	−	False Negative (FN)	True Negative (TN)

Terminology	Equation	Definition
Sensitivity	TP/(TP+FN)	Probability that a person having a disease will be correctly identified
Specificity	TN/(TN+FP)	Probability that a person who does not have a disease will be correctly identified
Positive predictive value	TP/(TP+FP)	Probability that an individual who tests positive has disease
Negative predictive value	TN/(TN+FN)	Probability that an individual who tests negative does not have the disease
Prevalence	TP+FN/(TP+FP+TN+FN)	Total number of cases in a population at a given time
Incidence	Generally calculated by: Prevalence × Length of disease process	Number of new cases of disease in the population over a given time

High sensitivity tests are better suited for screening purposes, while high specificity tests are used as confirmatory tests.

For chronic conditions (e.g., diabetes or cirrhosis), the prevalence is higher than the incidence because the long length of disease process increases prevalence. For conditions that resolve quickly (i.e., strep throat) or are rapidly fatal (i.e., pancreatic cancer), the incidence and prevalence are approximately equal.

The most rigorous form of a clinical trial is the **double-blind study** where neither the subject nor the examiner knows which drug the subject is receiving. Single-blind, double-blind, crossover, and placebo studies are done to reduce bias.

II. Cohort Studies
A. Prospective and observational
B. After assessment of exposure to a risk factor, subjects are compared to each other over a period of time
C. Clinical treatment trial
 1. Highest quality cohort study
 2. Compares the therapeutic benefits of 2 or more treatments
D. **Relative Risk**
 1. Calculated only for cohort studies
 2. Compares incidence rate in exposed group to incidence rate in unexposed individuals

III. Case-control studies
A. Retrospective and observational
B. Subjects with and without disorder are identified and information on exposure to risk factors is assessed
C. **Odds ratio**
 1. Used to determine relative risk in case-control studies

2. Based on disease occurring with or without exposure
3. Odds ratio = TP × TN/FP × FN

where: TP = True Positives
             TN = True Negatives
             FP = False Positives
             FN = False Negatives

IV. Testing and Statistical Methods

A. Reliability versus validity
1. **Reliability** refers to the reproducibility of test results either between examiners or between test-takers
2. **Validity** refers to the appropriateness of a test's measurements (i.e., the test measures what it is supposed to)
3. **Sensitivity** and **specificity** comprise validity

B. Bell curve (Figure 10-16)

FIGURE 10-16   The Bell Curve

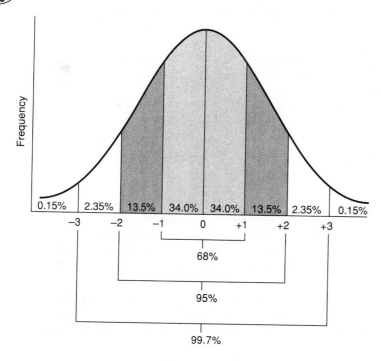

1. In a **normal distribution,** the mean, median, and mode are **equal.**
   a. Mean: average
   b. Median: middle value in a sequentially ordered group of numbers
   c. Mode: number that appears most often in a group
2. A bimodal distribution has two peaks.
3. Skew refers to the way a peak may be offset.
   a. **Positive skew:** peak is to the left (most scores at low end; mean > median > mode)
   b. **Negative skew:** peak is to the right (most scores at high end; mean < median < mode)

C. The **Null hypothesis** (H$_0$)
1. Postulates that there is no difference between groups
2. **Probability (p) value:** the chance of a type I error occurring (rejecting the null hypothesis when the null hypothesis is actually true)

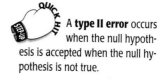

A type II error occurs when the null hypothesis is accepted when the null hypothesis is not true.

3. If p < 0.05, then the null hypothesis can be rejected
4. Example
   a. A study is conducted on the influence of medical school on dating frequency.
   b. The null hypothesis would be that medical school students, when compared to 22- through 26-year-olds in the working population, have no difference in dating frequency.
   c. If the p value of the study is less than 0.05 (meaning that there is a statistical difference), then the null hypothesis can be rejected.
   d. Furthermore, it can be stated that medical school decreases dating frequency.

V. General statistics

A. Leading causes of mortality
   1. Ages 1–14 years: injuries
   2. Ages 15–24 years: accidents (majority are motor vehicle)
   3. Ages 25–64 years: cancer (lung > breast/prostate > colon)
   4. Ages 65+ years: heart disease
   5. AIDS is the leading cause of death in males between 25 and 44 years of age.

B. Aging
   1. The elderly comprise 12% of the United States population.
      a. They incur 30% of health care costs.
      b. 5% are in nursing homes.
      c. **25% of suicides** are committed by the elderly population.
      d. 15% suffer from dementia.
   2. 75% of men and 50% of women 60–65 years of age have continued interest in sex.
   3. Life expectancy is 8 years longer for women.

C. Family
   1. 95% of people in the U.S. marry.
   2. Approximately 50% of marriages end in divorce.
   3. 50% of children live in an environment with two working parents.
   4. 20% of all families are single-parent households, while 50% of black families are single-parent households.
   5. Abuse
      a. 32% of children under 5 years of age are physically abused.
      b. 25% of children under 8 years of age are sexually abused.
   6. First sexual intercourse usually occurs around 16 years of age.

D. Disorders
   1. At least 25% of the people in the U.S. are obese.
   2. Insomnia occurs in 30% of people.
   3. Alcohol
      a. Highest use is by people 21–34 years of age.
      b. 13% of adults abuse alcohol.
   4. 1.5% chance of becoming schizophrenic (equal occurrence rate in men and women and whites and blacks)
   5. 10% of men and 15%–20% of women get unipolar disorder (depression).
   6. 1% of all individuals get bipolar disorder.

QUICK HIT Hard and fast statistical numbers are rarely sought after as answers on the USMLE Step 1 Exam. However, having a general idea of some select statistics may assist one in answering the vignette style questions.

QUICK HIT Suicide is the second leading cause of death for people 15–24 years of age.

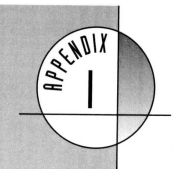

APPENDIX

1

Drug Index

The therapeutic agents shown in boldface type are those which are often emphasized in the classroom and the clinic. Particular attention should be paid to the information about these agents.

Therapeutic Agent (common name, if relevant) [Trade name, where appropriate]	Class—Pharmacology and Pharmacokinetics	Indications	Side or Adverse Effects	Contraindications or Precautions to Consider; Notes
5-Fluorouracil (5-FU)	*Antineoplastic*—inhibits thymidylate synthetase; inhibits RNA synthesis	Colon and breast cancer	Delayed toxicity: nausea, oral and GI ulcers, bone marrow depression	
6-Thioguanine	*Antineoplastic*—inhibits purine synthesis; disrupts DNA and RNA synthesis	Adult leukemias	Bone marrow suppression	
Acarbose [Precose]	*Hypoglycemic agent*—inhibits α-glucosidase; delays absorption of glucose from gut	Oral treatment for NIDDM (type II diabetes)	Flatulence, cramps, diarrhea; may reduce absorption of iron	
Acebutolol [Sectral]	*Antiarrhythmic (Class II)*—antihypertensive; β-blocker			
Acetaminophen [Tylenol]	*Analgesic, antipyretic*— unknown mechanism; not anti-inflammatory	Pain; fever	Liver toxicity in high doses	Overdose treated with N-acetylcysteine
Acetazolamide [Diamox]	*Diuretic*—carbonic anhydrase inhibitor on PCT and DCT; decreases production of aqueous humor in the eye	Diuresis; glaucoma; high altitude	Metabolic acidosis	
Acetohexamide [Dymelor]	*Hypoglycemic agent*—sulfonylurea; reduces K^+ efflux, increases Ca^{2+} influx, increases secretion of insulin	Oral treatment for NIDDM (type II diabetes)	Hypoglycemia; GI disturbances; muscle weakness; mental confusion	Contraindicated in patients with renal and liver impairment
Acetylcholine	*Muscarinic agonist*	Eye surgery (miotic)		
Acetylsalicylic acid (aspirin)	*Anti-inflammatory, antipyretic, analgesic*—acetylates COX irreversibly	Articular, musculoskeletal pain; chronic pain; acute gout	Irritates GI; inhibits platelet aggregation; causes hypersensitivity reactions	Contraindicated for patients with peptic ulcer, asthma, hyperthyroidism, or Parkinsonism
Aciretin	Vitamin A analog	Severe psoriasis	Teratogenic	Contraindicated for children with the flu (leads to Reye's syndrome), gouty patients
ACTH (corticotropin)	Increases production of steroids by the adrenal gland (zona fasciculata)			

Therapeutic Agent (common name, if relevant) [Trade name, where appropriate]	Class—Pharmacology and Pharmacokinetics	Indications	Side or Adverse Effects	Contraindications or Precautions to Consider; Notes
Acyclovir [Zovirax]	*Antiviral*—guanosine analog; inhibits DNA polymerase	Herpes, varicella, EBV, CMV (at high doses)	GI disturbances; CNS; renal problems; headache; tremor; rash	
Adenosine [Adenocard]	*Antiarrhythmic*—short duration; decreases conduction velocity; prolongs refractory period	Supraventricular tachycardia	Flushing; chest pain; hypotension	
Albendazole [Albenza]	*Anthelminthic*	Ascaris (roundworm), Ancylostoma (hookworm), Trichuris (whipworm), Strongyloides	Teratogenic; embryotoxic	Contraindicated in pregnant patients
Albuterol [Proventil, Ventolin]	*Bronchodilatation*—β_2-agonist	Asthma		
Alcohol (EtOH)	Acts at $GABA_a$ receptor	Sedative; hypnotic; depressive action on brain		
Alendronate [Fosamax]	*Bone stabilizer*—pyrophosphate analog; reduces hydroxyapatite crystal formation, growth, and dissolution, which reduces bone turnover	Hypercalcemia of malignancy; Paget's disease; osteoporosis; hyperparathyroidism		
Alfentanil [Alfenta]	*Opioid analgesic*	General anesthetic		
Allopurinol [Zyloprim]	*Antigout*—competitive inhibitor of xanthine oxidase	Chronic gout (due to renal obstruction or impairment or overproduction); rheumatic arthritis	Rash; fever; GI problems; hepatotoxicity; inhibition in the metabolism of other drugs; enhance effect of azathioprine	
α_2-macroglobulin	Inhibits fibrinolysis			
α_2-antiplasmin	Inhibits fibrinolysis			
α-bungarotoxin	Post-synaptic neuromuscular junction blocker; irreversibly binds nicotinic receptor			
Alprazolam [Xanax]	*Antianxiety*—benzodiazepine	Panic attack		
Alprostadil [Vasoprost]	Impotency therapy; prostaglandin E_1	Impotency; maintain patent ductus arteriosus	Penile pain; prolonged erection; flushing, bradycardia, tachycardia, hypotension, apnea	
Aluminum hydroxide	Antacid	Gastric irritability		Constipation

Drug	Mechanism / Class	Uses	Side Effects	Notes
Amantadine [Symmetrel]	*Antiviral—anti-Parkinsonian;* inhibits fusion of lysosomes; inhibits uncoating; increases release of endogenous dopamine	Influenza A; Parkinson's disease	Anti-cholinergic; nervousness; insomnia; drowsiness; GI disturbances	Oral administration
Amicar (EACA)	Competitive inhibition of plasminogen activation	Inhibits fibrinolysis; promotes thrombosis		
Amikacin [Amikin]	*Antibiotic*—aminoglycoside; binds 30s ribosome subunits; bacteriostatic at low concentration; bactericidal at high concentration	Proteus, Pseudomonas, Enterobacter	Ototoxicity; neurotoxicity	
Amiloride [Midamor]	*Diuretic*—K+ sparing; inhibits Na+ transport in the DCT	Diuresis	Hyperkalemia	
Aminoglutethimide [Cytadren]	*Antineoplastic*—aromatase inhibitor; inhibits adrenal steroid synthesis	Cancer		
Aminoglycosides	*Antibiotic*—binds 30s ribosome subunits; bacteriostatic at low concentration; bactericidal at high concentration	Broad spectrum: gram positive and negative; good for bone infections	Auditory, vestibular, renal toxicity; nausea; vomiting; vertigo; allergic skin rash; super-infections	
Amiodarone [Cordarone]	*Antiarrhythmic (Class III)*—K+ channel blocker	Ventricular/supraventricular arrhythmias	Bradycardia; heart block/failure; pulmonary fibrosis; photodermatitis	Also functions as class IA, 2, and 4
Amitriptyline [Elavil]	*Antidepressant*—TCA; blocks 5-HT and NE reuptake	Sedative; anti-depressant; prophylaxis for migraines		
Amobarbital [Amytal sodium]	*Sedative*—hypnotic; barbiturate; prolong IPSP duration	Anti-epileptic; cerebral edema; anesthetic		
Amodiaquine	*Anti-malarial*—uncertain mechanism	Suppression and treatment of acute attacks	Headache; GI and visual disturbances; pruritus; prolonged therapy may lead to retinopathy	
Amoxicillin + Clavulanic acid [Augmentin]	*Antibiotic*—inhibits β-lactamase; synergistic with penicillins			
Amphetamine	*Stimulant*—releases norepinephrine, serotonin, dopamine	Narcolepsy; attention deficit disorder; weight reduction	Psychosis; hallucinations	
Amphotericin B [Fungizone]	*Antifungal*—binds to cell membrane sterols (esp. ergosterol); forms pores in membrane; fungicidal	Candida, Histoplasma, Cryptococcus, Sporothrix	Hypersensitivity; flushing; chills; fever; headache; pain; hypotension; convulsions; thrombophlebitis; anemia; vomiting; impairment of renal function	

Therapeutic Agent (common name, if relevant) [Trade name, where appropriate]	Class—Pharmacology and Pharmacokinetics	Indications	Side or Adverse Effects	Contraindications or Precautions to Consider; Notes
Amrinone [Inocor]	*Inotropic agent*—phosphodiesterase inhibitor; increases contractility via increase in intracellular Ca^{2+}	CHF	Thrombocytopenia	
Anistreplase (APSAC) [Eminase]	*Thrombolytic*—plasminogen activator	Lysis of clots	Hemorrhage	Active compound via deacylation by esterase
Anthraquinones	*Laxative*—reduce absorption of electrolytes and water from gut	Stimulant laxative		
Antiprogesterone [RU-486, Mifepristone]	*Abortive agent*—progesterone receptor blocker	Abortion		
Aprotinin [Trasylol]	*Hemostatic agent*—anti-plasmin activator	Inhibits fibrinolysis; promotes thrombosis		
Asparaginase [Elspar]	*Antineoplastic*—deprives cells of asparagine	Cancer	Fever; mental depression; coma; hepatotoxicity	
Atenolol [Tenormin]	**Antihypertensive**—**β$_1$-blocker**	**Hypertension, angina**		
Atorvastatin [Lipitor]	**Lipid lowering agent**—**inhibits HMG-CoA reductase; lowers LDL**	**Hyperlipidemia (esp. type II)**	**Liver toxicity; myopathy; mild GI disturbances**	**Contraindicated in pregnant or lactating women and children**
Atracurium [Tracrium injection]	Non-depolarizing neuromuscular blocker			Minimal histamine release
Atropine	Cholinergic blocker	Dries salivary secretions; Parkinson's disease; peptic ulcer; diarrhea; GI spasm; bladder spasm; COPD; asthma; cholinomimetic poisoning; anti-diarrheal; anti-emetic; high dose: vasodilatation due to histamine release	**Dry mouth; hyperthermia; mydriasis; tachycardia; hot and flushed skin; agitation; delirium**	**Contraindicated in patients with glaucoma and elderly men with BPH**
Auranofin [Ridaura]	*Anti-rheumatic*—gold salt (oral)	Rheumatic arthritis	Skin eruption; itching; toxic nephritis; bone marrow suppression	
Aurothioglucose [Solganal]	*Anti-rheumatic*—gold salt	Rheumatic arthritis	Skin eruption; itching; toxic nephritis; bone marrow suppression	
Aurothiomalate	*Anti-rheumatic*—gold salt	Rheumatic arthritis	Skin eruption; itching; toxic nephritis; bone marrow suppression	
Azathioprine [Imuran]	*Immunosuppressant*—purine antagonist; inhibits nucleic acid metabolism; blocks both CMI and humoral response	Transplant (esp. kidney); acute glomerulonephritis; renal component of lupus; rheumatoid arthritis	Bone marrow depression; rash; fever; nausea; vomiting; hepatotoxicity; malignancy; GI intolerance	Metabolized by xanthine oxidase
Azlocillin	*Antibiotic*—β-lactam	Pseudomonas; Proteus		IV

Drug	Class/Mechanism	Clinical use	Adverse effects	Notes
Aztreonam [Azactam]	*Antibiotic*—inhibits transpeptidase and cell wall synthesis; monocyclic β lactam	Gram-negative bacteria		
Bacitracin	*Antibiotic*—inhibits cell wall formation; bactericidal	Gram-positive bacteria	Nephrotoxic	Topical only
Baclofen [Lioresal]	*Skeletal muscle relaxant*—GABA mimetic; works at the GABA$_b$ receptor	Muscle spasms; tetanus contractions; orthopedic manipulation		
BCNU (Carmustine)	*Antineoplastic*—DNA alkylation	Cancer	Delayed bone marrow suppression; lung and kidney damage	
Benserazide	*Anti-Parkinson's*—inhibits decarboxylase (L-DOPA to dopamine) in periphery	Parkinson's disease		
Benztropine [Cogentin]	*Anti-Parkinson's*—muscarinic blocker; H$_1$ blocker	Parkinson's disease		
Bephenium hydroxynaphthoate	*Antihelmintic*—cholinergic agonist causing contraction, then relaxation in worm	Necator and Ancylostoma (hookworms)	Vomiting	
Bethanechol [Urecholine, Duvoid]	**Muscarinic agonist**	**Atony of bladder; paralytic ileum**	**Contraindicated in patients as peptic ulcer, asthma, hyperthyroid, Parkinson's**	
Bis-chloroethylamines (nitrogen mustards) [Mustargen]	*Antineoplastic*—**DNA alkylation and cross-linking**	**Cancer**	**Nausea; vomiting; bone marrow suppression; alopecia; teratogenicity; carcinogenicity**	
Bismuth (colloidal) [Pepto-Bismol]	*Anti-ulcer, antidiarrheal*—cytoprotective	**Bactericidal for H. pylori (with ranitidine and clarithromycin)**		
Black widow spider venom	*Presynaptic neuromuscular junction blocker*—overstimulates ACh release			
Bleomycin [Blenoxane]	*Antineoplastic*—**binds, intercalates, and cuts DNA**	**Cancer**	**Fever; blistering; stomatitis; pulmonary fibrosis**	
Botulinum [Botox, Dysport]	*Neuromuscular blocker*—pre-synaptic neuromuscular junction blocker; prevents ACh release			
Bretylium [Bretylol]	*Antiarrhythmic (Class III)*—K$^+$ channel blocker		**Arrhythmias; orthostatic hypotension; nausea; vomiting**	

Therapeutic Agent (common name, if relevant) [Trade name, where appropriate]	Class—Pharmacology and Pharmacokinetics	Indications	Side or Adverse Effects	Contraindications or Precautions to Consider; Notes
Bromocriptine [Parlodel]	**Anti-Parkinson's—agonist at D_2; partial antagonist at D_1**	**Parkinson's disease; acromegaly (paradoxical effect—releases growth hormone from normal pituitary)**	**Inhibits prolactin release**	
Buclizine	*Anti-emetic*		Sedation; Parkinsonism	
Bumetanide [Bumex]	*Loop diuretic*—inhibits $Na^+/K^+/Cl^-$ reabsorption in the Loop of Henle	Congestive heart failure; diuresis	Ototoxicity; hyperuricemia; acute hypovolemia; hypokalemia; metabolic alkalosis; hyperglycemia	
Bupivacaine	*Anesthetic*—blocks Na^+ channel intracellularly	Local anesthetic	Sleepiness; light-headedness; visual/audio disturbances; restlessness; nystagmus; shivering; tonic clonic convulsions; death	
Buprenorphine [Buprenex]	*Opioid analog*—mixed agonist/antagonist action	Treatment of opioid/cocaine dependence		
Bupropion [Wellbutrin, Zyban]	***Antidepressant*—agonist at Da, 5-HT**	**Depression; smoking cessation**		
Buspirone [BuSpar]	*Antidepressant*—benzodiazepine-like agonist	Depression		
Butorphanol [Stadol]	***Opioid analog*—mixed agonist/antagonist action**	**Similar to pentazocine**		
Caffeine [NoDoz]	***Stimulant*—phosphodiesterase inhibitor, resulting in increased cAMP; stimulates CNS and cardiac smooth muscle; relaxes smooth muscle; produces diuresis; increases cerebrovascular resistance**	**Acute migraine attack**		
Calcitonin [Calcimar, Miacalcin]	***Hypocalcemic agent*—anti-osteoporotic agent; lowers plasma Ca^{2+} and phosphate; inhibits bone and kidney reabsorption**	**Hypercalcemia; Paget's disease; osteoporosis**		
Calcium carbonate [Caltrate]	*Dietary Ca^{2+} supplement*	Ca^{2+} deficiency		

Drug	Mechanism/Class	Use	Side effects	Notes
Calcium citrate	*Dietary Ca²⁺ supplement*	Ca^{2+} deficiency		
Calcium gluconate	*Dietary Ca²⁺ supplement*	Ca^{2+} deficiency		
Calcium lactate	*Dietary Ca²⁺ supplement*	Ca^{2+} deficiency		
Captopril [Capoten]	**Antihypertensive–heart failure agent; post-MI agent; vasodilator; ACE inhibitor**	**Congestive heart failure**	**Postural hypotension; renal insufficiency; hyperkalemia; persistent dry cough**	**Contraindicated in pregnancy**
Carbachol [Isopto carbachol]	*Anti-glaucoma agent-*muscarinic agonist	Miotic; glaucoma		Contraindicated in patients by peptic ulcer, asthma, hyperthyroid, and Parkinson's disease
Carbamazepine [Tegretol]	*Anti-epileptic-*Na⁺ channel blocker; decreases glutamate (and other excitatory neuro-transmitters)	Epilepsy (partial and tonic-clonic); trigeminal neuralgia	**Agranulocytosis**	Induces cytochrome P450
Carbidopa [Sinemet]	*Anti-Parkinson's—*inhibits decarboxylase (L-DOPA to dopamine) in periphery	Parkinson's disease; used with levodopa as Sinemet		
Carboplatin [Paraplatin]	*Antineoplastic-* cross-links DNA	Cancer	Bone marrow and renal toxicity; cystitis; peripheral neuropathy; ototoxicity; alopecia (severe)	Platinum containing
Carboprost [Prostin]	*Abortive agent-*PGF₂α	Therapeutic abortion		
Castor oil	*Laxative—*Reduce absorption of electrolytes and water from gut; active component is ricinoleic acid	Stimulant laxative	Nausea; vomiting; diarrhea	
Cephalosporins	*Antibiotic–*inhibits transpeptidase and cell wall synthesis	3rd generation cephalosporins are used for meningitis, Klebsiella, Lyme disease, and gram-negative bacteria	**Allergic reactions; pain at injection site; thrombophlebitis; bleeding disorders**	**1st generation: cefazolin, cephalexin; 2nd generation: cefaclor, cefoxitin, cefuroxime; 3rd generation: ceftriaxone; 4th generation: cefepime**
Chloral hydrate	*Anesthetic agent*	Sedative; hypnotic		Inexpensive
Chlorambucil [Leukeran]	*Antineoplastic-*DNA alkylation and cross-linking	Cancer	Nausea; vomiting; bone marrow suppression (mild); alopecia, teratogenicity, carcinogenicity, pulmonary fibrosis	
Chloramphenicol [Chloromycetin]	*Antibiotic—*binds 50s ribosome subunits; bacteriostatic, but bactericidal versus *Haemophilus influenzae* and *Neisseria meningitidis*	Broad-spectrum versus gram-negatives; typhoid fever; salmonella; Rocky Mountain spotted fever in children	Red cell anemia; bone marrow aplasia; gray baby syndrome	Interactions with phenytoin, warfarin, or coumarin; inhibits P450

Therapeutic Agent (common name, if relevant) [Trade name, where appropriate]	Class–Pharmacology and Pharmacokinetics	Indications	Side or Adverse Effects	Contraindications or Precautions to Consider; Notes
Chlordiazepoxide [Libritabs]	*Anti-anxiety*–benzodiazepine; enhances GABA; increases IPSP amplitude	Sedative; hypnotic; anti-anxiety; anti-epileptic		
Chloroquine phosphate [Aralen]	*Anti-malarial* —uncertain mechanism	**Suppression of malaria and treatment of acute attack; amebiasis; clonorchis;rheumatoid arthritis; SLE**	**Headache; GI disturbances; visual disturbances; pruritus; prolonged therapy may lead to retinopathy**	
Chlorpheniramine [Chlor-Trimeton]	*Antihistamine*–H$_1$ blocker	Allergies; motion sickness	Sedation; CNS depression; atropine-like effects; allergic dermatitis; blood dyscrasias; teratogenicity; acute anti-histamine poisoning	
Chlorpromazine [Thorazine]	*Anti-emetic,anti-psychotic*— blocks D$_2$ receptors	Anti-psychotic; anti-emetic; hiccups	Parkinsonism; tardive dyskinesia; orthostatic hypotension; anti-cholinergic effects; sedation; jaundice; photosensitivity, teratogenic	
Chlorpropamide [Diabinese]	*Hypoglycemic agent*–sulfonylurea; reduces K$^+$ efflux, increases Ca^{2+} influx, increases secretion of insulin	Oral treatment for NIDDM (type II diabetes)	Hypoglycemia; GI disturbances; muscle weakness; mental confusion	
Cholestyramine [Questran]	*Lipid lowering*–impedes fat absorption; lowers LDL; binds cholesterol metabolites	**Reduction of cholesterol**	**Steatorrhea; constipation; impairment of absorption of drugs/vitamins**	**Inhibits warfarin absorption**
Chlorguanide	*Antimalarial*—**inhibits dihydrofolate reductase**	**Prophylaxis for falciparum; suppression of vivax**	**Minor GI upset**	
Chlorprocaine	*Anesthetic*—Block Na$^+$ channel intracellularly	Local anesthetic	Sleepiness; light-headedness; visual/audio disturbances; restlessness; nystagmus; shivering; tonic-clonic convulsions, death	
Chorionic gonadotropin [Pregnyl]	*Infertility therapy*—LH-like in action	Treat infertility; induces ovulation; induces masculinization in infertile men; diagnostic for cryptorchidism in young boys		

Drug [brand]	Class / mechanism	Clinical use	Side effects / notes
Cimetidine [Tagamet]	*H₂ blocker*	Inhibition of gastric acid secretion (esp. ulcers)	Gynecomastia; rare: headache, dizziness, fatigue, CNS, weak anti-androgenic effect, leukopenia, reduced sperm count	Inhibits metabolism and/or absorption of some drugs; inhibits cytochrome P450
Ciprofloxacin [Cipro]	*Quinolone antibiotic*—blocks DNA synthesis by inhibiting DNA gyrase	Gram-negative infections (esp. UTI and bone): Pseudomonas, Enterobacteriaceae, Neisseria; gram positive infections; intracellular: Legionella	GI disturbances; headache; dizziness; phototoxicity; cartilage damage	May elevate theophylline to toxic levels causing seizure
Cisapride [Propulsid]	*GI stimulant*—agonist at 5-HT₄; pro-kinetic	Increases stomach motility		Arrhythmias; taken off the market
Cisplatin [Platinol]	*Anti-neoplastic*—cross-links DNA	Cancer	Bone marrow and renal toxicity; cystitis; peripheral neuropathy; ototoxicity; alopecia (severe)	
Clavulanic acid	*Antibiotic*—β-lactamase inhibitor; synergistic with penicillins			
Clindamycin [Cleocin]	*Antibiotic*—binds to 50s subunits; bacteriostatic or bactericidal	Gram-positive bone infections; anaerobic infections	Severe diarrhea; potentially fatal pseudomembranous colitis due to *Clostridium difficile*	
Clofazimine [Lamprene]	*Antibiotic*—anti-leprosy; unknown mechanism	Mycobacterium leprae	Turns skin red-brown or black	
Clofibrate [Atromid-S]	*Lipid lowering agent*—lowers VLDL, TG, cholesterol; increases activity of LPL; inhibits lipolysis; increases HDL	Hyperlipidemia (esp. type III)	Increased risk of GI and liver cancer; potentiates anticoagulant drugs; myositis; gallstones; mild GI disturbances	LDL may rise, thus no change in total cholesterol
Clomiphene [Clomid]	*Ovulation stimulant*—partial estrogen receptor agonist; decreases estrogen feedback inhibition of GnRH; leads to increase in gonadotropin secretion	Stimulates ovulation in infertility	Ovarian enlargement	
Clonazepam [Klonopin]	*Antiepileptic*—benzodiazepine	Epilepsy (absence seizures)		
Clonidine [Catapres]	*Antihypertensive*—α₂-agonist	Hypertension; smoking withdrawal; heroin and cocaine withdrawal	Drowsiness; dry mouth; rebound hypertension after abrupt withdrawal	

Therapeutic Agent (common name, if relevant) [Trade name, where appropriate]	Class—Pharmacology and Pharmacokinetics	Indications	Side or Adverse Effects	Contraindications or Precautions to Consider; Notes
Clotrimazole [Lotrimin, Mycelex]	*Antifungal*—inhibit ergosterol synthesis, so cell membrane can't form	Topical use against dermatophytes, ringworm, fungi, mold, and oral candidiasis in AIDS		
Cloxacillin [Apo-cloxi, Cloxapen]	*Antibiotic*—β-lactam; penicillinase resistant	Staph infections		
Clozapine [Clozaril]	*Antipsychotic*—blocks D_2 and 5-HT_2 receptors; also blocks D_4	Anti-psychotic	Orthostatic hypotension; sedation; agranulocytosis	
Cocaine	*CNS stimulant*—blocks norepinephrine, serotonin, and dopamine reuptake	Local anesthetic	Vasoconstriction; hypertension; nasal mucus ischemia	
Codeine	Opioid agonist	Good anti-tussive; moderate for pain		
Colchicine	*Antigout*—inhibits phagocytosis and secretion of inflammatory mediators; decreases LTB_4	Acute gout	Nausea; diarrhea; vomiting; abdominal cramps	Contraindicated in elderly and feeble patients and in patients with GI disturbances, cardiac anomalies, or renal problems
Colestipol [Colestid]	*Lipid lowering agent*—impedes fat absorption; lowers LDL; binds cholesterol metabolites	Reduction of cholesterol	Steatorrhea; constipation; impaired absorption of drugs and vitamins	
Corticotropin-releasing hormone (CRH)	Increases ACTH production by anterior pituitary	Used in diagnosis of Cushing's syndrome		
Cortisol (hydrocortisone) [Hydrocortone, Nutracort]	*Glucocorticoid*—induces new protein synthesis; increases gluconeogensis and lipolysis; reduces peripheral glucose use; catabolism effect on muscle, bone, skin, fat, lymph tissue; anti-inflammatory; immunosuppressant	Adrenal insufficiency; congenital adrenal hyperplasia; diagnosis of pituitary-adrenal disorder; reduce inflammation (esp. chronic); leukemia; decrease hypercalcemia	Iatrogenic Cushing's syndrome; redistribution of fat; acne; insomnia; weight gain; hypo-kalemia; decrease in skeletal muscle; osteoporosis; hyper-glycemia; ulcers; psychosis; cataracts; increased susceptibility to infections; growth suppression in children	
Cosyntropin [Cortrosyn]	*ACTH analog*—increases production of steroids by adrenal	Used in diagnosis of adreno-cortical insufficiency		
Cromolyn [Nasalcrom, Gastrocrom]	*Anti-asthmatic*—anti-allergic; inhibits histamine release from mast cells	Prophylaxis for asthma	Laryngeal edema (rare)	

Drug	Class/Mechanism	Clinical Use	Toxicity/Side Effects
Cyanocobalamine (Anacobin)	Supplies vitamin B₁₂	B₁₂ deficiency	
Cyclizine [Marezine]	*Anti-emetic*—H₁ blocker	Nausea and vomiting	
Cyclobenzaprine [Flexeril]	*Centrally acting muscle relaxant*	Muscle spasms; tetanus contractions; orthopedic manipulation	Teratogenic; Anti-muscarinic effects
Cyclophosphamide [Cytoxan]	*Immunosuppressant*—**alkylating agent; destroys proliferating lymphoid cells; alkylates resting cells**	**Transplant rejection; rheumatic arthritis**	**GI and bone marrow toxicity; hemorrhagic cystitis**
Cycloserine [Seromycin]	*Antibiotic*—analog of D-alanine; interferes with cell wall synthesis	Mycobacterium	Psychotic reactions
Cyclosporine [Sandimmune]	*Immunosuppressant*—**inhibits T-helper cell activity; inhibits IL-2, IL-3 and INF-γ formation by T-helper cells**	**Transplant rejection**	**Nephrotoxic; hepatotoxic; hypertension; increased incidence of viral infection and lymphoma**
Cyproheptadine [Periactin]	*Antihistamine*—antipruritic; 5-HT₃ agonist; histamine blocker	Decreases diarrhea in carcinoid tumors; decreases dumping syndrome	Weight gain
Cytosine arabinoside [Cytosar-U]	*Antineoplastic*—inhibits DNA replication and RNA polymerization; competitive inhibitor of dCTP; inhibits chain elongation	Cancer; AML	Severe myelosuppresion; stomatitis; alopecia
Dacarbazine (DTIC-Dome)	*Antineoplastic*—DNA alkylation; strand breakage; inhibits nucleic acid and protein synthesis	Cancer	
Dactinomycin [Cosmegen]	*Antineoplastic*—cross-links DNA; intercalates into DNA	Cancer	Skin eruptions; hyperkeratosis
Danazol [Danocrine]	*Testosterone derivative*—**weak agonist for androgen, progesterone, and glucocorticoid receptors**	**Endometriosis and fibrocystic disease**	**Masculinization in females; gynecomastia in males**
Dantrolene [Dantrium]	*Non-centrally acting muscle relaxant*—**decrease Ca²⁺ from sarcoplasmic reticulum**	**Malignant hypertension**	**Hepatotoxic**
Dapsone [Dapsone]	*Antibiotic*—related to sulfonamides	Mycobacterium leprae	GI disturbances; hemolysis; methemoglobinemia
Daunorubicin [DaunoXome, Cerubidine]	*Antineoplastic*—**oxidizes free radicals; breaks DNA; intercalates into DNA; affects plasma membrane**	**Cancer**	**Cardiac changes resulting in cumulative cardiotoxicity**

Therapeutic Agent (common name, if relevant) [Trade name, where appropriate]	Class—Pharmacology and Pharmacokinetics	Indications	Side or Adverse Effects	Contraindications or Precautions to Consider; Notes
Deferoxamine [Desferal]	*Metal chelator*	**Acute toxicity of iron**	**Hypotensive shock; neurotoxic if long-term use**	
Desflurane [Suprane]	*Anesthetic*	General anesthetic	Irritating to airway	
Desipramine [Norpramin]	*Antidepressant*—TCA; blocks norepinephrine, 5-HT, muscarinic, α₁, and histamine receptors	Depression	Tremors (due to NE block); anorexia (5-HT block); anti-cholinergic (muscarinic block); hypotension (α_1 block); drowsiness (histamine block)	
Desmopressin (DDAVP)	*Antidiuretic*—recruits water channels to luminal membrane in collecting duct	**Anti-diuresis**	**Overhydration; allergic reaction; larger doses result in pallor, diarrhea, hypertension; coronary constriction; chronic rhinopharyngitis**	**Synthetic analog to vasopressin; intranasal administration**
Dexamethasone [Decadron, Maxidex]	*Corticosteroid*—reduces lymph node and spleen size; inhibits cell cycle activity of lymphoid cells; lyses T-cells; suppresses antibody, prostaglandin, and leukotriene synthesis; blocks monocyte production of IL-1	**Anti-emetic; autoimmune disorders; allergic reactions; asthma; organ transplant (esp. during rejection crisis)**	**Insomnia; epigastric disturbances; Cushingoid reaction; psychosis; glucose intolerance; infection; hypertension; cataracts**	
DHEA	Androgen and estrogen precursor		Acne; hair loss; hirsutism; deepening of voice	
Diazepam [Valium]	*Anti-anxiety, benzodiazepine*—enhances GABA; increase IPSP amplitude	**Sedative; hypnotic; anti-anxiety; anti-epileptic (status epilepticus, grand mal)**	**Sedation**	
Diazepam binding inhibitor (DBI)	Benzodiazepine receptor antagonist			
Diclofenac [Cataflam, Voltaren]	*NSAID*—enteric coated			
Dicloxacillin [Dynapen, Pathocil]	*Antibiotic*—β-lactam; penicillinase resistant	Staph infections		
Dicyclomine [Bentyl]	*Anti-muscarinic*	Bladder/GI spasm; decreases acid in ulcer		
Dideoxyinisine [ddI], Didanosine [ddA] [Videx]	*Antiviral*—reverse transcriptase inhibitor	**AIDS**	**Abdominal cramps; diarrhea; peripheral neuropathy; acute pancreatitis**	

Drug	Classification / Mechanism	Clinical Use	Side Effects	Notes / Contraindications
Diethylcarbamazine [Hetrazan]	*Antihelmintic*—sensitizes helminthes to phagocytosis by macrophages	Filariasis	Headache; malaise; joint pain; anorexia; death of filaria causes: swelling and edema of skin, enlarged lymph nodes, hyper-pyrexia, tachycardia	
Diflunisal [Dolobid]	*Anti-inflammatory, antipyretic*	Long-acting pain relief		
Digitoxin [Crystodigin]	*Inotropic agent*—cardiac glycoside; increases cardiac contractility	Severe left ventricular systolic dysfunction	Progressive dysrhythmia; anorexia; nausea; vomiting; headache; fatigue; confusion; blurred vision; altered color perception; halos around dark objects	Contraindicated in patients by right-sided heart failure, diastolic failure, or Wolf-Parkinson-White syndrome; ECG changes: increases PR, decreases QT, depresses ST, inverts T
Digoxin [Lanoxin]	***Inotropic agent—cardiac glycoside; increases cardiac contractility***	**Severe left ventricular systolic dysfunction; antiarrhythmic**	**Progressive dysrhythmia; anorexia; nausea; vomiting; headache; fatigue; confusion; blurred vision; altered color perception; haloes around dark objects**	**Contraindicated in patients by right-sided heart failure, diastolic failure; ECG changes: increases PR, decreases QT, depresses ST, inverts T**
Diiodohydroxyquin [Yodoxin]	*Anti-protozoal; direct action*	Amebae	Subacute myelo-optic neuropathy	
Diltiazem [Cardizem, Dilacor]	***Antiarrhythmic (Class IV)*—Ca^{2+} blocker**	**Angina; AV nodal arrhythmia; decreases blood pressure**		
Dimenhydrinate [Dramamine]	*Anti-vertigo*—anti-emetic; H$_1$ blocker	Emesis; dizziness		
Dimercaprol [BAL in oil, British antlewisite, dimercaptopropanol]	*Metal chelator*	Arsenic, mercury, or cadmium poisoning	Hypertension; tachycardia; headaches; nausea; vomiting; pain at injection site	
Dinoprostone [Cervidil, Prepidil]	*Antihemorrhagic (oxytocin agonist)*—PGE$_2$; increases collagenase	Softening, ripening, dilation of cervix (induces labor)		
Diphenhydramine [Benadryl]	***Anti-Parkinson's*—antihistamine; anti-emetic; muscarinic blocker; H$_1$ blocker**	**Parkinson's disease; asthma; motion sickness; anti-emetic**	**Sedation; CNS depression; atropine-like effects; allergic dermatitis; blood dyscrasias; teratogenicity; acute anti-histamine poisoning**	
Disopyramide [Norpace]	*Antiarrhythmic (Class IA)*—Na$^+$ channel blocker	Wolf-Parkinson-White	Heart failure	Contraindicated in patients with sick sinus syndrome
Disulfiram [Antabuse]	***Anti-alcoholic agent*—inhibits aldehyde dehydrogenase**	**Alcohol ingestion**	**Tachycardia; hyperventilation; nausea**	
Dobutamine [Dobutrex]	***Inotropic agent*—β agonist; positive inotropic effects on the heart and vasodilatation**	**Acute heart failure; increases cardiac output**		

Therapeutic Agent (common name, if relevant) [Trade name, where appropriate]	Class–Pharmacology and Pharmacokinetics	Indications	Side or Adverse Effects	Contraindications or Precautions to Consider; Notes
Doxazosin [Cardura]	Antihypertensive—α_1 blocker	Hypertension		
Doxepin [Sinequan]	Antidepressant, antianxiety—TCA; blocks norepinephrine, 5-HT, muscarinic, α_1, histamine receptors	Antidepressant	Tremors (due to NE block); anorexia (5-HT block); anti-cholinergic (muscarinic block); hypotension (α1 block); drowsiness (histamine block)	
Doxorubicin [Adriamycin]	Antineoplastic—oxidizes free radicals; breaks DNA; intercalates into DNA; affects plasma membrane	Cancer	Cardiac changes resulting in cumulative cardiotoxicity	
Dronabinol [Marinol]	Antiemetic—unknown mechanism; binds opiate receptors and directly inhibits vomiting center in medulla	Antiemetic	Dry mouth; dizziness; inability to concentrate; disorientation; anxiety; tachycardia; depression; paranoia; psychosis	THC derivative
d-Tubocurarine [Tubarine]	Non-depolarizing neuromuscular blocker			
Echothiophate [Phospholine Iodide]	Anti-glaucoma—inhibits cholinesterase; nicotinic receptor stimulator; irreversible	Closed angle glaucoma	Open angle glaucoma	
Edetate calcium disodium (calcium EDTA) [Calcium disodium versenate]	Metal chelator	Lead toxicity	Nephrotoxic	
Edrophonium [Enlon, Tensilon]	Cholinesterase inhibitor	Diagnosis of myasthenia gravis; emergency anesthetic		
Emetine	Anti-protozoal—causes degeneration of nucleus and reticulation of cytoplasm; directly lethal	Severe amebae infection	Diarrhea; nausea; vomiting; abdominal pain; cardiac effects: hypotension, precordial pain, ECG changes	
Enalapril [Vasotec]	Antihypertensive—vasodilator; ACE inhibitor	Congestive heart failure	Postural hypotension; renal insufficiency; hyperkalemia; persistent dry cough	Pregnancy
Encainide	Antiarrhythmia (Class IC)—Na^+ channel blockers	Wolf-Parkinson-White syndrome		No anti-muscarinic action; no effect on action potential
Enflurane [Ethrane]	Anesthetic agent	General anesthetic	Seizure	Abnormal ECG or seizures

Drug	Mechanism	Clinical use	Side effects / Notes	Additional
Ephedrine [Broncholate]	*Bronchodilation*—mixed adrenergic agonist	Stimulates norepinephrine release; anti-tussive; myasthenia gravis	Increases BP	
Epinephrine [Primatene mist]	*Nonspecific adrenergic agonist*—vasoconstrictor	Acute asthma, anaphylactic shock		Activates both α and β receptors, but is preferential for β
Epoprostenol [Flolan]	*Prostacyclin*—increases cardiac index, stroke volume; decreases pulmonary vascular resistance and mean systemic pressure	Pulmonary hypertension		
Ergotamine [Ergomar]	*Anti-migraine*—vasoconstriction	Acute attack of migraine	Gangrene due to vasoconstriction	Contraindicated in pregnant patients or patients with cardiovascular disease or coronary artery disease
Erythromycin [E-Mycin]	*Antibiotic*—binds to the 23s of the 50s ribosome subunits	First choice for cell wall deficient bugs: Mycoplasma, Rickettsia, Chlamydia, Legionella; Cornybacterium diphtheria		
Erythropoietin (EPO) [Procrit, Epogen]	Colony stimulating factor	Anemia; renal defects; AIDS	Hypertension	
Esmolol [Brevibloc]	*Antiarrhythmic (Class II)*—β blocker	Block effect of catecholamines on heart; decreases activity of nodal tissue; slows sinus rate; depress AV conduction	Asthma; negative inotrope	
Estrogen [Estratab, Premarin]	Growth and development of female organs; linear bone growth; epiphyseal closure; endometrial growth; maintain responsiveness of breasts, uterus, and vagina; inhibits bone reabsorption; increases hepatic production of α-2-globulins, coagulation factors II, VII, IX, X, and HDL; decreases antithrombin III and cholesterol	Osteoporosis; contraception; can be used in combination with progesterone	May lead to sodium and water retention; nausea; breast tenderness; hyperpigmentation; increased risk of bleeding, gallbladder disease, migraines, hypertension	
Ethacrynic acid [Edecrin]	*Loop diuretic*—inhibits Cl⁻ transport in ascending limb and PCT; works on K/Cl transporter and Cl⁻ channel	Diuresis	Ototoxicity; metabolic alkalosis; hypokalemia; hyperglycemia; hyperuricemia	
Ethambutol [Myambutol]	*Antibiotic*—unknown mechanism	Mycobacterium	Visual disturbances; tolerance develops	
Ethanosuxamide	*Anti-epileptic*—decrease Ca²⁺ conduction	Epilepsy (absence seizures)		

Therapeutic Agent (common name, if relevant) [Trade name, where appropriate]	Class–Pharmacology and Pharmacokinetics	Indications	Side or Adverse Effects	Contraindications or Precautions to Consider; Notes
Ether	**Anesthetic agent**	**General anesthetic**		
Etidocaine [Duranest]	Anesthetic agent—block Na$^+$ intracellularly	Local anesthetic	Sleepiness; lightheadedness; visual/audio disturbances; restlessness; nystagmus; shivering; tonic-clonic convulsions; death; greater toxicity than other local anesthetics	
Etidronate [Didronel]	Bone stabilizer—pyrophosphate analog; reduce hydroxyapatite crystal formation, growth, and dissolution, which reduces bone turnover	Hypercalcemia of malignancy; Paget's disease; osteoporosis; hyperparathyroidism		
Etomidate [Amidate]	Anesthetic agent	Induce stage 3 anesthesia	Painful injection; myoclonic movements	
Etretinate	Vitamin A analog	Severe acne; psoriasis		
Famotidine [Pepcid]	**H$_2$ blocker**	**Inhibits gastric acid secretion (esp. ulcer)**	**Gynecomastia; rare: headache, dizziness, fatigue, CNS, leukopenia, reduced sperm count**	**Inhibits metabolism and/or absorption of some drugs**
Fentanyl [Duragesic]	**Opioid agonist**	**Analgesic; general anesthetic**	**Prolonged recovery; nausea**	
Fexofenadine hydrochloride [Allegra]	Antihistamine			
Finasteride [Proscar]	**Androgen hormone inhibitor—inhibits 5-α reductase**	**Benign prostatic hyperplasia**		
Flecainide [Tambocor]	Antiarrhythmic (Class IC)—Na$^+$ channel blocker			
Fluconazole [Diflucan]	**Antifungal—inhibits ergosterol synthesis, preventing cell membrane formation**	**Cryptococcal meningitis; oral candidiasis in AIDS**	**Abdominal pain; nausea**	
Flucytosine [Ancobon]	Antifungal—competitive inhibitor of thymidylate synthetase; impairs DNA synthesis	Candida; Cryptococcus; aspergillus	Nausea; vomiting; diarrhea; rash; bone marrow and liver toxicity; enterocolitis	Imported in the fungus via permease
Fludrocortisone [Florinef]	Mineralocorticoid—aldosterone analog	Used with cortisol in adrenal insufficiency		

Drug [brand]	Class / Mechanism	Clinical use	Toxicity / Side effects	Notes
Flumazenil [Romazicon]	Benzodiazepine receptor antagonist	Alcohol abuse; anxiety		IV only
Flunarizine [Sibelium]	Weak Ca^{2+} channel blocker	Prophylaxis for migraine		
Fluoride	Stabilizes hydroxyapatite crystal structure; stimulates new growth of bone (unknown mechanism)		Nausea; vomiting; neurologic symptoms; arthralgias; arthritis	
Fluoxetine [Prozac]	*Antidepressant—antianxiety; SSRI*	**Depression; anxiety; obsessive-compulsive disorder**	**Agitation; tremors; mania; pre-occupation with suicide; nausea; headache; insomnia**	
Fluphenazine [Prolixin]	*Antipsychotic*—blocks D$_2$ receptors	Psychosis	Parkinsonism; tardive dyskinesia	
Flurazepam [Dalmane]	*Benzodiazepine*—enhances GABA; increases IPSP amplitude	Sedative; hypnotic; anti-anxiety; anti-epileptic		
Flutamide [Eulexin]	*Antineoplastic*—competitive androgen receptor blocker	**Metastatic prostate cancer**		
Fluvastatin [Lescol]	*Lipid lowering agent*—inhibits HMG-CoA reductase; lowers LDL	Hyperlipidemia (esp. type II)	Liver toxicity; myopathy; mild GI disturbances	Contraindicated: pregnant/lactating women or children
Fluvoxamine [Luvox]	*Antidepressant-SSRI*	Anxiety; obsessive-compulsive disorder		
Foscarnet [Foscavir]	*Antiviral*—non-nucleoside inhibitor of DNA polymerase	CMV, herpes in AIDS	Hypocalcemia; CNS, cardiac and renal toxicity; anemia	
Fosinopril [Monopril]	*Antihypertensive*—ACE inhibitor; vasodilator	Congestive heart failure	Postural hypotension; renal insufficiency; hyperkalemia; persistent dry cough	Contraindicated in pregnant women
Furosemide [Lasix]	*Loop diuretic*—inhibits Na$^+$/K$^+$/Cl$^-$ reabsorption in the Loop of Henle	**Congestive heart failure; diuresis**	**Ototoxicity; hyperuricemia; acute hypovolemia; hypokalemia; metabolic alkalosis; hyperglycemia**	
Gabapentin [Neurontin]	*Anti-epileptic*—block Na$^+$ channels	Add on drug for epilepsy		
Gallamine [Flaxedil]	*Non-depolarizing neuromuscular blocker*			No histamine release; affects cardiac receptors
Ganciclovir [Cytovene]	*Antiviral*—guanosine analog; inhibits DNA polymerase	**CMV (esp. CMV retinitis in AIDS)**	**Bone marrow suppression; renal impairment; seizures**	
Gemfibrozil [Lopid]	*Lipid lowering agent*—lowers VLDL, TG, cholesterol; increases activity of LPL; inhibits lipolysis; increases HDL	Hyperlipidemia	Potentiates anticoagulant drugs; myositis; gallstones; mild GI disturbances	Contraindicated in patients with impaired renal or hepatic function, and in pregnant or lactating women

Therapeutic Agent (common name, if relevant) [Trade name, where appropriate]	Class—Pharmacology and Pharmacokinetics	Indications	Side or Adverse Effects	Contraindications or Precautions to Consider; Notes
Gentamicin [Garamycin]	Antibiotic—aminoglycoside; binds 30s ribosome subunits; bacteriostatic at low concentration; bactericidal at high	Gram-negative meningitis		Contraindicated in neonates; peak and trough levels must be measured
Glipizide [Glucotrol]	Hypoglycemic agent—sulfonylurea; reduces K+ efflux, increases Ca2+ influx, increases secretion of insulin	Oral treatment for NIDDM (type II diabetes)	Hypoglycemia; GI disturbances; muscle weakness; mental confusion	
Glyburide [Diabeta, Micronase]	Hypoglycemic agent—sulfonylurea; reduces K+ efflux, increases Ca2+ influx, increases secretion of insulin	Oral treatment for NIDDM (type II diabetes)	Hypoglycemia; GI disturbances; muscle weakness; mental confusion	
Glyceryl guaiacolate [Fenesin]	Expectorant—increases bronchial secretion	Promotes cough		
Glycopyrrolate [Robinul]	Antimuscarinic	Bladder/GI spasm; decreases acid in ulcer		
GnRH	Controls release of FSH, LH	Stimulates pituitary function		
Gonadorelin [Lutrepulse]	Analog of GnRH—controls release of FSH, LH	Stimulates pituitary function		
Griseofulvin [Fulvicin, Grifulvin, Grisactin]	Antifungal—inhibit cell mitosis by disrupting mitotic spindles; binds to tubulin	Dermatophytes (esp. Trichophyton rubrum)	Headache; lethargy; mental confusion; fever; rash; nausea; vomiting; diarrhea; hepatotoxic; photosensitivity	
Growth hormone (somatotropin) [Somatrem]	Causes liver to produce insulin-like growth factors (somatomedins)	Replacement therapy in children and burn victims		
Growth hormone releasing hormone (GH-RH)	Stimulates release of GH	Dwarfism		
Guanethidine [Ismelin]	Antihypertensive—interferes with norepinephrine release	Severe hypertension	Postural hypotension; impotence; Pain at injection	Contraindicated in patients taking TCAs
Haloperidol [Haldol]	Antipsychotic—blocks D2 receptors	Psychosis	Parkinsonism; tardive dyskinesia	
Haloprogin [Halotex]	Antifungal—unknown mechanism; fungistatic	Topical for tinea pedis		

266

Drug	Class/Mechanism	Clinical use	Side effects	Notes
Halothane [Fluothane, Somnothane]	*Anesthetic agent*	General anesthetic	Hepatotoxic; malignant hyperthermia (w/succinylcholine); arrhythmia	Contraindicated in adults
Heparin	Increases PTT by joining with antithrombin-III	Deep vein thrombosis; pulmonary vein thrombosis	Overdose reversed by IV protamine sulfate; osteoporosis	Fast acting; does not cross placenta
Heroin	Metabolized to morphine			More lipid soluble than morphine
Hexafluorenium	Degrades pseudocholinesterase; potentiates non-depolarizing muscular blockers			
Hexamethonium	Nicotinic ganglionic blocker	Hypertensive emergency		
Hydralazine [Apresoline]	*Antihypertensive*—vasodilator	Congestive heart failure, hypertension	Lupus-like reaction	
Hydrochlorothiazide [Esidrix, Hydrodiuril]	*Diuretic*—decrease Na⁺ absorption in the distal tubule by inhibiting the Na⁺/Cl⁻ transport; reduced peripheral resistance	Hypertension, CHF	Hypokalemia; hyperuricemia; hypovolemia; hyperglycemia (especially in diabetics); hypercalcemia; hypersensitivity reaction	
Hydrocodone [Bancap-HC]	*Opioid agonist*	Antitussive; analgesic		
Hydromorphone [Dilaudid]	Opioid agonist	Antitussive; analgesic		
Hydroxychloroquine [Plaquenil]	*Antiprotozoal*—antirheumatic	Rheumatic arthritis; malaria	Ocular toxicity (blurred vision)	Contraindicated in patients with psoriasis
Hydroxyurea [Hydrea]	*Antineoplastic*—binds ribonucleotide reductase; inhibits formation of deoxyribose nucleic acid	Melanoma; chronic myelogenous leukemia; sickle cell disease	Nausea; vomiting; bone marrow suppression	
Ibuprofen [Advil, Motrin]	*NSAID*		Fewer than aspirin	
Ibutilide [Corvert]	*Antiarrhythmic (Class III)*—K⁺ channel blocker	Terminate atrial fibrillation and flutter	Prolongs Q-T interval	
Idoxuridine [Herplex Liquiflim]	*Antiviral*—thymidine analog; inhibits DNA polymerase; inhibits DNA synthesis	Topical for HSV keratitis	Local irritation; allergic contact keratitis	
Idozoxan	*Antihypertensive*—α₂ blocker			
Ifosfamide [Ifex]	*Antineoplastic*—DNA alkylation and cross-linking	Cancer	Cystitis; nephrotoxicity; nausea; vomiting; bone marrow suppression; alopecia; teratogenicity; carcinogenicity	

Therapeutic Agent (common name, if relevant) [Trade name, where appropriate]	Class—Pharmacology and Pharmacokinetics	Indications	Side or Adverse Effects	Contraindications or Precautions to Consider; Notes
Imipenem [Primaxin]	*Antibiotic*—inhibits trans-peptidase and cell wall synthesis; monocyclic β-lactam	Dormant bacteria	Seizure	
Imipramine [Tofranil]	*Antidepressant*—TCA; blocks norepinephrine, 5-HT, muscarinic, α₁, histamine receptors; antiarrhythmic (class IA)	Antidepressant; bed wetting	Tremors (due to NE block); anorexia (5-HT block); anti-cholinergic (muscarinic block); hypotension (α₁ block); drowsiness (histamine block)	
Indecainide	*Antiarrhythmic (Class IC)*—Na$^+$ channel blockers			No anti-muscarinic action; no effect on action potential
Indinavir [Crixivan]	*Antiviral*—protease inhibits	AIDS		
Indomethacin [Indocin]	*NSAID*	Closes PDA; gout		
Interferon, α2a (Roferon-A) and α2b (Intron A) and αn3 (Alferon-N)	*Antiviral*—decrease protein synthesis	**Genital warts; chronic hepatitis B and C; AIDS related Kaposi's sarcoma; laryngeal papillomatosis; hairy cell leukemia**	**Flu-like symptoms; tachycardia; fever; neutropenia; headache; somnolence; malaise**	
Ipratropium [Atrovent]	*Bronchodilator*—anti-muscarinic	Bronchodilates for asthma		
Isocarboxazid [Marplan]	*Antidepressant*—MAO inhibitor; non-selective but isoenzyme A most important; irreversible	Depression		
Isoflurane	*Anesthetic*	General anesthetic		Best muscle relaxer; most widely used
Isoniazid [INH, Nydrazid]	*Antibiotic*—inhibits synthesis of mycolic acids	**Mycobacterium (M. tuberculosis and M. kansasii) treatment**	**Peripheral and CNS effects due to pyroxidine deficiency; liver damage; hemolytic anemia in G-6-PD deficient**	
Isoproterenol [Isuprel]	*Bronchodilator*—β agonist (non-selective)	Asthma		
Isosorbide dinitrate [Isordil]	*Anti-anginal*—stimulates synthesis of cGMP leading to muscle relaxation via NO formation; vasodilator	Angina; congestive heart failure	Headache; orthostatic hypotension; syncope	Long acting
Isotretinoin [Accutane]	**Vitamin A analog**	**Severe acne; psoriasis**	**Keratinization; teratogenic**	

Drug	Class / Mechanism	Clinical Use	Toxicity	Notes
Itraconazole [Sporanox]	*Antifungal*—inhibits ergosterol synthesis, preventing cell membrane formation	Oral for fungal infections (esp. dermatophytoses and onychomycosis)	GI disturbances; hepatotoxicity	
Kanamycin [Kantrex]	*Antibiotic*—aminoglycoside; binds 30s ribosome subunits; bacteriostatic at low concentration; bactericidal at high	Reduction of gut flora	Ototoxicity; neurotoxicity	
Ketamine [Ketalar]	**Anesthetic agent**	**General anesthetic**	**Dissociative anesthesia; catatonia; hallucinations**	
Ketoconazole [Nizoral]	**Antifungal**—inhibits ergosterol synthesis, preventing cell membrane formation; inhibits gonadal steroid synthesis	**Chronic mucocutaneous candidiasis; blastomycosis; histoplasmosis; prostate carcinoma**	**Nausea; vomiting; diarrhea; rash; headache; anorexia; thrombocytopenia; gynecomastia; hepatotoxic**	**Inhibits cytochrome P450**
Labetalol [Normodyne, Trandate]	**Antihypertensive**—β and α_1 blocker	**Hypertension**		
Lactulose [Chronulac]	Osmotic laxative	Decreases ammonia in hepatic encephalopathy		
Lamivudine [Epivir]	*Antiviral*—reverse transcriptase inhibitor	AIDS		
Lamotrigine [Lamictal]	*Antiepileptic*—block Na^+ channels	Add on drug for epilepsy		
Leucovorin	Allows stem cells to bypass the inhibition of dihydrofolate reductase caused by methotrexate	Treat acute toxicity of methotrexate		
Leuprolide [Lupron]	**GnRH agonist**—suppression of FSH, LH when given continuously	**Prostate cancer; polycystic ovary disease; uterine fibroids; endometriosis**		
Levallorphan	Mixed agonist/antagonist of opioids	Similar to nalorphine		
Levamisole [Ergamisol]	*Antihelminthic*—immunostimulatory to host; helps rid host of parasite	Ascaris (roundworm); Ancylostoma (hookworm); therapy for immunodeficiency	GI disturbances; rashes; neutropenia	
Levodopa [Larodopa]	**Anti-Parkinsonian agent**—precursor of dopamine; administered with carbidopa (most often) or benserazide to inhibit carboxylase deactivation of levodopa in periphery	**Parkinson's disease**		**Inhibited by Vitamin B6; do not give with MAOI or pyridoxine**

Therapeutic Agent (common name, if relevant) [Trade name, where appropriate]	Class—Pharmacology and Pharmacokinetics	Indications	Side or Adverse Effects	Contraindications or Precautions to Consider; Notes
Levofloxacin [Levaquin]	*Quinolone antibiotic*—blocks DNA synthesis by inhibiting DNA gyrase	Gram-negative infections (esp. UTI and bone): Pseudomonas, Entero-bacteriaceae; Neisseria; gram-positive infections; intracellular: Legionella	GI disturbances; headache; dizziness; phototoxicity; cartilage damage	May elevate theophylline to toxic levels causing seizure
Levomethadyl	*Opioid agonist*	Long lasting maintenance therapy for heroin addiction		
Levorphanol [Levo-Dromoran]	*Opioid agonist*		Less than morphine	
Levothyroxine (T₄) [Levothroid]	Synthetic analog of thyroid hormone T₄	Replacement therapy for thyroid hormone		
Lidocaine [Xylocaine]	*Antiarrhythmic (Class IB)*, *anesthetic agent*—block Na⁺ channels intracellularly	Local anesthetic; ventricular tachycardia; post-MI ventricular tachycardia	Sleepiness; light-headed; visual/audio disturbances; restlessness; nystagmus; shivering; tonic-clonic convulsion; death	Given with epinephrine to maintain locality and increase duration of anesthetic properties via epinephrine mediated vasoconstriction
Lisinopril [Prinivil, Zestril]	*Antihypertensive*—vasodilator; ACE inhibitor	Congestive heart failure	Postural hypotension; renal insufficiency; hyperkalemia; persistent dry cough	Pregnancy
Lithium carbonate [Eskalith, Lithobid, Lithotab, Lithonate]	*Antimanic agent*	Manic-depression; cluster headache	Diabetes insipidus; ataxia; tremors; confusion; seizures	
Loperamide [Imodium]	*Antidiarrheal*—similar to opioid agonist	Oral antidiarrheal		
Loratadine [Claritin]	*Antihistamine*	Seasonal allergies	Gynecomastia; rare: headache, dizziness, fatigue, CNS, weak anti-androgenic effect, leukopenia, reduced sperm count	Inhibits metabolism and/or absorption of some drugs
Lorazepam [Ativan]	*Antianxiety*—benzodiazepine; enhances GABA; increases IPSP amplitude	Sedative; hypnotic; antianxiety; anti-epileptic; panic attack		
Losartan [Cozaar]	*Antihypertensive*—angiotensin II receptor antagonist	Hypertension	Dizziness; upper respiratory infection; headache	
Lovastatin [Mevacor]	*Lipid lowering agent*—inhibits HMG-CoA reductase; lowers LDL	Hyperlipidemia (esp. type II)	Liver toxicity; myopathy; mild GI disturbances	Contraindicated: pregnant/lactating women or children
Magnesium hydroxide [Milk of Magnesia]	*Laxative*—antacid	Constipation		Diarrhea

Drug	Classification/Mechanism	Indication	Side Effects	Notes
Magnesium salts	*Osmotic laxative*			
Malathion	*Organophosphate*—inhibits cholinesterase			Least toxic organophosphate
Mannitol [Osmitrol]	Osmotic diuretic—affects the PCT	Diuresis		
Mebendazole [Vermox]	*Antihelminthic*—irreversible; inhibits glucose uptake	Hookworm; roundworm; threadworm; some cestodes		
Mecamylamine [Inversine]	*Antihypertensive*—nicotinic ganglionic blocker	Hypertension emergency; smoking cessation	Decreases GI motility; cycloplegia; hypotension; xerostomia	
Mechlorethamine (nitrogen mustard) [Mustargen]	*Antineoplastic*—DNA alkylation and cross-linking	Cancer	Nausea; vomiting; bone marrow suppression; alopecia; teratogenicity; carcinogenicity	
Meclizine [Antivert, Bonine]	*Antiemetic agent*—H$_1$ blocker	Emesis	Teratogenic	
Mefloquine [Lariam]	*Antimalarial*—uncertain mechanism	Treatment of acute attack of chloroquine-resistant organisms	CNS—dizziness, disorientation, hallucinations, seizure, depression; GI disturbances; nausea; vomiting; abdominal pain	
Melatonin		Promotes sleep		
Melphalan [Alkeran]	*Antineoplastic*—DNA alkylation and cross-linking	Cancer	Nausea; vomiting; bone marrow suppression (serious); alopecia; teratogenicity; carcinogenicity; pulmonary fibrosis; hypersensitivity	
Menotropin [Pergonal]	Mixture of FSH and LH	Secondary hypogonadism with infertility		
Meperedine [Demerol]	*Opioid agonist*	**Analgesic; acute migraine attacks**	**CNS excitation at high doses; histamine release**	**Contraindicated in patients with MAO inhibitors (results in hyperpyrexia)**
Mephenesin	Centrally acting muscle relaxant	Muscle spasms; tetanus contractions; orthopedic manipulation	Sedation	
Mepivacaine [Isocaine]	*Anesthetic agent*—blocks Na$^+$ channels intracellullarly	Local anesthetic	Sleepiness; light-headed; visual/audio disturbances; restlessness; nystagmus; shivering; tonic-clonic convulsion; death	
Mercaptopurine [Purinethol]	*Antineoplastic*—inhibits purine synthesis; disrupts DNA and RNA synthesis	Childhood leukemias	Bone marrow suppression	
Mercurial diuretics	*Diuretic*—unclear mechanism of diuresis; may be on ascending limb and DCT	Diuresis	Metabolic alkalosis, kidney damage	

Therapeutic Agent (common name, if relevant) [Trade name, where appropriate]	Class—Pharmacology and Pharmacokinetics	Indications	Side or Adverse Effects	Contraindications or Precautions to Consider; Notes
Metformin [Glucophage]	*Hypoglycemic agent*—decreases glucose production in liver; increases glucose uptake	Oral treatment of NIDDM (type II)	Lactic acidosis	
Methadone [Dolophine]	*Opioid agonist*—**synthetic**	**Maintenance therapy for heroin addiction**		
Methicillin [Staphcillin]	*Antibiotic*—β-lactam; penicillinase resistant	Staph infections		
Methimazole [Tapazole]	*Thyrotoxic agent*—**inhibits peroxidase enzyme in thyroid; decreases synthesis of thyroid hormone**	**Hyperthyroidism**	**Agranulocytosis**	
Methohexital [Brevital]	*Anesthetic agent*—barbiturate; prolongs IPSP duration	Anti-epileptic; cerebral edema; anesthetic (stage 3 anesthetic)		Ultra-short acting
Methotrexate [Rheumatrex]	*Antineoplastic*—**dihydrofolate reductase inhibitor; immunosuppressant**	**Rheumatic arthritis; bone marrow transplant; acute lymphocytic and myelogenous leukemia; chorio-carcinoma; lung cancer**	**Oral and GI ulceration; bone marrow suppression; thrombo-cytopenia; leukopenia; hepatotoxic**	**Leucovarin is given as an adjuvant after treatment**
Methoxyflurane [Penthrane]	*Anesthetic agent*	General anesthetic	Nephrotoxic	
Methylcelluose [Citrucel]	*Dietary fiber*	Laxative		
Methyldopa [Aldomet]	*Antihypertensive*—**inhibits sympathetic outflow; centrally acting**	**Hypertension**	**Hemolytic anemia**	**Positive Coombs' test**
Methylphenidate [Ritalin]	*CNS stimulant*—amphetamine; release neurotransmitter from synapse	Stimulant; treatment of choice for Attention-Deficit Hyperactivity Disorder		
Methysergide [Sansert]	*Anti-migraine*—**5-HT antagonist and weak vasoconstrictor**	**Prophylaxis of migraine**	**GI distress; inflammatory fibrosis of kidney, lung and cardiac valves**	**Contraindicated in patients by periph-eral vascular disease, coronary artery disease, and pregnancy; patient placed on a drug holiday to prevent side effects**
Metoclopramide [Reglan]	*GI stimulant*—**stimulates Ach (D$_2$ and 5-HT$_3$ antagonists); pro-kinetic**	**Anti-emetic; relief of nausea from migraine; increases stomach motility**	**Sleepiness; fatigue; headache; insomnia; dizziness; nausea**	

Metocurine [Metubine Iodide]	Non-depolarizing neuromuscular blocker			
Metolazone [Mykrox, Zaroxolyn]	*Diuretic*—decrease Na+ in the distal tubule by inhibiting the Na+/Cl--cotransporter; reduced peripheral resistance	Hypertension, CHF	Hypokalemia; hyperuricemia; hypovolemia; hyperglycemia (especially in diabetics); hypercalcemia; hypersensitivity reaction; Na+ excretion in advanced renal failure	
Metoprolol [Toprol XL]	*Antihypertensive, antiarrhythmic (Class II)*—β blocker	Hypertension; angina; MI		
Metronidazole [Flagyl]	**Antibiotic—penetrates cell membrane and gives off nitro moiety; reacts with DNA; inhibits replication; bactericidal**	***B. fragilis* (esp. for endocarditis and CNS); amebiasis; giardiasis**	**Nausea; vomiting; disulfiram-like reaction to alcohol; metallic taste; paresthesia; stomatitis; carcinogenic and mutagenic**	**Contraindicated in pregnancy**
Metyrapone [Metopirone]	Inhibits cortisol synthesis	Diagnosis of pituitary dysfunction		
Mevastatin	*Lipid lowering agent*—inhibits HMG-CoA reductase; lowers LDL	Hyperlipidemia (esp. type II)	Liver toxicity; myopathy; mild GI disturbances	Contraindicated in pregnant/lactating women or children
Mexiletine [Mexitil]	*Antiarrhythmic (Class IB)*—Na+ channel blocker			
Mezlocillin [Mezlin]	*Antibiotic*—β-lactam	Pseudomonas; Proteus		IV
Miconazole [Monistat IV]	*Antifungal*—inhibits ergosterol synthesis, preventing cell membrane formation	Broad spectrum, including yeasts and dermatophytes	Burning, itching, and redness when used topically; thrombophlebitis; nausea; vomiting; anaphylaxis when used IV	
Milrinone [Primacor]	*Inotropic agent*—phosphodiesterase inhibitor; increase contractility via increase in intracellular Ca²+	Congestive heart failure		
Mineral oil [Fleet Mineral Oil Enema]		Laxative	May interfere with absorption of fat-soluble vitamins	
Minoxidil [Loniten, Rogaine]	*Antihypertensive*—hair growth stimulant; vasodilator	Congestive heart failure, hypertension	Hypertrichosis (hair growth)	
Misoprostol [Cytotec]	*Anti-ulcer*—PGE₁	Protects against ulcers	Diarrhea; nausea; miscarriages	
Molindone [Moban]	*Antipsychotic*—blocks D₂ receptors	Psychosis	Parkinsonism; tardive dyskinesia	
Moricizine [Ethmozine]	*Antiarrhythmic (Class IC)*—Na+ channel blockers	Ventricular arrhythmia	Dizziness; nausea	

Therapeutic Agent (common name, if relevant) [Trade name, where appropriate]	Class—Pharmacology and Pharmacokinetics	Indications	Side or Adverse Effects	Contraindications or Precautions to Consider; Notes
Morphine [Astramorph, Duramorph, Infumorph, Kadian, MS Contin, Oramorph, MSIR, Roxanol]	*Opioid agonist*—converted to more potent morphine-6-glucose	Severe pain; general anesthetic; anti-tussive; antidiarrheal	Histamine release; constipation; nausea	
Muromonab (OKT3)	*Immunosuppressant*—monoclonal antibody against CD_3 on T-lymphocytes	Acute rejection of renal transplants		
Muscarine	*Muscarinic agonist*		Abdominal pain; diarrhea; bronchoconstriction	Contraindicated in patients with peptic ulcer, asthma, hyperthyroid, Parkinson's disease
Nabilone [Cesamet]	*Anti-emetic*—unknown mechanism; binds opiate receptors and directly inhibits vomiting center in medulla	Emesis	Dry mouth; dizziness; inability to concentrate; disorientation; anxiety; tachycardia; depression; paranoia; psychosis	THC derivative
n-Acetylcysteine [Mucomyst]	*Mucolytic*—replenish glutathione	Overdose of acetaminophen; liquefy sputum to assist expulsion		
Nadolol [Corgard]	*Antihypertensive*—antianginal; β blocker	Hypertension; angina		
Nafcillin [Unipen]	*Antibiotic*—β-lactam; penicillinase resistant	Staph infections		
Naftifine [Naftin]	*Antifungal*—inhibits squalene-2,3-epoxidase	Topical for tinea cruris and tinea corporis		
Nalbuphine [Nubain]	Mixed agonist/antagonist of opioids	Similar to pentazocine		
Nalidixic acid [Neg-Gram]	*Antibiotic*—urinary antiseptic; unknown mechanism of action	Coliform UTIs		
Nalorphine	Mixed agonist/antagonist of opioids	Antagonizes effects of morphine	Respiratory depression; analgesia	
Naloxone [Narcan]	Antagonist of all opioids	Drug of choice for opioid antagonism		Ineffective to use against barbiturate overdose, but safe
Naltrexone [ReVia]	Antagonist of all opioids	Longer action than naloxone; can be used orally		
Naproxen [Naprosyn]	*NSAID*			

Drug	Action	Use	Notes
Natamycin [Natacyn]	*Antifungal*—binds to cell membrane sterols (esp. ergosterol); forms pores in membrane; fungicidal	Topical for fungal keratitis (eye)	
Nefazodone [Serzone]	*Antidepressant*—post-synaptic 5-HT$_2$ antagonist	Depression	
Nelfinavir	*Antiviral*—protease inhibitor	AIDS	
Neomycin [Mycifradin, Neosporin]	*Antibiotic*—*lipid lowering agent*; lowers LDL; inhibits resorption of cholesterol and bile acids; aminoglycoside; binds 30s ribosome subunits; bacteriostatic at low concentration; bactericidal at high	Hyperlipidemia; reduction of gut flora	Inhibits absorption of digitalis
Neostigmine [Prostigmin]	**Inhibits cholinesterase**	**Paralytic ileus; neurogenic bladder; myasthenia gravis**	
Niclosamide [Niclocide]	*Antihelminthic*—inhibits anaerobic metabolism	Tapeworms: T. solium, T. saginata, H. nana	
Nicotine [Habitrol Nicoderm, Nicotrol]	***Nicotinic agonist***	**Stop smoking**	
Nifedipine [Adalat, Procardia]	***Antianginal*—Ca^{2+} blocker**	**Angina**	**Dizziness; nausea; headache; gingival problems**
Niridazole	*Antihelminthic*—induces breakdown of glycogen; inhibits glucose uptake	Schistosomes	CNS; inhibits spermatogenesis; ECG changes; GI disturbances
Nitrofurantoin [Furadantin]	*Antibiotic*—urinary antiseptic; unknown mechanism of action	Gram positive and negative bacteria	Contraindicated in patients by renal insufficiency
Nitroglycerin [Deponit, Minitran]	***Antianginal*—stimulates synthesis of cGMP leading to muscle relaxation via NO formation**	**Angina**	**Headache; orthostatic hypotension; syncope** **Monday disease; short acting**
Nitrosoureas	*Antineoplastic*—alkylating agent; lipid soluble	CNS tumors	Contraindicated in patients with hepatosplenic form of disease—more likely to cause CNS problems
Nitrous oxide	*Anesthetic agent*	General anesthetic	Hypoxia
Nizatidine [Axid]	H$_2$ blocker	Inhibits gastric acid secretion (esp. ulcer)	Gynecomastia; rare: headache, dizziness, fatigue, CNS, weak anti-androgenic effect, leukopenia, reduced sperm count	Inhibits metabolism and/or absorption of some drugs

Therapeutic Agent (common name, if relevant) [Trade name, where appropriate]	Class–Pharmacology and Pharmacokinetics	Indications	Side or Adverse Effects	Contraindications or Precautions to Consider; Notes
Nortriptyline [Pamelor]	*Antidepressant*—TCA; blocks norepinephrine, 5-HT, muscarinic, α_1, histamine receptors	Depression	Tremors (due to NE block); anorexia (5-HT block); anticholinergic (muscarinic block); hypotension (α_1 block); drowsiness (histamine block)	
Nystatin [Mycostatin]	*Antifungal*—binds to cell membrane sterols (esp. ergosterol); forms pores in membrane; fungicidal	**Mucosal candida infections (skin, vaginal, GI)**	Few	
Octreotide [Sandostatin]	*Analog of somatostatin*—decreases release of GH, gastrin, secretin, VIP, CCK, glucagon, insulin, calcitonin, PTH, renin, and TSH	**Acromegaly; glucagonoma; insulinoma**	Nausea; cramps; gallstones	
Ofloxacin [Floxin]	*Quinolone antibiotic*—blocks DNA synthesis by inhibiting DNA gyrase	Gram-negative infections (esp. UTI and bone): Pseudomonas, Enterobacteriaceae, Neisseria; gram-positive infections; intracellular: Legionella	GI disturbances; headache; dizziness; phototoxicity; cartilage damage	May elevate theophylline to toxic levels causing seizure
Olanzapine [Zyprexa]	*Antipsychotic*	Psychosis		
Omeprazole [Prilosec]	*Anti-ulcer*—proton pump inhibitor; blocks H^+/K^+ ATPase	**Reduce acid secretion**		**Inhibits cytochrome P450: Given with clarithromycin and amoxicillin for *H. pylori***
Ondansetron [Zofran]	*Anti-emetic*—5-HT$_3$ (serotonin) blocker	**Emesis (due to cancer therapy)**	Headache; constipation; dizziness	
Oxacillin [Bactocill]	*Antibiotic*—β-lactam; penicillinase resistant	Staph infections		
Oxaprozin [Daypro]	*NSAID*—mildly uricosuric	Acute gout		Contraindicated in patients with kidney stones
Oxazepam [Serax]	*Antianxiety*—benzodiazepine; enhances GABA; increase IPSP amplitude	Sedative; hypnotic; anti-epileptic		
Oxybutynin [Ditropan]	*Antimuscarinic*	Bladder/GI spasm; decrease acid in ulcer		

Drug	Class / Mechanism	Indication	Side Effects	Notes
Oxytocin [Syntocinon]	**Stimulates uterine contraction; contraction of breast myo-epithelial cells; milk letdown reflex**	**Induce labor**		
Paclitaxel [Taxol]	*Antineoplastic*—polymerizes tubules	Ovarian and breast cancer		
Pamidronate [Aredia]	*Bone stabilizer*—pyrophosphate analog; reduce hydroxyapatite crystal formation, growth and dissolution, which reduces bone turnover	Hypercalcemia of malignancy; Paget's disease; osteoporosis; hyperparathyroidism		
Pancuronium [Pavulon]	Non-depolarizing neuromuscular blocker			Minimal histamine release
Paroxetine [Paxil]	*Antidepressant*—SSRI	Depression; anxiety	Nausea; headache; insomnia	
Penicillamine [Cuprimine, Depen]	*Anti-arthritis*—anti-gold medicine; not specific; unknown mechanism; arthritis relief	Rheumatic arthritis; copper poisoning; metal chelator	Decreases Vitamin B6; bone marrow suppression; proteinuria; autoimmune syndrome	
Penicillin	***Antibiotic*—inhibits transpeptidase and cell wall synthesis**	**Gram positive bacteria-aerobic, some anaerobic, and spirochetes**	**Allergic reactions; platelet aggregation problems; direct CNS toxicity; superinfections**	
Pentazocine [Talwin]	Mixed agonist/antagonist of opioids	Analgesia		Only mixed agonist/antagonist available orally
Pentobarbital [Nembutal sodium]	*Barbiturate*—prolongs IPSP duration	Cerebral edema; anesthetic		
Pergolide [Permax]	*Anti-Parkinson's*—dopamine agonist; inhibits prolactin release	Treat breast engorgement; inhibits lactation		
Phenazocine	*Opioid agonist*			
Phenobarbital	***Barbiturate*—prolongs IPSP duration**	**Anti-epileptic (partial and tonic-clonic); cerebral edema; anesthetic**		
Phenolphthalein [Ex-Lax]	*Laxative*—reduce absorption of electrolytes and water from gut	Stimulant laxative	Tumorogenic	
Phenoxybenzamine [Dibenzyline]	*Antihypertensive*—α blocker; long acting; irreversible	Pheochromocytoma	Nasal congestion; miosis; orthostatic hypotension	
Phentolamine [Regitine]	***Antihypertensive*—α blocker**	**Diagnosis of pheochromocytoma; hypertension (especially tyrosine induced)**		
Phenylbutazone [Butazolidin]	***NSAID***	**Rheumatic arthritis; acute gout**	**Agranulocytosis; aplastic anemia**	

Therapeutic Agent (common name, if relevant) [Trade name, where appropriate]	Class–Pharmacology and Pharmacokinetics	Indications	Side or Adverse Effects	Contraindications or Precautions to Consider; Notes
Phenylephrine [Neo-Synephrine, Nostril]	*Nasal decongestant*—α_1-agonist	Tachycardia		
Phenylzine	*Antidepressant*—MAO inhibitor; non-selective but isoenzyme A most important; irreversible	Depression		
Phenytoin [Dilantin]	*Anti-epileptic*—decreases Na^+ flux	**Epilepsy (partial and tonic-clonic); digitalis-induced arrhythmia**	**Decreases folic acid; gingival hyperplasia; hirsutism; nystagmus**	Induces cytochrome P450
Physostigmine [Eserine]	Inhibits cholinesterase	**Intestinal or bladder atony; glaucoma**		
Pilocarpine [Ocusert]	*Anti-glaucoma*—muscarinic agonist	**Xerostomia; narrow and open angle glaucoma**	**Focusing problems; nausea; abdominal pain; sweating; high dose: bradycardia, hypotension**	**Contraindicated in patients by peptic ulcer, asthma, hyperthyroid, Parkinson's disease**
Pindolol [Visken]	*Antihypertensive antiarrhythmic (Class II)*—β-blocker	Hypertension		
Piperacillin [Pipracil]	*Antibiotic*—β-lactam	Pseudomonas; Proteus		IV
Piperazine [Entacyl]	*Antihelminthic*—causes flaccid paralysis in worm	Ascariasis (roundworm); Oxyuriasis (pinworm)	GI disturbances; urticaria; minor CNS	
Piroxicam [Feldene]	*NSAID*			Long acting; contraindicated in the elderly
Platelet activating factor [PAF]	Activation of platelets and PMN aggregation; increase vascular permeability			
Plicamycin [Mithracin]	*Antineoplastic*—inhibits DNA directed RNA synthesis; decreases protein synthesis needed for bone reabsorption	Paget's disease; hypercalcemia		
Polymyxins [Aerosporin]	*Antibiotic*—disrupts cell membranes; bactericidal	**Gram-negative bacteria: Pseudomonas and Coliform; topical only; intrathecal for Pseudomonas meningitis**	**Neurotoxic; nephrotoxic**	
Potassium iodide [Thyro-Block]	*Expectorant*—increase bronchial secretions; high doses decrease release of thyroid hormone	Promote cough; hyperthyroidism		

Drug [Brand]	Mechanism / Class	Clinical Use	Side Effects	Notes / Contraindications
Pralidoxime [Protopam]	**Acetylcholine esterase reactivator**	**Overdose of malthion/parathion organophosphates; must be used before aging occurs**		
Pravastatin [Pravachol]	*Lipid lowering agent*—inhibits HMG-CoA reductase; lowers LDL	Hyperlipidemia (esp. type II)	Liver toxicity; myopathy; mild GI disturbances	Contraindicated in pregnant/lactating women or children
Praziquantel [Bitricide]	*Antihelminthic*—increases membrane permeability causing loss of Ca^{2+}	Schistosomes; flukes	GI disturbances; headache; fever; urticaria	
Prazosin [Minipress]	**Antihypertensive**—α_1-**blocker**	**Pheochromocytoma; hypertension**	**Postural hypotension**	
Prednisone [Deltasone]	*Glucocorticoid*—inhibits protein synthesis; reduce lymph node and spleen size; inhibits cell cycle activity of lymphoid cells; lyse T-cells; suppress antibody, prostaglandin, and leukotriene synthesis; block monocyte production of IL-1	Rheumatic arthritis; autoimmune disorders; allergic reaction; asthma; organ transplant (esp. during rejection crisis)	Osteoporosis; cushingoid reaction; psychosis; glucose intolerance; infection; hypertension; cataracts	
Prilocaine [Citanest]	*Anesthetic agent*—blocks Na^+ channels intracellularly	Local anesthetic	Sleepiness; light-headedness; visual/audio disturbances; restlessness; nystagmus; shivering; tonic-clonic convulsion; death	
Primaquine phosphate [Primaquine Phosphate]	*Antimalarial*—unknown mechanism	Cures vivax malaria; prophylaxis for falciparum malaria	GI disturbances; mild anemia; marked hemolysis in G-6-PD deficient individuals; prolongs QT interval	
Probenecid [Benemid]	*Antigout*—small dose inhibits tubule excretion; large dose inhibits tubule reabsorption (e.g., promotes excretion) of uric acid	Chronic gout	Rash; GI disturbances; drowsy	**Acute gout**
Probucol [Bifenabid, Lesterol]	*Lipid lowering agent*—lowers HDL and LDL; mechanism unknown	Hyperlipidemia	Prolongs Q-T interval; GI disturbances	Contraindicated in patients with heart disease
Procainamide [Pronestyl, Procanbid]	*Antiarrhythmic (Class IA)*—Na^+ **channel blocker**	**Ventricular arrhythmia**	**Lupus-like syndrome**	
Procaine [Novocain]	*Anesthetic agent*—blocks Na^+ intracellularly	Local anesthetic	Sleepiness; light-headedness; visual/audio disturbances; restlessness; nystagmus; shivering; tonic-clonic convulsion; death	

Therapeutic Agent (common name, if relevant) [Trade name, where appropriate]	Class–Pharmacology and Pharmacokinetics	Indications	Side or Adverse Effects	Contraindications or Precautions to Consider; Notes
Procarbazine [Matulane]	*Antineoplastic*—DNA alkylation and strand breakage; inhibits nucleic acid and protein synthesis	Cancer		
Prochlorperazine [Compazine]	*Antiemetic*—D_2 receptor antagonist	Counteract nausea of migraine; anti-emetic	Teratogenic	
Progesterone [Progestasert]	*Hormone*—secretory changes in endometrium and breast; necessary to maintain pregnancy	Treat primary hypogonadism; relief of menopause; decrease osteoporosis; suppress dysmenorrhea and excess androgen secretion by ovary; used in combination with estrogen for oral contraception	Long-lasting suppression of menses; endometriosis; hirsutism; bleeding disorders; nausea; breast tenderness; hyperpigmentation; gallbladder disease; migraines; hypertension	
Prolactin	Stimulates lactation of breast			
Promethazine [Phenergan]	*Antihistamine*—anti-emetic; D_2 receptor antagonist; H_1 blocker	Counteract nausea of migraine; allergies; motion sickness	Sedation; CNS depression; atropine-like effects; allergic dermatitis; blood dyscrasias; teratogenicity; acute antihistamine poisoning	
Propafenone [Rythmol]	*Antiarrhythmic (Class IC)*—Na^+ channel blocker			
Propofol [Diprivan]	Anesthetic agent	General anesthetic; fast-acting for ambulatory or outpatients	Seizure	
Propranolol [Inderal]	*Antihypertensive; anti-anginal; antiarrhythmic (Class II)*—anti-migraine; β-blocker	Hypertension; angina; MI; arrhythmias; prophylaxis of migraine	Reduces renin secretion	
Propylthiouracil [Propyl-Thyracil]	Inhibits peroxidase enzyme in thyroid; decreases synthesis of thyroid hormone	Hyperthyroidism	Agranulocytosis	
Protriptyline [Vivactil]	*Antidepressant*—TCA; blocks norepinephrine, 5-HT, muscarinic, α^1, and histamine receptors	Depression	Tremors (due to NE block); anorexia (5-HT block); anticholinergic (muscarinic block); hypotension (α_1 block); drowsiness (histamine block)	
Psyllium [Perdiem Fiber]	*Laxative*—dietary fiber	Constipation		

Drug	Classification / Mechanism	Clinical Use	Adverse Effects	Notes
PTH	Increases plasma Ca^{2+} levels by increasing reabsorption in kidney; activates Vitamin D which aids in Ca^{2+} absorption from gut; resorbs Ca^{2+} from bone; plasma phosphate reabsorption is decreased by kidney	Used to distinguish between hypoparathyroidism and pseudo-hypoparathyroidism		
Pyrantel [Antiminth, Reese's Pinworm Medicine]	*Antihelminthic*—depolarizing neuromuscular blocker causing spastic paralysis in worms	Ascaris (roundworm); Ancylostoma (hookworm); Threadworm		
Pyrazinamide [Tebrazid]	*Antibiotic*	Mycobacterium	Impairs liver function	
Pyridostigmine [Mestinon]	Inhibits cholinesterase	**Myasthenia gravis**		
Pyrimethamine [Daraprim]	*Antimalarial*—inhibits dihydrofolate reductase	Malaria	Large doses cause megaloblastic anemia	
Quetiapine	*Antipsychotic*	Psychosis		
Quinacrine [Atabrine]	*Antiprotozoal*—unknown mechanism	Giardia	Headache; nausea; vomiting; blood dyscrasias; yellow staining of skin; exfoliative dermatitis; retinopathy	
Quinapril [Accupril]	*Antihypertensive*—vasodilator; ACE inhibitor	Congestive heart failure	Postural hypotension; renal insufficiency; hyperkalemia; persistent dry cough	Contraindicated in pregnancy
Quinidine [Quinaglute]	*Antiarrhythmic (Class IA)*—Na^+ channel blocker	Arrhythmias; acute malarial infection	**May precipitate arrhythmias at high doses; nausea; vomiting; diarrhea; cinchonism: tinnitus, headache, nausea, disturbed vision; renal damage; hemolytic anemia; purpura; agranulocytosis**	**Torsades des Pointes**
Quinine	*Antimalarial*—unknown mechanism	**Suppression and treatment of acute attack of chloroquine-resistant organism**	Cinchonism: tinnitus, headache, nausea, disturbed vision; renal damage; hemolytic anemia; purpura; agranulocytosis	
Quinolones	*Antibiotic*—blocks DNA synthesis by inhibiting DNA gyrase	Gram-negative infections (esp. UTI and bone): Pseudomonas, Enterobacteriaceae, Neisseria; gram-positive infections; intracellular: Legionella	GI disturbances; headache; dizziness; phototoxicity; cartilage damage	May elevate theophylline to toxic levels causing seizure
Radioiodide [I-131]	Destroys thyroid gland	Hyperthyroidism	Hypothyroidism	

Therapeutic Agent (common name, if relevant) [Trade name, where appropriate]	Class—Pharmacology and Pharmacokinetics	Indications	Side or Adverse Effects	Contraindications or Precautions to Consider; Notes
Ranitidine [Zantac]	H₂ blocker	Inhibits gastric acid secretion (esp. ulcer)	Gynecomastia; rare: headache, dizziness, fatigue, CNS, leuko-penia, reduced sperm count	Inhibits metabolism and/or absorption of some drugs
Reserpine [Reserfia]	*Antihypertensive*—prevents storage of monoamines in synaptic vesicle	Hypertension	Mental depression	
RhoGam	Rh immunoglobulin	Prevents hemolytic disease of the newborn		
Ribavirin [Virazid, Virazole]	*Antiviral*—guanosine analog; inhibits DNA polymerase	Broad spectrum against DNA (herpes) and RNA (influenza A and B); RSV in children	Headache; rash; fatigue; dyspnea	
Rifampin [Rifadin]	*Antibiotic*—inhibits DNA dependent RNA polymerase	Mycobacterium	Orange body fluids	Interferes with birth control pills by increasing estrogen metabolism; induces cytochrome P450
Risperidone [Risperdal]	*Antipsychotic*—blocks D₂ and 5-HT₂ receptors	Psychosis		
Ritodrine [Yutopar]	β2 agonist	Inhibit preterm labor; relax uterus		
Ritonavir [Norvir]	*Antiviral*—protease inhibitor	AIDS		
Ropivacaine	*Anesthetic agent*—blocks Na⁺ intracellularly	Local anesthetic	Sleepiness; light-headed; visual/ audio disturbances; restlessness; nystagmus; shivering; tonic-clonic convulsion; death	
Saquinavir [Invirase]	*Antiviral*—protease inhibitor	AIDS		
Sarin/Somin	Inhibits cholinesterase		Rapidly fatal	
Scopolamine [Transderm Scop]	Cholinergic blocker	Motion sickness; Parkinson's disease, anti-emetic		
Scorpion toxin	Pre-synaptic neuromuscular junction blocker; overstimulates ACh release			
Secobarbital [Novosecobarb, Seconal]	*Anti-epileptic*—anesthetic agent; barbiturate; prolong IPSP duration	Epilepsy, cerebral edema		
Selegiline [Eldepryl]	*Anti-Parkinson's*—increases dopamine by inhibiting MAO_b irreversibly	Parkinson's disease		

Drug	Class / Mechanism	Clinical use	Side effects / toxicity	Notes
Sertraline [Zoloft]	*Antidepressant*—SSRI	Depression	Nausea; headache; insomnia	
Sevoflurane [Sevorane, Ultrane]	Anesthetic agent	General anesthetic		
Sildenafil [Viagra]	**Phosphodiesterase type 5 inhibitor (cGMP specific)**	**Erectile dysfunction**	**Abnormal vision; UTI's; cardiovascular events; priapism; dyspepsia**	Contraindicated in pregnant/lactating women or children
Simvastatin [Zocor]	*Lipid lowering agent*—inhibits HMG-CoA reductase; lowers LDL	Hyperlipidemia (esp. type II)	Liver toxicity; myopathy; mild GI disturbances	
Sodium nitroprusside	*Antianginal*—antihypertensive; vasodilator	Congestive heart failure		
Somatostatin [Zecnil]	*Hormone*—**decreases release of GH, gastrin, secretin, VIP, CCK, glucagon, insulin, calcitonin, PTH, renin, and TSH**	Acromegaly; glucagonoma; insulinoma	**Nausea; cramps; gallstones**	
Sotalol [Betapace]	*Antiarrhythmic (Class III)*—K+ channel blocker		Torsades de pointes	
Spectinomycin [Trobicin]	*Antibiotic*—aminoglycoside; binds 30s ribosome subunits; bacteriostatic at low concentration; bactericidal at high	Used to treat gonorrhea in those allergic to penicillin		
Spironolactone [Aldactone]	K+ sparing diuretic; aldosterone antagonist acts at DCT	Diuresis	**Hyperkalemia; gynecomastia; impotence; GI disturbances**	
Streptokinase [Streptase]	*Thrombolytic*—plasminogen activator	Lysis of clots	**Hemorrhage**	
Streptomycin	*Antibiotic*—aminoglycoside; binds 30s ribosome subunits; bacteriostatic at low concentration; bactericidal at high	Tuberculosis and other mycobacteria		
Strychnine	Acts on the post-synaptic Renshaw cell; binds to glycine receptor (mimics effect of tetanus)	Depression		
Succinylcholine [Anectine]	Depolarizing neuromuscular blocker		**Increases intra-ocular pressure; scoline apnea in genetically defective pseudocholinesterse; malignant hyperthermia if given with halothane**	**Contraindicated in patients with glaucoma, antibiotics**
Sucralfate [Carafate]	*Anti-ulcer*—protective coating of GI lining	Reduces effect of gastric acid on mucosa	Constipation	
Sufentanil [Sufenta]	*Opioid agonist*	Pain; general anesthetic		

Therapeutic Agent (common name, if relevant) [Trade name, where appropriate]	Class—Pharmacology and Pharmacokinetics	Indications	Side or Adverse Effects	Contraindications or Precautions to Consider; Notes
Sulfinpyrazone [Anturane]	*Antigout*—uricosuric (similar to probenecid)	Chronic gout	GI irritation; hypersensitivity reaction; agranulocytosis	
Sulfonamides	**Antibiotic**—competitive inhibitor of dihydropteroate synthetase (blocks folic acid synthesis)	**Broad spectrum; gram-positive UTI; Chlamydia infection of genital tract and eye; treatment of nocardiosis**	**Form crystals in kidney and bladder causing damage, nausea, vomiting, headache**	
Sulindac [Clinoril]	*Anti-inflammatory*—pro-drug sulfide	Chronic inflammation (arthritis)		
Sumatriptan [Imitrex]	**Antimigraine**—agonist at 5-HT$_{1d}$ receptors	**Acute attack of migraine**		
Syrup of Ipecac [Quelidrine]	*Expectorant*—increase bronchial secretion	Promotes cough		
Tacrine [Cognex]	**Alzheimer's agent**—noncompetitive cholinesterase inhibitor; muscarinic agonist	**Alzheimer's disease**		
Tacrolimus (FK506) [Prograf]	*Immunosuppressant*—blocks activation of T-cell transcription factors; involved in interleukin synthesis	Transplant rejection	Nephrotoxic; neurotoxic; hyperglycemia; GI disturbances	
Tamoxifen [Nolvadex]	**Antineoplastic**—competitive estrogen receptor blocker	**Treats estrogen dependant breast cancer in post-menopausal women; reduce contralateral breast cancer**	**May increase risk of other cancer; hot flashes; flushing**	
Temazepam [Restoril]	*Benzodiazepine*—enhances GABA; increases IPSP amplitude	Sedative; hypnotic; anti-anxiety; anti-epileptic		
Terazosin [Hytrin]	*Antihypertensive*—α$_1$ blocker	Pheochromocytoma; hypertension; benign prostatic hyperplasia	Postural hypotension	
Terbinafine [Lamisil]	Antifungal—inhibits squalene-2,3-epoxidase	Orally for onychomycosis; topically for dermatophytes		
Terbutaline [Brethine, Bricanyl, Brethaire]	**Bronchodilator**—β$_2$ agonist	**Bronchodilates to treat asthma; inhibit pre-term labor; relax uterus**		
Tetanus toxin		Acts at the pre-synaptic Renshaw cell; prevents glycine release		

Drug [brand]	Class/Mechanism	Use	Side effects	Notes
Tetracaine [Pontocaine]	*Anesthetic agent*—blocks Na^+ channels intracellularly	Local anesthetic	Sleepiness; light-headedness; visual/audio disturbances; restlessness; nystagmus; shivering; tonic-clonic convulsion; death	
Tetracycline [Achromycin, Sumycin, Topicycline]	***Antibiotic***— binds 30s ribosome subunits; bacteriostatic	**Broad spectrum including Chlamydia, Rickettsia, and Mycoplasma**	**Liver toxicity; depression of bone/teeth development; phototoxic reactions; superinfections due to broad spectrum; Fanconi's syndrome**	**Contraindicated in pregnancy and children**
THC (active ingredient in marijuana)	Unknown mechanism; binds opiate receptors and directly inhibits vomiting center in medulla	Anti-emetic	Dry mouth; dizziness; inability to concentrate; disorientation, anxiety; tachycardia, depression, paranoia; psychosis	
Theobromine	Unknown mechanism; stimulates CNS, cardiac muscle; relaxes smooth muscle; produces diuresis; increases cerebral vascular resistance			
Theophylline [Aerolate, Elixophyllin, Resbid, Slo-bid, Slo-Phyllin, Theo-24, Theo-Dur, Theolair, T-Ohyl, Uniphyl]	***Bronchodilator***—unknown mechanism; stimulates CNS, cardiac muscle; relaxes smooth muscle; produces diuresis; increases cerebral vascular resistance	**Asthma**		**Tolerance develops**
Thiabendazole [Mintezol]	***Antihelminthic***	**Strongyloides; Ancylostoma (hookworm); Enterobius (pinworm); Trichuris (whipworm)**	**Vomiting; diarrhea; dizziness; bradycardia; hypotension; paresthesias; yellow vision; angioneurotic edema; perianal rashes**	
Thiopental [Pentothal]	*Anesthetic agent*—barbiturate; prolongs IPSP duration	Anti-epileptic; cerebral edema; anesthetic (stage 3 anesthetic)	Laryngospasm during stage 3 induction	
Thioridazine [Mellaril]	*Antipsychotic*—blocks D_2 receptors	Psychosis	Orthostatic hypotension; anti-cholinergic effects; sedation	
Thiotepa [Thioplex]	*Antineoplastic*—unknown mechanism	Cancer		
Thiothixene [Navane]	*Antipsychotic*—blocks D_2 receptors	Psychosis	Anti-cholinergic effects	
Ticarcillin [Ticar]	*Antibiotic*—β-lactam	Pseudomonas; Proteus		*IV*; given with clavulanic acid

Therapeutic Agent (common name, if relevant) [Trade name, where appropriate]	Class–Pharmacology and Pharmacokinetics	Indications	Side or Adverse Effects	Contraindications or Precautions to Consider; Notes
Ticlopidine [Ticlid]	**Inhibits ADP-induced platelet aggregation; acts on ADP receptor**	**Transient ischemic attack (TIA); stroke**		
Timentin	Inhibits β-lactamase; synergistic with penicillins		Asthma	
Timolol [Betimol, Blocadren, Timoptic]	*Anti-glaucoma—antihypertensive;* β blocker	Hypertension; MI; glaucoma		
Tizanadine [Zanaflex]	*Centrally acting muscle relaxant*—presynaptic inhibition of motor neurons; acts like clonidine on α_2	Muscle spasms from spinal cord injury; multiple sclerosis		
Tobramycin [Tobrex]	*Antibiotic*—binds 30s ribosome subunits; bacteriostatic at low concentration; bactericidal at high	Similar to gentamicin		
Tocainide [Tonocard]	*Antiarrhythmic (Class IB)*—Na^+ channel blocker			
Tolazamide [Tolinase]	*Hypoglycemic agent*—sulfonylurea; reduces K^+ efflux, increases Ca^{2+} influx, increases secretion of insulin	Oral treatment for NIDDM (type II diabetes)	Hypoglycemia; GI disturbances; muscle weakness; mental confusion	
Tolbutamide [Orinase]	*Hypoglycemic agent*—sulfonylurea; reduces K^+ efflux, increases Ca^{2+} influx, increases secretion of insulin	Oral treatment for NIDDM (type II diabetes)	Hypoglycemia; GI disturbances; muscle weakness; mental confusion	
Tolnaftate [Tinactin, Desenex]	*Antifungal*—unknown mechanism; bactericidal	Topical against: T. rubrum, T. tonsurans, T. versicolor, T. mentagrophytes		
Topiramate [Topamax]	*Anti-epileptic*—blocks Na^+ channels	Add on drug for epilepsy		
Torsemide [Demadex]	Loop diuretic; inhibits Na/K/Cl channel	Diuresis	Ototoxicity; metabolic alkalosis; hypokalemia; hyperglycemia; hyperuricemia	
t-PA [Activase]	***Thrombolytic*—plasminogen activator**	**Lysis of clots**	**Hemorrhage**	

Drug	Class/Mechanism	Use	Notes/Side effects
Tramadol [Ultram]	*Analgesic*—similar to opioid agonist	Chronic pain of osteoarthritis	
Tranexamic acid (AMCHA) [Cyklokapron]	*Thrombotic agent*—competitive inhibitor of plasminogen activation	Inhibits fibrinolysis; promotes thrombosis	
Tranylcypromine [Parnate]	*Antidepressant*—MAO inhibitor; non-selective, but isoenzyme A most important; reversible	Depression	Only reversible MAOI
TRH [protirelin] [Relefact TRH]	Stimulates TSH, prolactin, and GH release	Diagnosis of thyroid disease	
Triamterene [Dyrenium]	*Diuretic*—K$^+$ sparing diuretic; decreases K$^+$ secretion by inhibiting Na$^+$ resorption in DCT	Diuresis	Hyperkalemia
Triazolam [Halcion]	*Benzodiazepine*—enhances GABA; increase IPSP amplitude	Sedative; hypnotic; anti-anxiety; anti-epileptic	Paranoia; violent behavior
Tricalcium phosphate	Dietary Ca^{2+} supplement	Ca^{2+} deficiency	
Trientine [Cuprid, Syprine]	*Metal chelator*	Copper poisoning; Wilson's disease	
Trifluridine [Viroptic]	*Antiviral*—thymidine derivative; inhibits DNA polymerase; inhibits DNA synthesis	DNA viruses	
Trihexyphenidyl [Artane]	*Anti-Parkinson's*—muscarinic blocker	Parkinson's disease	
Trimethaphan [Arfonad]	*Antihypertensive*—non-depolarizing nicotinic blocker	Hypertension (short term)	
Trimethoprim [Proloprim, Trimpex]	**Antibiotic—competitive inhibition of dihydrofolate reductase (blocks folic acid synthesis)**	**Gram-negative UTI; combined with sulfonamides to treat UTI, otitis media, chronic bronchitis, shigellosis, and PCP**	
Troglitazone [Rezulin]	*Hypoglycemic agent*—reduces insulin resistance by increasing transcription of insulin response genes; increases glucose uptake	Type II diabetes	
Trovafloxacin [Trovan]	*Quinolone antibiotic*—blocks DNA synthesis by inhibiting DNA gyrase	Gram-negative infections (esp. UTI and bone): Pseudomonas, Enterobacteriaceae, Neisseria; gram-positive infections; intracellular: Legionella	GI disturbances; headache; dizziness; phototoxicity; cartilage damage

Therapeutic Agent (common name, if relevant) [Trade name, where appropriate]	Class—Pharmacology and Pharmacokinetics	Indications	Side or Adverse Effects	Contraindications or Precautions to Consider; Notes
TSH (thyrotropin) [Thyrogen]	Increases output of thyroid hormone	Assess thyroid function; increase uptake of I-131 in thyroid carcinoma		
Undecylenic acid [Desenex]	*Antifungal*—unknown mechanism; fungistatic	Topical for dermatophytes (esp. Tinea pedis)		
Urofollitropin [Metrodin]	FSH analog	Infertility		
Urokinase [Abbokinase]	*Thrombolytic agent*—plasminogen activator	Lysis of clots	Hemorrhage	
Valacyclovir [Valtrex]	*Antiviral*—guanosine analog; inhibits DNA polymerase	Herpes; Varicella; EBV and CMV at high doses	GI disturbances; CNS and renal problems; headache; tremor; rash	Longer lasting than acyclovir
Valproic acid [Depakene]	*Anti-epileptic*—blocks Na^+ channels and increases GABA	Epilepsy: partial, absence, and tonic-clonic	Liver toxicity; pancreatitis; potentially fatal	
Vancomycin [Vancocin]	*Antibiotic*—disrupts cell wall and cell membrane; bactericidal	Serious infections by gram-positive bacteria: strep, staph, pneumococcus and some anaerobes (esp. *C. difficile*)	Ototoxicity; nephrotoxicity; "red man syndrome" due to histamine release	
Vasopressin [Pitressin]	*Anti-diuretic*—recruits water channels to lumenal membrane in collecting duct	Anti-diuresis; treats pituitary diabetes insipidus	Overhydration; allergic reaction; larger doses: pallor, diarrhea, hypertension; coronary constriction; chronic rhinopharyngitis	Also known as ADH, AVP
Vecuronium [Norcuron]	Non-depolarizing neuromuscular blocker			
Verapamil [Calan, Isoptin]	*Antiarrhythmic (Class IV)*—Ca^{2+} blocker	Atrial tachyarrhythmia; decreases reperfusion injury	AV block; constipation; hypotension; GI distress	
Vidarabine [Vira-A]	*Antiviral*—adenosine analog; inhibits DNA polymerase	Herpes (also topical for HSV keratitis); varicella	GI disturbances; CNS, bone marrow suppression; liver and kidney dysfunction	
Vinblastine [Velban]	*Antineoplastic*—depolymerizes microtubules	Hodgkin's	Peripheral neuritis	

Drug	Class / Mechanism	Clinical Use / Function	Symptoms	Notes
Vincristine [Oncovin]	*Antineoplastic*—depolymerizes microtubules	Acute leukemia	Peripheral neuritis	
Vitamin A (Retinol) [Aquasol A]	*Vitamin*	Night blindness, xerophthalmia	Hyperkeratosis	
Vitamin B_1 (thiamine)	*Vitamin*	**Alcoholics (prophylaxis for Wernicke-Korsakoff)**		**Decrease results in beriberi**
Vitamin B_{12} [Anacobin, Cyanocobalamine, Shovite]	*Vitamin*	**Megaloblastic anemia**		
Vitamin B_2 (riboflavin)	*Vitamin*—component of flavin compounds: FMN, FAD			Inhibits chlorpromazine; decrease results in skin, oral, ocular lesions
Vitamin B_3 (nicotinic acid, Niacin) [Nia-bid, Niacels]	*Vitamin*—component of nicotinic compounds: NAD, NADH	Maintains integrity of skin; decreases VLDL and LDL		Decrease: dermatitis, diarrhea, dementia, death
Vitamin B_5 (pantothenic acid)	*Vitamin*—component of CoA			
Vitamin B_6 (pyridoxine) [Beesix, Doxine]	*Vitamin*	Protein metabolism; neurotransmitter synthesis	Neuritis; convulsions	Isoniazid decreases amount
Vitamin C (ascorbic acid)	*Vitamin*	Maintains collagen; oxidation-reduction reactions		Decrease: scurvy
Vitamin D (calcitriol) [Rocaltrol]	***Vitamin*—binds to receptors in cytoplasm; alters gene expression and protein synthesis; increases bone reabsorption of Ca^{2+}; increases renal and intestinal absorption of Ca^{2+} and phosphate**	**Rickets; osteomalacia; hypocalcemia; hypoparathyroidism; osteoporosis**		
Vitamin E (tocopherol)	*Vitamin*—antioxidant	Prophylaxis for heart disease		Decrease: abortion, creatinuria, ceroid pigment
Vitamin K (mephyton)	*Vitamin*—enhances clotting factors	Bleeding disorders		Decreased in children of mothers taking phenytoin or phenobarbital
Vitamin M (folic acid) [Folvite]	*Vitamin*—one carbon carrier	Nucleic acid synthesis; given to pregnant mothers		Decrease: neural tube defects in utero; decreased in pregnancy or with use of phenytoin, isoniazid
Warfarin [Coumadin]	*Anticoagulant*—inhibits potassium epoxide regeneration	Thrombosis	Bleeding	Contraindicated in patients with liver, CNS, hemostatic disease; 99% exists protein bound

Therapeutic Agent (common name, if relevant) [Trade name, where appropriate]	Class—Pharmacology and Pharmacokinetics	Indications	Side or Adverse Effects	Contraindications or Precautions to Consider; Notes
Yohimbine	*Impotence therapy—* α_2-antagonist			
Zafirlukast [Accolate]	***Anti-asthma agent—*blocks leukotriene receptors (LTD4)**	**Reduces bronchoconstriction and inflammatory cell infiltrate in asthma**		
Zidovudine [Retrovir]	***Antiviral—*thymidine analog; reverse transcriptase inhibitor**	**AIDS**	**Nausea; headache; bone marrow suppression; myalgias**	
Zileuton	***Anti-asthma agent—*5-Lipoxygenase inhibitor**	**Improves asthma**		
Zolpidem [Ambien]	Binds to benzodiazepine receptor, but is not a benzodiazepine	Hypnotic		

5HT=5-hydroxytryptamine (serotonin); *ACE*=angiotensin-converting enzyme; *ACh*=acetylcholine; *ACTH*=adrenocorticotropic hormone; *ADP*=adenosine diphosphate; *AML*=acute myelocytic leukemia; *ATPase*=adenosine triphosphatase; *AV*=atrioventricular; *BP*=blood pressure; *BPH*=benign prostatic hypertrophy; *cAMP*=cyclic adenosine monophosphate; *CCK*=cholecystokinin; *cGMP*=cyclic guanosine monophosphate; *CHF*=congestive heart failure; *CMI*=cell-mediated immunity; *CMV*=cytomegalovirus; *CNS*=central nervous system; *CoA*=coenzyme A; *COPD*=chronic obstructive pulmonary disease; *COX*=cyclo-oxygenase; *DCT*=distal convoluted tubule; *dCTP*=deoxycytidine triphosphate; *DHEA*=dehydroepiandrosterone; *EBV*=Epstein-Barr virus; *ECG*=electrocardiogram, electrocardiography; *FAD*=flavin adenine dinucleotide; *FMN*=flavin mononucleotide; *FSH*=follicle stimulating hormone; *GABA*=γ-aminobutyric acid; *GH*=growth hormone; *GI*=gastrointestinal; *GnRH*=gonadotropin-releasing hormone; *HDL*=high-density lipoprotein; *HMG-CoA*=3-hydroxy-3-methylglutaryl coenzyme A; *INF*=interferon; *IPSP*=inhibitory postsynaptic potential; *LDL*=low-density lipoprotein; *L-DOPA*=levodopa (levo-3, 4-dihydroxyphenylalanine); *LH*=luteinizing hormone; *LPL*=lipoprotein lipase; *LTB₄*=leukotriene B₄; *LTD₄*=leukotriene B₄; *MAO*=monoamine oxidase; *MAOb*=monoamine oxidase B; *MAOI*=monoamine oxidase inhibitor; *MHC*=major histocompatibility complex; *MI*=myocardial infarction; *NAD*=nicotinamide adenine dinucleotide; *NADH*=reduced nicotinamide adenine dinucleotide; *NE*=norepinephrine; *NIDDM*=non-insulin-dependent diabetes mellitus; *NO*=nitric oxide; *NSAID*=nonsteroidal anti-inflammatory drug; *PCP*=phencyclidine; *PCT*=proximal convoluted tubule; *PDA*=patent ductus arteriosus; *PGE₁*=prostaglandin E₁; *PGE₂*=prostaglandin E₂; *PGF₂-α*=prostaglandin F₂₋α; *PMN*=polymorphonuclear; *PTH*=parathyroid hormone; *PTT*=partial thromboplastin time; *Rh*=rhesus [factor]; *RSV*=respiratory syncytial virus; *SLE*=systemic lupus erythematosus; *SSRI*=selective serotonin reuptake inhibitor; *TCA*=tricyclic antidepressant; *TG*=triglycerides; *THC*=tetrahydracannabinol; *TNF*=tumor necrosis factor; *TSH*=thyroid-stimulating hormone; *UTI*=urinary tract infection; *VIP*=vasoactive intestinal peptide; *VLDL*=very low density lipoprotein

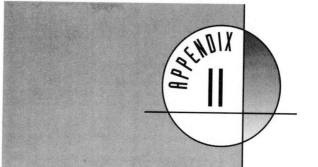

APPENDIX

II

Bug Index

Bacteria

Name	Morphology	Pathogenesis	Description of Disease	Laboratory Findings, Notes	Transmission	Prevention and Therapy
Actinomyces israelii	Gm⁺; filamentous; anaerobic	Unknown	Actinomycosis—abscesses with draining sinus tracts	Forms filaments; sulfur granules	Dental disease or trauma	Penicillin and drainage
Bacillus anthracis	Gm⁺; rod with square ends; capsule of D-glutamate (only protein capsule); non-motile; spore-former; aerobic	Anthrax toxin—edema factor (exotoxin); protective antigen for cell entry; lethal factor (mode of action unknown)	Anthrax—cutaneous eschar (malignant pustules), pulmonary disease, septicemia	Medusa-head colonies	Spores from animals (usually cattle);	Attenuated strain human vaccine; penicillin
Bacillus cereus	Gm⁺; rod; spore-former; aerobic	Spores germinate when rice is reheated; entero-toxins—emetic toxin, diarrheal toxin	Food poisoning—early vomiting and late diarrhea		Enter through the GI tract via reheated rice	Avoid refried rice and beans; treatment is symptomatic; cephalosporin
Bacteroides fragilis	Gm⁻; bacilli; anaerobic; capsulated	Capsule; weak endotoxin	Sepsis; peritonitis; bacteremia; foul-smelling abscess	Mixed infections	Deep penetrating wounds; wound débridement	Metronidazole
Bordetella pertussis	Gm⁻; coccobacilli; capsule	Noninvasive infection of bronchial epithelium; pertussis toxin (2 subunits)—"A" subunit ADP ribosylates adenylate cyclase increasing cAMP, while B subunit causes attachment	Whooping cough	Culture nasopharynx onto 10%–15% blood agar (Bordet-Gengou agar); slide agglutination test	Droplet nuclei	Acellular pertussis vaccine (at 2, 4, and 6 months) or whole inactive cells; erythromycin
Borrelia burgdorferi	Spirochete; microaerophilic; flagella	Invasion and replication in the bloodstream	Lyme disease—erythema chronicum migrans with involve-ment of the heart, joints, and CNS	Common in the Northeast, Midwest, and Western U.S.	Deer ticks	Avoid ticks, wear long pants in wooded areas; doxycycline and penicillin
Brucella	Gm⁻; coccobacillus; facultative intracellular	Catalase; LPS; inhibits release of peroxidase in macrophages	Undulating fever—macrophages engulf and then re-release into the bloodstream; granulomas		Contaminated milk and cheese	Pasteurization of dairy products; tetracycline
Campylobacter jejuni	Gm⁻; comma-shaped bacilli; motile	Enterotoxin with anti-genic diversity stimulates cAMP	Gastroenteritis—blood and pus in stool	Microaerophilic; Campy plate; diarrhea in college students	Milk, water, poultry	Symptomatic

BUG INDEX

293

Name	Morphology	Pathogenesis	Description of Disease	Laboratory Findings, Notes	Transmission	Prevention and Therapy
Chlamydia psittaci	Obligate intracellular	Unknown	Psittacosis—dry cough with CNS symptoms	Giemsa stain; inactive form extracellular (elementary body) and metabolically active form intracellular (reticulate body)	Aerosol of dried bird feces	Tetracycline
Chlamydia trachomatis	Obligate intracellular	Unknown	Strains A–C—blindness; Strains D–K: chlamydia, nongonococcal urethritis, cervicitis; strains L1-L3: lymphogranuloma venereum	Leading cause of preventable blindness in the world; inactive form extracellular (elementary body) and metabolically active form intracellular (reticulate body)	Sexual contact or via birth canal	Tetracycline
Clostridium botulinum	Gm⁺; rod; spore former; anaerobic	Botulinum toxin inhibits release of acetylcholine; exotoxins A, B, and E	Botulism (weakness and respiratory paralysis); food, wound, and infant types; floppy baby syndrome; dysphagia; constipation	Toxin	Spores from contaminated food	Sterilization of canned foods; cook to inactivate toxin; trivalent antitoxin; respiratory support
Clostridium difficile	Gm⁺; rod; spore former, anaerobic	Exotoxins A and B—A (cholera like) causes fluid release, B (diphtheria like) damages mucosa and causes pseudomembrane formation	Antibiotic-associated pseudomembranous colitis; bloody diarrhea	ELISA detects toxin B in the stool sample	Hospital workers	Withdraw causative antibiotics (usually clindamycin); vancomycin
Clostridium perfringens	Gm⁺; rod; spore former; anaerobic	α-Toxin (damages cell membranes); γ-toxin (tissue necrosis and hemolysis); cholera-like heat-labile enterotoxin (food poisoning—watery diarrhea)	Gas gangrene; food poisoning; anaerobic cellulitis	Large rods found in food; double-zone of hemolysis	Grows in traumatized tissue (muscle); spores in food and soil germinate in reheated foods	Clean and débride wounds; cook food well
Clostridium tetani	Gm⁺; rod; spore-former (tennis racquet shaped); anaerobic	Tetanus toxin (exotoxin)—blocks release of inhibitory neurotransmitters	Tetanus: lockjaw (trismus), spastic paralysis (opisthotonos), sardonic grin (risus sardonicus)		Spore entry via wound (e.g., a rusty nail)	Toxoid vaccine (2, 4, 6, 18 months) booster every 10 years; tetanus immunoglobulin (passive immunity); penicillin

Organism	Characteristics	Toxin/Virulence	Disease	Lab ID	Transmission	Treatment/Vaccine
Corynebacterium diphtheriae	Gm+; rod; club shaped; arranged in V or L; non-spore former	Exotoxin—A ADP ribosylates EF-2 and B binds toxin to the cell; phage conversion	Diphtheria—pseudomembrane forms in the throat; bull neck; systemic toxemia	Tellurite plate (Löffler's medium) grows black colonies	Airborne droplets	Inactivated toxoid vaccine; antitoxin (neutralizes unbound toxin); penicillin
Coxiella burnetii	Obligate intracellular	Unknown	Q fever	Only rickettsia not transmitted to humans by an arthropod vector	Inhalation of aerosols of urine, feces; transplacental	Tetracycline
Enterococci faecalis	Gm+; cocci	Lipoteichoic acid	Urinary, biliary, and cardiovascular infections; endocarditis	Catalase-negative; bacitracin resistant; variable hemolysis; grows in 6.5% NaCl/Lancefield group D	Normal flora of gut gaining access to blood	Penicillin and an aminoglycoside
Escherichia coli	Gm−; bacilli	Endotoxin—septic shock; heat-labile (LT) enterotoxin: increased cAMP leads to diarrhea; heat-stable (ST) stimulates guanylate cyclase to cause diarrhea; pili; adhere to epithelium especially in UTIs; Verotoxin (O157:H7); shiga-like toxin in EHEC that inhibits 28S rRNA to cause bloody diarrhea	UTIs; sepsis; neonatal meningitis; enteropathogenic *E. coli* (EPEC); traveler's diarrhea; enterotoxigenic *E. coli* (ETEC): watery diarrhea; enteroinvasive *E. coli* (EIEC): dysentery; enterohemorrhagic *E. coli* (EHEC): bloody diarrhea, hemolytic uremic syndrome	Transplacental; fecal-oral route	UTIs: ampicillin or sulfonamides; sepsis: cephalosporins; traveler's diarrhea: rehydration
Francisella tularensis	Gm−; rod; intracellular	Capsular; intracellular within macrophages	Painful lymph nodes; glandular and ocular ulcers	Cysteine agar	Zoonotic via rabbits	Live attenuated vaccine; streptomycin; thorough cooking of meat
Gardnerella vaginalis	Gm− variable; bacillus	Unknown	Vaginosis—watery discharge, fishy odor	Clue cells	Sexually transmitted	Metronidazole
Haemophilus ducreyi	Gm−; bacilli	Virulence via pili	Chancroid with pain and purulent exudate	Lesions similar to those of syphilis	Sexually transmitted	Nafcillin
Haemophilus influenzae	Gm−; coccobacilli; polysaccharide capsule (polyribitol phosphate)	IgA protease degrades antibody and attaches to respiratory tract; capsule (type B) prevents phagocytosis	Infantile meningitis; epiglottitis; otitis media	Needs heme (factor X) and NAD (factor V) to grow; chocolate agar; check CSF	Respiratory droplets	Hib vaccine (B type capsule conjugated to diphtheria toxoid as a carrier protein); ceftriaxone
Helicobacter pylori	Gm−; bacilli; motile; urease +; flagella	Urease results in ammonia production and subsequent gastric damage	Peptic ulcers (type B gastritis)	Microaerophilic; Campy plate; urea breath test	Ingestion	Triple therapy regimens—(1) amoxicillin, metronidazole, bismuth; (2) amoxicillin, omeprazole, ranitidine

Name	Morphology	Pathogenesis	Description of Disease	Laboratory Findings, Notes	Transmission	Prevention and Therapy
Klebsiella pneumoniae	Gm⁻; bacilli; capsule	Large capsule hinders phagocytosis	Pneumonia; UTI; bacteremia	Pneumonia, particularly in malnourished alcoholics	Aspiration of respiratory droplets	Cephalosporins
Legionella pneumophila	Gm⁻; bacilli	Endotoxin affects smokers, alcoholics, and those older than 55 years of age	Legionnaire's disease (atypical pneumonia)	Dieterle silver stain; cysteine required for culture	Aerosol from environmental water sources	Erythromycin
Listeria monocytogenes	Gm⁺; rod; arranged in V or L; tumbling motility; non-spore-former — COLD GROW -	Grows intracellularly in macrophages; listeriolysin-O cytotoxic * ONLY G+ LPS *	Meningitis and sepsis in newborns and immunocompromised	Small gray colonies; β-hemolysis; motility	Transferred to humans by animals or their feces; unpasteurized milk; contaminated vegetables	Ampicillin
Mycobacterium avium-intracellulare (MAC)	Acid-fast bacilli	Unknown	Tuberculosis-like disease in the immunocompromised		From the soil and water to the immunocompromised individuals	Amikacin plus doxycycline
Mycobacterium leprae	Acid-fast; bacilli; obligate intracellular	Tuberculoid: cell-mediated response causes damage; lepromatous: anergy of CD8 cells leads to uncontrolled replication	Leprosy—tuberculoid and lepromatous; lesions in cool parts of body	Cannot be grown in culture but is harvested in the footpads of armadillos	Prolonged contact, especially with the lepromatous form	Dapsone and rifampin for tuberculoid form; clofazamine, dapsone, rifampin for lepromatous form; 2-year treatment
Mycobacterium tuberculosis	Acid-fast bacilli; aerobic; high lipid cell walls (mycolic acids and wax D)	Cord factor; granulomas and caseation	Tuberculosis	Ziehl-Neelsen stain; slow-growing (3–8 weeks) on Lowenstein-Jensen medium; niacin +; PPD + if >10 cm after 48 hours	Droplets from coughing	BCG vaccine with live, attenuated organisms (rarely used in the U.S.); isoniazid, rifampin, pyrazinamide for 6–9 months
Mycoplasma pneumoniae	Obligate intracellulare; not seen on a Gram stain; smallest free-living organism; only bacteria with cholesterol in membrane (no cell wall)	Hydrogen peroxide and lytic enzymes resulting in damage to the respiratory tract	Walking pneumonia; bullous myringitis (inflamed tympanic membrane)	Positive cold-agglutinin; highest incidence in 5 to 15 year olds	Respiratory droplets	Erythromycin
Neisseria gonorrhoeae (gonococcus)	Gm⁻; cocci; coffee bean shape; no polysaccharide capsule	Endotoxin (lipid A); pili with variation; proteins I, II, III (porin, adhesin, autoagglutination); deficiencies in late-acting complement components	Urethral and vaginal infections; discharge; salpingitis and PID; neonatal conjunctivitis; septic arthritis	Thayer-Martin agar; only glucose fermentation; oxidase +; also check for chlamydia due to common coinfection	Sexual contact; newborns; symptomatic in men but not usually in women	Condoms; erythromycin or silver nitrate in neonates; ceftriaxone; spectinomycin and tetracycline

Organism	Morphology	Virulence/Mechanism	Disease	Lab/Diagnosis	Transmission	Treatment
Neisseria meningitidis (meningococcus)	Gm⁻; cocci; coffee-bean shaped; polysaccharide capsule (anti-phagocytic)	Endotoxin (LPS) contains lipid A; capsule; IgA protease; pili variation; deficiencies in late-acting complement components; asplenic patients	Meningitis; petechial rash; pharyngitis	Glucose and maltose fermentation; oxidase +; lumbar puncture with high protein and low glucose; grows on Thayer-Martin agar	Respiratory droplets	Vaccine, rifampin; penicillin G
Nocardia asteroides	Acid-fast; bacillus; aerobic	Unknown; immuno-compromised at risk	Nocardiosis—lung, heart, and brain abscesses	Forms filaments	Airborne particles	Sulfonamides
Pseudomonas aeruginosa	Gm⁻; coccobacilli	Pili; A/B toxin similar to diphtheria; flagella; hemolysin	UTI; septicemia; burn infections *Pneumonia External otitis*	Fruity smell; green, water-soluble pigment	Water; environment; opportunistic: catheters, leukemia patients, burns, cystic fibrosis	Very resistant to antibiotics *aminoglycoside + extended PCN*
Rickettsia prowazekii	Obligate intracellular	Invasion of the endothelial lining; possible endotoxin	Epidemic typhus		Human-to-human spread	Tetracycline
Rickettsia rickettsii	Obligate intracellular	Invasion of endothelial lining	Rocky Mountain spotted fever: vasculitis, rash spreads from periphery inward	Weil-Felix reaction (agglutination when patient's serum mixed with OX strain of *Proteus vulgaris*)	Dermacentor ticks	Tetracycline
Rickettsia typhi	Obligate intracellular	Invasion of endothelial lining; possible endotoxin	Endemic typhus—rash spreads from the trunk outward		Spread by fleas	Tetracycline
Shigella	Gm⁻; rod; nonmotile; non-spore-formers	Invades mucosa; ulceration and PMN infiltrate; shiga toxin (A/B toxin): works on 28S ribosome and removes the base; low infective dose	Bacterial dysentery (shigellosis): ulcerative colitis of large intestine, fever, chills, cramps, tenesmus, bloody stool	Rectal swab; three types: *dysenteriae* (rare), *sonnei* (most common, day-care), *flexneri* (gay men)	Fecal-oral route	Public health measures; significant resistance; fluids; ampicillin
Staphylococcus aureus	Gm⁺; cocci; capsule; protein A in the cell wall; yellow, creamy, grape-like clusters on culture	Rapid growth; protein A (anti-phagocytic); enterotoxin (watery diarrhea); toxic shock syndrome toxin; exfoliation; α-toxin; coagulase	Abscesses; pyogenic infections (endocarditis, osteomyelitis); food poisoning; toxic shock syndrome; scalded skin syndrome	Coagulase +; catalase +; β-hemolytic; novobiocin-sensitive; ferment mannitol	Via the hands from the skin, nasal mucosa	Hand washing; 80% *PCNase* penicillin-resistant (make β-lactamase); vancomycin; cephalosporin

Name	Morphology	Pathogenesis	Description of Disease	Laboratory Findings, Notes	Transmission	Prevention and Therapy
Staphylococcus epidermidis	Gm+; cocci; white, creamy, grape-like clusters on culture	Surface glycocalyx	Endocarditis; infection on catheters and implant sites; sepsis in neonates	Coagulase −; catalase +; no hemolysis; novobiocin-sensitive	On skin; IV drug users	Vancomycin
Staphylococcus saprophyticus	Gm+; cocci; creamy, grape-like clusters	Selectively adheres to transitional epithelium	UTIs in young women	Coagulase −; catalase +; no hemolysis; novobiocin resistant	Many sexual partners	Quinolones
Streptococcus agalactiae	Gm+; cocci; diploid	Capsular antigen	Neonatal sepsis and meningitis	Catalase −; bacitracin resistant; β-hemolysis; Lancefield group B	Genital tract of some women	Ampicillin before delivery; penicillin G
Streptococcus pneumoniae	Gm+; cocci; lancet shaped; in pairs; polysaccharide capsule (85 different types)	Capsule prevents phagocytosis; IgA protease; adheres to mucosa	Pneumonia; meningitis; bacteremia; upper respiratory infection; otitis media	Catalase −; α-hemolysis; bile soluble; inhibited by optochin; quelling reaction (capsular swelling)	Non-communicable	Polysaccharide capsular vaccine available for high-risk groups; penicillin and erythromycin
Streptococcus pyogenes	Gm+; cocci; chains or pairs; rough or smooth hyaluronic acid capsule	M protein (pili); streptokinase (dissolves fibrin); DNase; hyaluronidase; hemolysins: erythrogenic toxin (scarlet fever rash); streptolysin O and S; exotoxin A (superantigen causing TSS-like syndrome)	Pharyngitis; cellulitis; rheumatic fever; acute glomerulonephritis; pharyngitis; TSS-like syndrome	Catalase −; bacitracin (A disk) sensitive; β-hemolytic; antistreptolysin-O for serotyping; Lancefield group A	Normal flora of skin, throat causing disease when in blood	Penicillin G
Treponema pallidum	Spirochete	Multiplication followed by blood vessel involvement	Syphilis—primary with painless sores, purulent exudate, and induration; secondary with a rash; tertiary (rare) includes CNS involvement and aortitis	Dark-field microscopy; RPR (or VDRL) test for cardiolipin; systemic illness can occur with treatment (Jarisch-Herxheimer reaction)	Sexually transmitted; transplacental	Penicillin

Organism						
Tropheryma whippelli	Gm⁻; rod	Foamy macrophages found in the lamina propria of the jejunum	Whipple's disease—steatorrhea, lymphadenopathy, fever, and cough	Visualization of the organism in a biopsy of the small bowel	Unknown	Trimethoprim-sulfamethoxazole
Vibrio cholerae	Gm⁻; comma-shaped rod; polar flagella	Pili adhere to gut mucosa; phage-coated cholera toxin: 2 A active subunits and 5 B binding units (A subunit ADP ribosylates G protein increasing in cAMP and causing movement of ions and water out of the cell)	Rice-water stools		Fecal-oral route via water and food	Vaccine not effective; rehydration; tetracycline
Vibrio parahaemolyticus	Gm⁻; bacilli	Toxin	Explosive diarrhea; cramps; nausea	High infective dose required	Shellfish	Self-limiting
Yersinia pestis	Gm⁻; bacillus; intracellular	V and W antigens (active within macrophages); fibrinolysin; F1 protein inhibits phagocytosis	Bubonic plague (with lymph node swelling and bubo); fever; conjunctivitis	Cultures are hazardous and precautions must be taken	Zoonotic via rat fleas	Vaccine; streptomycin

ADP=adenosine diphosphate; *bCG*=bacille Calmette-Guérin; *cAMP*=cyclic adenosine monophosphate; *CNS*=central nervous system; *CSF*=cerebrospinal fluid; *DNase*=deoxyribonuclease; *EHEC*=enterohemorrhagic *Escherichia coli*; *EIEC*=enteroinvasive *Escherichia coli*; *ELISA*=enzyme-linked immunosorbent assay; *EPEC*=enteropathogenic *Escherichia coli*; *ETEC*=enterotoxigenic *Escherichia coli*; *GI*=gastrointestinal; *Gm−*=gram-negative; *Gm+*=gram-positive; *Hib*=Haemophilus influenza type B; *IgA*=gamma A immunoglobulin; *IV*=intravenous; *NAD*=nicotinamide-adenine dinucleotide; *PID*=pelvic inflammatory disease; *PPD*=purified protein derivative; *LPS*=lipopolysaccharide; *PMN*=polymorphonuclear neutrophils; *RPR*=rapid plasma reagin; *TSS*=toxic shock syndrome; *UTI*=urinary tract infection; *U.S.*=United States; *VDRL*=Venereal Disease Research Laboratory.

Viruses

Name	Morphology	Description of Disease	Laboratory Findings, Notes	Pathogenesis	Transmission	Prevention; Therapy
Adenovirus	Non-enveloped DNA virus; double-stranded	Pharyngitis or pneumonia	Complement fixation	Infects the epithelium of the eyes and respiratory tract	Respiratory droplets; hand-to-eye	Live vaccine to high-risk populations; no treatments
Coxsackie B virus	Non-enveloped RNA virus; single-stranded; linear; + polarity	Myocarditis, pericarditis	Isolating virus in cell culture; rise in convalescent antibody	Replicates in the pharynx and GI tract and spreads to other tissues	Fecal-oral and respiratory	No therapy or prevention
Cytomegalovirus	Enveloped DNA virus; linear; double-stranded	Pneumonia and hepatitis in immunocompromised; mononucleosis in transplant patients	"Owl's eye" nuclear inclusions	Infects the oropharynx initially; involves lymphocytes	Human body fluids transplacental, organ transplant	Ganciclovir
Ebola virus	Enveloped RNA virus; single-stranded; linear; -polarity	African hemorrhagic fever—often rapidly fatal	Virus isolation; rise in antibody titer	Viral replication in all organs leads to necrosis	Contact with blood and body secretions	None
Epstein-Barr virus	Enveloped DNA virus; linear; double-stranded	Infectious mononucleosis; may cause Burkitt's lymphoma	Atypical lymphocytes; + heterophil antibody (Monospot test); common infection of college students	Spreads via the lymph nodes and bloodstream to the liver and spleen from the pharyngeal epithelium	Saliva	None
Hanta virus	Enveloped, RNA virus; single-stranded; circular, segmented; -polarity	Hanta pulmonary syndrome—influenza-like followed by acute respiratory failure	PCR assay of viral RNA from lung tissue	Invasion of the respiratory epithelium	Airborne (inhalation of rodent urine and feces); found in southwestern U.S.A	None
Hepatitis A virus	Non-enveloped RNA virus; single stranded; + polarity	Hepatitis A	Detect IgM antibody	Replicates in the GI tract; spreads to the liver; hepatocellular injury via cytotoxic T cell response	Fecal-oral route; killed viral vaccine; immune globulin during the incubation period may hinder disease	None
Hepatitis B virus	Enveloped DNA virus; incomplete circular double-stranded; polymerase in virion (virion called the Dane particle); surface antigen (HbsAg); core antigen (HbcAg); "e" envelope antigen	Hepatitis B; arthritis; rash; glomerulonephritis; may result in carcinoma of the liver	Serologic tests for HbsAg, HbsAb, and HbcAb	Immune response (CD8 cells) to the virus results in hepatocellular injury; Ag-Ab complexes form	Blood, sexual, and transplacental	Vaccine; no treatment

Virus	Properties	Disease	Diagnosis	Pathogenesis	Transmission	Treatment
Hepatitis C virus	Enveloped RNA virus; single-stranded; + polarity	Hepatitis C; possible predisposition to hepatocellular carcinoma	Serologic; most common cause of transfusion-related hepatitis	Cytotoxic T cells result in hepatocellular injury	Blood, transplacental, sexual	Alpha interferon
Hepatitis D virus	Enveloped defective RNA virus; circular; single-stranded; -polarity; no polymerase	Hepatitis D	Serologic testing for delta agent	Cytotoxic T cells result in hepatocellular injury; uses hepatitis B surface antigen as a protein coat and can only replicate in hosts already infected with hepatitis B virus	Blood, transplacental, sexual; prevention of hepatitis B	Alpha interferon
Herpes simplex virus type 1	Enveloped DNA virus; linear; double-stranded	Herpes labialis (fever blisters and cold sores); keratitis; encephalitis	Multinucleated giant cells in Tzanck smear	Lesions on the mouth and face initially; travels retrograde and becomes latent in the trigeminal ganglion; recurrences induced by sunlight, stress, fever	Saliva; direct contact with the lesion	Acyclovir; trifluorothymidine for keratitis
Herpes simplex virus type 2	Enveloped DNA virus; linear; double-stranded	Herpes genitalis; meningitis	Multinucleated giant cells on Tzanck smear	Vesicular lesions on the genitalia; retrograde passage through the axon and latency in the sacral ganglion; stress-induced recurrences	Sexual, transplacental	Acyclovir
Human herpes virus 6	Enveloped DNA virus; linear; double-stranded	Roseola infantum (exanthem subitum)—common disease of children characterized by high fever and rash	PCR or acute and convalescent antibody titers	Infects T and B cells	Saliva	Symptomatic
Human immuno-deficiency virus	Enveloped RNA virus; diploid; single-stranded; + polarity; reverse transcriptase	AIDS	Screen with ELISA; Western blot test confirms	Infects and kills helper T cells via the CD4 receptors and gp120 protein	Body fluids, transplacental; screen blood	AZT to HIV-infected mothers and newborns; AZT, ddI, ddC; treat opportunistic infections like pneumonia or Kaposi's sarcoma
Influenza virus	Enveloped RNA virus; segmented; single-stranded; -polarity; polymerase in virion	Influenza	Cell culture; hemagglutination inhibition; complement fixation	Infects the epithelium of the respiratory tract via hemagglutinin and neuraminidase on surface spikes; antigenic shift and drift of surface spikes lead to epidemics	Respiratory droplets; inactivated strains of current virus cause disease	Amantadine for both prevention and treatment

Name	Morphology	Description of Disease	Laboratory Findings, Notes	Pathogenesis	Transmission	Prevention; Therapy
Measles virus	Enveloped RNA virus; single-stranded; -polarity; polymerase in virion	Measles; subacute sclerosing panen-cephalitis (SSPE)	None	Infection spreads via the bloodstream from the upper respiratory tract to the organs; maculopapular rash due to an immune response	Respiratory droplets	Attenuated vaccine; no treatment.
Mumps virus	Enveloped RNA virus; single-stranded; -polarity; polymerase in virion	Mumps; sterility due to bilateral orchitis	Cell culture and hemadsorption	Spreads from the upper respiratory tract to the organs (parotid glands, testes, ovaries, CNS) via the bloodstream	Respiratory droplets	Attenuated vaccine; no treatment
Norwalk virus	Non-enveloped; RNA virus; single-stranded; linear; + polarity	Gastroenteritis	Not performed	Immune response to viral invasion results in the destruction of the small intestinal epithelium	Fecal-oral	Symptomatic treatment
Papillomavirus	Non-enveloped DNA virus; circular; double-stranded	Papillomas (warts); condylomata acuminata; cervical and penile carcinoma	Koilocytes (squamous cell with perinuclear clearing) in lesions	E6 and E7 early viral genes inhibit activity of p53 and rb tumor suppressor genes	Sexual via direct contact with genital lesions	Alpha interferon; liquid nitrogen for warts
Parvovirus B19	Non-enveloped; DNA virus; single-stranded; linear	Erythema infectiosum (fifth disease)—characterized by "slapped cheek" appearance; may have aplastic crisis in sickle cell disease	Parvovirus specific IgG/IgM antibody levels; laboratory analysis for viral DNA	Erythema infectiosum—virus causes immune-complex deposition; aplastic anemia: virus infects immature RBCs and kills them	Unknown, may be respiratory or direct contact	Self-limited
Poliovirus	Non-enveloped RNA virus; single-stranded; + polarity	Aseptic meningitis (more common); paralytic poliomyelitis	Isolation from CSF	Replicates in the pharynx and GI tract and spreads to the CNS; death of the anterior horn cells in the spinal cord	Fecal-oral	Salk vaccine: inactivated; Sabin vaccine: attenuated, given in childhood immunizations; no treatment

Virus	Genome/Structure	Disease	Diagnosis	Pathogenesis	Transmission	Treatment/Vaccine
Rabies virus	Enveloped RNA virus; bullet shape; singe-stranded; -polarity RNA; polymerase in virion	Rabies	Negri bodies (eosinophillic inclusion in nerve cell)	ACh receptor of neuron binds virus; the virus follows the retrograde direction to invade the CNS and brain, resulting in encephalitis	Animal (skunks, bats) bites	Pre-exposure: vaccine; post-exposure: inactivated vaccine from human cell culture; no treatment
Reovirus (Rotavirus)	Non-enveloped RNA virus; 11 segments; double-stranded; RNA polymerase in virion	Gastroenteritis in children	ELISA detects the virus in stool	Resistant to stomach acid, thus infects the small intestine	Respiratory droplets; fecal-oral route	None
Respiratory syncytial virus	Enveloped RNA virus; single-stranded; -polarity; polymerase in virion	Pneumonia or bronchiolitis in children	Multi-nucleated giant cells	Immune response to lower respiratory tract infection	Respiratory droplets	Ribavarin
Rhinovirus	Non-enveloped RNA virus; single-stranded; + polarity; numerous serotypes	Common cold	None	Upper respiratory tract mucosa and conjunctiva infected; replicates at temperature <37°C and killed by stomach acid	Aerosol droplets with hand-to-nose transmission	None
Rubella virus	Enveloped RNA virus; single-stranded; + polarity	Rubella; congenital: cardiovascular and neurologic malformations, especially if infection occurs during the first trimester	Growth in cell culture via interference of coxsackievirus; recent infection in the mother is detected by IgM or IgA	Spreads from the nasopharynx to the skin via the bloodstream; rash caused by replication and immune injury	Respiratory droplets	Attenuated vaccine; no treatment
Varicella-zoster virus	Enveloped DNA virus; linear; double-stranded	Chickenpox (varicella) in children; shingles (zoster) in adults	Intranuclear inclusions; shingles generally follows the distribution of the dermatomes	Infects respiratory tract and spreads to the liver and skin via the blood; an acute episode followed by latency in the sensory ganglia	Chickenpox—respiratory droplets; shingles: reactivation of the latent virus	Attenuated vaccine; no treatment

ACh=acetylcholine; *Ag-Ab*=antigen-antibody; *AZT*=azidothymidine; *CNS*=central nervous system; *CSF*=cerebrospinal fluid; *ddI*=dideoxyinosine; *DNA*=deoxyribonucleic acid; *ELISA*=enzyme-linked immunosorbent assay; *GI*=gastrointestinal; *HbcAb*=hepatitis B core antibody; *HbcAg*=hepatitis B core antigen; *HbsAb*=hepatitis B surface antibody; *HbsAg*=hepatitis B surface antigen; *HIV*=human immunodeficiency virus; *IgA*=gamma A immunoglobulin; *IgG*=gamma G immunoglobulin; *IgM*=gamma M immunoglobulin; *PCR*=polymerase chain reaction; *RBC*=red blood cell; *RNA*=ribonucleic acid; *SSPE*=subacute sclerosing panencephalitis.

Fungi

Name	Morphology	Pathogenesis	Description of Disease	Laboratory Findings, Notes	Transmission	Prevention: Therapy
Aspergillus fumigatus	Filamentous; septate hyphae and dichotomous branching	Opportunistic; growth of *Aspergillus* in a pre-existing cavitary lesion in the lung	Aspergilloma—hemoptysis; invasive aspergillosis in neutropenic individuals	Septate, branching hyphae; "fungus ball" seen on a radiograph	Airborne spores	Amphotericin B, itraconazole; surgery to remove a "fungus ball"
Blastomyces dermatitidis	Dimorphic fungus—mold in the soil, while a yeast in tissue	Invades the respiratory tract and may invade the skin or bone	Blastomycosis—granulomatous and suppurative infection of the respiratory tract	Tissue biopsy showing circular yeast with a broad-based bud	Airborne; endemic to North America	Itraconazole; amphotericin B for serious infections
Candida albicans	Pseudohyphae and hyphae on invasion; yeast in normal flora; germ tubes at 37°C	Opportunistic in the immunosuppressed and those with foreign bodies (e.g., catheters); muco-cutaneous lesions in children with a T cell defect	Thrush, chronic mucocutaneous candidiasis; vaginal candidiasis	Colonies on Sabouraud's agar; germ tube formation	Part of the normal flora	Oral form can be prevented by nystatin "swish and swallow"; treatment with nystatin; miconazole; amphotericin B
Coccidioides immitis	Dimorphic—mold in the soil, spherule in the tissue	Inhalation; spherules, releasing endospores within the respiratory tract	Coccidioidomycosis—an influenza-like illness with fever and cough	Tissue specimen showing spherules	Airborne; endemic to southwestern U.S. and Latin America	Amphotericin B; ketoconazole
Cryptococcus neoformans	Encapsulated; not dimorphic	Usually immuno-compromised; spread via the bloodstream	Cryptococcosis; cryptococcal meningitis	Organism with a capsule seen on an Indian ink preparation; latex agglutination test	Inhalation of airborne yeast cells	Oral fluconazole as preventative in AIDS patients; amphoteric in B with flucytosine
Histoplasma capsulatum	Dimorphic—a mold in the soil, a yeast in tissue	Inhaled spores are engulfed by macrophages and develop into yeast forms intracellularly	Histoplasmosis—granulomas in the lung tissue	Tissue biopsy showing yeast cells visible in macrophages; radio-immunoassay for histoplasma RNA and DNA	Airborne; endemic to Ohio and Mississippi River valley; found in bird droppings	Amphoteric in B; itraconazole
Mucor species	Nonseptate hyphae that branch at near right angles	Invade the sinuses, lungs, and GI tract	Tissue necrosis	Nonseptate hyphae seen microscopically	Airborne	Amphoteric in B; débridement of necrotic tissue
Sporothrix schenckii	Thermally dimorphic fungus	Inflammation and swelling of the lymph nodes and vessels	Sporotrichosis ("rose gardener's disease")	Cigar-shaped budding cells	Thorn prick	Protection during gardening; potassium iodide; ketoconazole

AIDS=acquired immunodeficiency syndrome; *DNA*=deoxyribonucleic acid; *GI*=gastrointestinal; *RNA*=ribonucleic acid

Parasites and Protozoa

Name	Morphology	Pathogenesis	Description of Disease	Laboratory Findings, Notes	Transmission	Prevention; Therapy
Ascaris lumbricoides	Intestinal parasite	Larvae in the lung and a heavy worm burden in gastrointestinal tract	Ascariasis—intestinal obstruction, abdominal pain, coughing, nausea	Eosinophilia; eggs in feces	Contaminated food or soil	Maintain sanitary conditions; mebendazole
Entamoeba histolytica	Intestinal protozoan; cigar-shaped cysts; 4 nuclei	Trophozoite form invades the colon	Amebic dysentery; liver abscess; flask-shaped ulcers	Trophozoites seen in stool	Fecal-oral	Maintain sanitary conditions; metronidazole with diloxanide; steroids exacerbate
Enterobius vermicularis	Intestinal parasite	Worms and eggs (passed in feces) result in perianal pruritus	Pinworm infection—anal pruritus, vaginal irritation, cystitis	Eggs on "Scotch tape" test (tape applied to the anus and then viewed under a microscope)	Reinfection by self; fecal-oral contact; egg ingestion	Mebendazole
Giardia lamblia	Intestinal protozoan; pear-shaped; flagella; tumbling motility; 4 nuclei	Interfere with fat and protein absorption	Giardiasis—acute diarrhea	Visible in stool	Fecal-oral	Maintain sanitary conditions; metronidazole
Leishmania donovani	Protozoa	Organs of the reticulo-endothelial system are destroyed by macro-phages infected with bacteria	Visceral leishmaniasis (kala-azar)—hyper-pigmentation of the skin, massive splenomegaly, fever, anemia, and malaise	Biopsy of reticulo-endothelial tissue shows the infected macrophages	Female *Phlebotomus* sandfly transmits the disease from the infected host to a human	Protection from sandfly bites; sodium stibogluconate (antimony compound)
Plasmodium species	Blood and tissue protozoan; signet-ring trophozoites in RBCs; Schüffner's dots (red-yellow dots in RBCs); "banana-shaped" gametocytes	Sporozoites from bite enter the bloodstream and invade hepatocytes (exoerythrocytic phase); merozoites invade the RBCs (erythrocytic phase)	Malaria—fever, chills, hepatomegaly, splenomegaly, symptoms in cyclical pattern (3 days for *malariae*; 2 days for *ovale, falciparum, vivax*); tissue anoxia	Blood smear shows organisms; *P. falciparum* is acute and needs immediate treatment	Female anopheles mosquito; chloroquine; insecticides	Protection from bites Chloroquine; quinine; mefloquine
Pneumocystis carinii	Respiratory pathogen	Alveolar inflammation	Pneumonia	Silver stain; confusion about classification: protozoan or fungus	Inhalation by immunocompromised individual	Trimethoprim-sulfamethoxa-zole; pentamidine
Schistosoma	Blood fluke; eggs have spine (*S. mansoni* has large lateral spine, *S. haematobium* has a terminal spine, *S. japonicum* has a small lateral spine); 2 sexes	Eggs lead to inflammation, fibrosis, and granuloma formation	Schistosomiasis—pipestem fibrosis of liver; *S. haematobium* affects the bladder; *S. mansoni* affects the colon	Eggs in the stool or urine	Penetration of the skin by cercariae	Maintain sanitary conditions; praziquantel

Name	Morphology	Pathogenesis	Description of Disease	Laboratory Findings, Notes	Transmission	Prevention; Therapy
Taenia sp.	Cestode: *T. solium*—pork tapeworm; *T. saginata*—beef; *Diphyllobothrium latum*—fish; 4 suckers and circle of hooks; 5–10 uterine branches	Encyst in tissue (eyes, brain, muscle) resulting in mass lesions	Taeniasis and cysticercosis	Gravid proglottids in stool	Eating raw or undercooked meat	Cook meat and maintain sanitary conditions; niclosamide
Toxoplasma gondii	Tissue protozoan	Infect macrophages; infect the brain, liver, eyes	Toxoplasmosis	Serologic; high morbidity and mortality	Ingestion of cysts; transplacental; cat feces	Cook meat; sulfonamides
Trichinella spiralis	Intestinal parasite	Muscle inflammation	Trichinosis—periorbital edema, myositis, fever, diarrhea	Larvae on muscle biopsy; eosinophilia by 14th day; double-barreled egg	Eating raw or undercooked meat	Cook meat; thiabendazole
Trichomonas vaginalis	Urogenital protozoan; pear-shaped; flagella	Attach to the wall of the vagina	Trichomoniasis—itching and burning with yellow discharge from the vagina (strawberry cervix)	Visible in secretions	Sexual transmission	Treat both partners; metronidazole
Trypanosomiasis brucei (African)	Blood and tissue protozoan	Infects the brain and leads to encephalitis	Sleeping sickness—Winterbottom's sign, blank look, fever, edema, epilepsy	Visible in the blood	Tstetse fly (in Africa);	Protection from bites; insecticide; Suramin
Trypanosomiasis cruzi (American)	Blood and tissue protozoan	Amastigotes attack cells, especially cardiac muscle cells	Chagas' disease—CHF; Romaña's sign	Visible in the blood	Reduvid bugs (in Latin America)	Protect from bites; insecticide; Nifurtimox

CHF=congestive heart failure; *RBC*=red blood cell

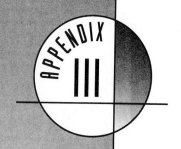

APPENDIX
III

At the Bedside

● Table of Contents for At the Bedside

● List of Abbreviated Terms for At the Bedside

Term	Meaning
AAO ×3	Awake, alert, and oriented to time, place, and person
Abd	Abdomen
ABG	Arterial blood gas
AXR	Abdominal X-ray
B/L	Bilateral
BP	Blood pressure
BUN	Blood urea nitrogen
c/c/e	Clubbing/cyanosis/edema
c/o	Complaining of . . .
c/w	Consistent with . . .
c/w/r	Crackles/wheezes/rhonchi
CBC	Complete blood count
Cr	Creatinine
CTA	Clear to auscultation
CVA	Costovertebral angle, cerebrovascular accident
CXR	Chest x-ray, chest radiograph
DOE	Dyspnea on exertion
DTR	Deep tendon reflexes
DVT	Deep vein thrombosis
ECG	Electrocardiogram
ED	Emergency Department
EOMI	Extraocular muscles intact
Ext	Extremities
GERD	Gastroesophageal reflux disease
h/o	History of
HC	Head circumference
Hct	Hematocrit
HEENT	Head, eyes, ears, nose, throat
Hgb	Hemoglobin
HJR	Hepatojugular reflex

Term	Meaning
HR	Heart rate
Ht	Height
HTN	Hypertension
IVDU	Intravenous drug use
JVD	Jugular venous distention
LFTs	Liver function tests
m/o	Months/old
m/r/g	Murmurs/rubs/gallops
NGT	Nasogastric tube
NPO	Nothing by mouth
PERRLA	Pupils equal round reactive to light and accommodate
PFTs	Pulmonary function tests
PMH	Past medical history
PMI	Point of maximal impulse
PMNs	Polymorphonuclear leukocytes
PND	Paroxysmal nocturnal dyspnea
PPD	Purified protein derivative (a tuberculosis test)
Pt	Patient
RR	Respiratory rate
RRR	Regular rate and rhythm
RUQ	Right upper quadrant
SOB	Shortness of breath
STD	Sexually transmitted disease
U/A	Urinalysis
URI	Upper respiratory infection
US	Ultrasound
VSD	Ventriculoseptal defect
WBC	White blood cell
WNL	Within normal limits
Wt	Weight
y/o	Year old

CASE 1   CC: "I vomited a lot of blood."

HISTORY: This 50 y/o white man presents to the ED and states that he has **vomited blood** 3 times in the past 24 hours. The volume of blood in the vomitus is increasing. He **drank 10 cans of beer a few hours before the vomiting began.** He denies retching, coughing, or any prior episodes of nonbloody vomiting. He states that he has never vomited blood before but does tend to vomit after consuming a large amount of alcohol. The patient has noted an **increase in the size of his abdomen** but denies any increase in appetite. He also states that he has "pins and needles" in his feet at night. He denies fever, chills, night sweats, pleurisy, abdominal pain, wheezing, or dyspnea and does not take aspirin or nonsteroidal anti-inflammatory drugs regularly. He has no history of peptic ulcer disease, HTN, or cancer. He denies bright red blood in his stool (hematochezia), dark black stool (melena), or fatty, bulky, foul-smelling, glistening stools (steatorrhea). The patient denies smoking and IVDU but has consumed 2 six-packs of beer/day for the past 30 years.

PHYSICAL: The patient appears emaciated and in acute distress. BP (supine):120/70; BP (standing): 90/50, HR (supine):100; HR (standing):110, RR:12, Temp 99.4°F. HEENT: sclera **(+) icterus,** conjunctiva pale, oral mucosa dry. Neck: (−) JVD, HJR. Lungs: CTA B/L, (−) c/w/r. Heart: tachycardic but regular, normal S1, S2, (−) S3, S4, (−) m/r/g. Skin: **(+) gynecomastia, (+) spider angiomas.** Abd: soft, distended, nontender, (−) guarding, rebound, (+) bowel sounds, (+) splenomegaly, **(+) caput medusae,** (+) shifting dullness (ascites), (−) hepatomegaly. Hemoccult test (−) for blood in stool. Ext: (+) palmar erythema, (+) flexion contracture of fingers B/L **(Dupuytren's contracture),** (−) telangiectasia. G/U: **testicular atrophy.** Neuro: decreased vibratory sensation B/L **(sensory neuropathy),** (−) asterixis.

DIFFERENTIAL: Mallory-Weiss tear; Boerhaave's syndrome; acute gastritis; peptic ulcer disease; variceal bleeding 2° to alcoholic cirrhosis.

DIAGNOSTICS: CBC: decreased Hb and Hct, platelets decreased. Blood alcohol level: elevated. ABG (PO_2, PCO_2, pH): WNL. CXR: (−) mediastinal air, (−) cardiomegaly, (−) pulmonary edema; (−) hiatal hernia. LFTs: AST, ALT-elevated with **AST/ALT > 2,** increased direct bilirubin, slightly increased alkaline phosphatase, slightly increased prothrombin time (PT), normal albumin level. Electrolytes: normal, BUN/Cr ratio >36, normal blood glucose. NGT: bright red blood in stomach. Upper endoscopy: bleeding esophageal varices.

DIAGNOSIS: Variceal bleeding 2° to alcoholic cirrhosis (see Figure).

ASSESSMENT/PLAN: A 50 y/o man presents to the ED c/o hematemesis. Variceal bleeding is a life-threatening emergency. The patient should have a blood type and cross match. He has evidence of decreased blood volume (tachycardia, decreased Hgb and Hct, orthostatic hypotension) and should be transfused with 2 units of whole blood. The variceal bleeding can be stopped with an upper endoscopy procedure—either **sclerotherapy, balloon tamponade, endoscopic ligation**). Give IV vasopressin to cause vasoconstriction and decrease blood flow to the portal venous system. The patient should be monitored for he-

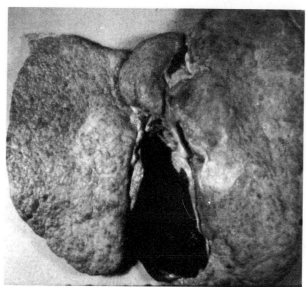

(continued)   **CASE 1** Cirrhosis of the liver in a chronic alcoholic.

CASE 1 CC: "I vomited a lot of blood." (Continued)

patic encephalopathy and acute renal failure. Give IV thiamine and glucose to prevent **Wernicke-Korsakoff syndrome.** Once the patient is stable, the portal hypertension can be managed by either transjugular intrahepatic portosystemic shunt (TIPS) or portosystemic surgery. β-Blockers will help prevent further variceal bleeding. The patient should be encouraged to enter a rehabilitation program to control his alcoholism. The patient should be instructed to eat a low-protein diet (to decrease ammonia production that may lead to encephalopathy), with multivitamin supplements.

Variceal Bleeding 2° to Alcoholic Cirrhosis: The jaundice, gynecomastia, spider angiomas, splenomegaly, caput medusa, ascites, palmar erythema, testicular atrophy, and Dupuytren's contracture are all signs of alcoholic cirrhosis. The cirrhosis is irreversible; however, abstinence from alcohol may prevent further degradation of liver function. The peripheral sensory neuropathy is caused by the toxic effects of alcohol as well as a **thiamine deficiency.** Complications of alcoholic cirrhosis include portal hypertension, variceal bleeding, spontaneous bacterial peritonitis, hepatic encephalopathy, hepatorenal syndrome, and coagulopathy (due to decrease in vitamin K–dependent clotting factors).

Mallory-Weiss tears: The hematemesis could have been the result of Mallory-Weiss tears. These tears, near the gastroesophageal junction of the stomach, are common in alcoholics after episodes of **vomiting** and **retching.** This patient did not retch or vomit prior to having hematemesis. Upper endoscopy would have shown Mallory-Weiss tears in the esophagus if they were present.

Boerhaave's syndrome (rupture of the esophagus): A patient with a ruptured esophagus would present with hematemesis and decreased blood volume. The CXR would show **mediastinal air.** Also, auscultation of the chest did not reveal any decreased breath sounds (indicating air in the chest). Blood in the stomach on gastric lavage is consistent with Boerhaave's syndrome. Upper endoscopy would have shown esophageal rupture if it had been present.

Acute gastritis: Alcohol-induced acute gastritis could have resulted in hematemesis. The patient stated that he had been drinking prior to hematemesis. Gastric lavage positive for blood is consistent with acute gastritis. However, the patient had no complaints of **epigastric burning or pain.** Also, upper endoscopy would have revealed evidence of acute gastritis (ulceration, inflammation, and friability). Upper endoscopy is the method of differentiating between acute gastritis and variceal bleeding 2° to alcoholic cirrhosis.

Peptic ulcer disease (PUD): A patient with a perforated ulcer would present with hematemesis and hypovolemia. However, this patient had no history of PUD or epigastric pain after meals. CXR would have shown air under the diaphragm (indicating a perforation). Also, upper endoscopy would have demonstrated a bleeding ulcer.

CASE 2 CC: "My stomach really hurts and I have this awful pain in my side."

HISTORY: 28 y/o man presents complaining of a sudden onset of **epigastric/periumbilical pain** that was dull and poorly localized since 6 PM. The pain was accompanied by the urge to defecate, **nausea,** and **vomiting.** Defecation brought no relief of any of the patient's symptoms. The patient did not have diarrhea. In the next 5 hours, the pain became more localized to the patient's **right lower quadrant.** The pain is now stabbing and severe. The patient **has not eaten** since lunch and stated that he "doesn't want to even think about eating." The patient's past medical history includes exercised-induced asthma when he was young and an allergy to penicillin, but no history of any gastrointestinal disease. The family history is noncontributory.

PHYSICAL: The patient appears toxic (decreased interest in the environment), leaning to his right side in an effort to guard his lower right quadrant. Temp: 38.3°C; HR: 100; RR: 22. Lungs: CTA. Abd: nondistended, increased **guarding,** positive bowel sounds. Point tenderness at **McBurney's point.** Positive **Rovsing's sign.** Positive **rebound tenderness** upon cessation of palpation of the lower right quadrant. Positive **psoas sign.** No abdominal masses.

DIFFERENTIAL: Perforated peptic ulcer, acute gangrenous cholecystitis, acute intestinal obstruction, Meckel's diverticulum, Crohn's disease, mesenteric adenitis, *Yersinia enteritis* (in females also pelvic inflammatory disease, ectopic/tubal pregnancy, ovarian cyst, salpingitis).

DIAGNOSTICS: CBC: **leukocytosis.** U/A: WNL. AXR (supine and upright): no air-fluid levels on upright and no enlarged loops of bowel. Ultrasound: increased thickness of the appendiceal wall, liver/gallbladder—WNL, in female ovary/fallopian tubes—WNL.

DIAGNOSIS: Acute appendicitis.

ASSESSMENT/PLAN: 28 y/o man with an 8-hour history of dull periumbilical pain that increased in intensity and localized to the lower right quadrant. The patient has had nausea, vomiting, and anorexia since the pain began. The patient demonstrates lower right quadrant point tenderness at McBurney's point upon palpation, rebound tenderness localized to the right side, positive Rovsing's sign, and psoas sign. Treatment is immediate **laparotomy** to remove the appendix and IV antibiotics (third-generation cephalosporin).

Diagnosis of appendicitis is made on clinical presentation. Clinical diagnosis and operation must be rapid to avoid possible perforation, peritonitis, and even death.

Crohn's disease: This diagnosis is not likely because of the lack of a gastrointestinal history. Although there was a history of nausea and vomiting, there was no history of diarrhea or gastrointestinal disorders in the past.

Yersinia enteritis: This diagnosis would have been more likely if more than one family member was ill.

Acute intestinal obstruction: This diagnosis is unlikely because of the lack of **distended loops of bowel** and **air-fluid levels** on upright abdominal x-ray films. Tinkles (high-pitched bowel sounds) are also expected.

Perforated peptic ulcer: There is no history of ulcer pain and no **air under the diaphragm** on an upright abdominal film. Presentation may include right lower quadrant pain.

Many other diagnoses such as PID, ectopic pregnancy, salpingitis, ovarian cyst, Meckel's diverticulum, or mesenteric adenitis cannot be adequately ruled in or out by clinical presentation. If a normal appendix is found on laparoscopy, these other diagnoses must be considered.

CASE 3 — CC: "I threw up and my side really hurts."

HPI: A 40 y/o **obese woman** presents at the ED with **RUQ pain** and **nausea.** The patient states that the pain is intermittent and sharp and has been getting worse. The pain has lasted for about 4 hours. The day before admission, she had a similar episode as well as similar episodes during the past year. The pain is **worse after eating a high-fat meal** and nothing makes the pain better. Pt has vomited twice in the past 2 days. The patient denies diarrhea, constipation, change in diet, peptic ulcer, hepatitis, chills, recent infection, or STD. The patient does not smoke, drinks socially, and denies IVDU. She is married and monoga-

(continued)

CASE 3 CC: "I threw up and my side really hurts." (Continued)

mous with **three children;** her last menstrual period was 10 days ago; and she is **using oral contraceptive pills** (OCPs).

PHYSICAL: Obese patient who is uncomfortable, anxious, and writhing in pain. **Temp=100.5°F,** HR=90, RR=12, BP=140/80. No orthostatic hypotension. HEENT: sclera anicteric, conjunctiva pink. Lungs: CTA. Abd: moves with each breath, (+) abdominal distention, (−) stria, RUQ is tender to palpation, **(+) Murphy's sign,** localized rebound tenderness, (−) guarding, (−) organomegaly, ascites could not be assessed. Stool: (−) occult blood. Pelvic: WNL.

DIFFERENTIAL: Acute cholecystitis; acute cholangitis; sclerosing cholangitis; hepatitis; liver neoplasm; acute pancreatitis; gallstone in the pancreatic duct; pyelonephritis; perforated ulcer; diabetic ketoacidosis (DKA); ectopic pregnancy.

DIAGNOSTICS: CBC: **elevated WBC,** normal RBC, Hgb and Hct normal. Electrolytes: serum glucose, serum amylase, serum lipase—all normal. LFTs: serum total bilirubin mildly elevated, creatine kinase—normal. Cardiac troponins—normal. β-HCG levels undetectable. BUN / Cr—normal. Urine dip and U/A—normal. US of abdomen: (+) calculus in the gallbladder (see Figure). HIDA scan: (+) obstruction in cystic duct.

DIAGNOSIS: Acute cholecystitis due to cholelithiasis.

ASSESSMENT/PLAN: 40 y/o obese, multiparous woman with RUQ pain and nausea with history of OCP use. Treat the patient with NPO; perform nasogastric suction to prevent gastric contents from stimulating the gallbladder to release bile. Give meperidine for pain; administer IV antibiotics (amoxicillin/clavulanate, ceftazidime, metronidazole). After the patient is stable, perform a laparoscopic cholecystectomy.

Acute Cholecystitis due to Cholelithiasis: Charcot's triad of **sudden onset RUQ pain, fever, leukocytosis.** Serum bilirubin is mildly elevated and a stone is present in the gallbladder on US, with an obstruction of the cystic duct on a HIDA scan.

Acute cholangitis: HIDA scan shows a gallstone in the gallbladder but not in the **common bile duct.** Also, serum bilirubin is only mildly elevated.

Sclerosing cholangitis: Patients with this disease present with acute cholangitis, jaundice, pruritus, and RUQ pain. This patient demonstrates only RUQ pain.

Liver neoplasm: LFTs are not elevated (except for total bilirubin), with no liver masses demonstrated on abdominal US.

Acute pancreatitis: Pain would **radiate to the patient's back;** serum **amylase** and **lipase** would be **elevated;** serum calcium would be decreased.

Gallstone in pancreatic duct: HIDA scan showed only an obstruction in the cystic duct, not the pancreatic duct or ampulla of Vater.

Pyelonephritis: U/A and urine dipstick are normal. **WBC casts** are often seen in this disease. Pain pres-

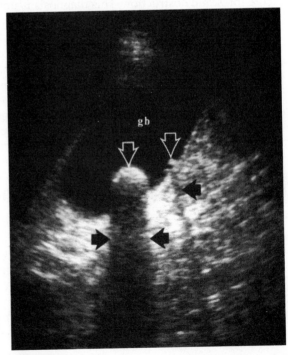

CASE 3 Gallstones shown on ultrasound.

ent at the costovertebral angles that does not worsen with inspiration is not consistent with pyelonephritis. Bowel sounds would not be diminished because the kidneys are retroperitoneal and not in contact with the small intestine and colon. Pyelonephritis would not present with rebound tenderness.

Perforated ulcer: This would result in peritonitis (which the patient does not have) and decreased blood volume. This patient has normal Hgb, Hct, and electrolytes. Also, there is no orthostatic hypertension.

DKA: Usually the abdominal pain due to DKA is **diffuse pain.** Also, this patient has normal serum glucose, and there are no **ketones** in the urine. The anion gap is normal, and she is not dehydrated.

Ectopic pregnancy: The patient's last menstrual period was 10 days ago with normal flow and duration, and her β-hCG was undetectable.

CASE 4 — CC: "My son is wheezing and can't breathe."

HISTORY: 5 y/o white male infant who presents to the ED with an acute attack of shortness of breath and wheezing. Over the last 4 days, the patient has experienced about five episodes of shortness of breath, wheezing, and coughing. These episodes have been getting progressively worse. These periods happen generally at **night** and tonight, they woke the patient. The cough is nonproductive. Six days earlier, the patient developed an **upper respiratory infection.** The patient has been afebrile and complains of no syncope, changes in appetite, urination, diarrhea, constipation, or other constitutional symptoms. The patient has had two past episodes of wheezing and shortness of breath that occurred once after being exposed to **extremely cold air** and the other after **strenuous exercise** playing soccer. Both episodes resolved within minutes. The patient also has a history of multiple upper respiratory infections in the winter that subsequently "go to the chest" and take about 2 weeks to fully recover. The patient has never been diagnosed with asthma or reactive airway disease. The patient has no known drug allergies, but is allergic to cats. The patient has a family history of a mother and sister with **eczema.** There have been no changes in the home environment such as new carpets or new animals. The patient's **father smokes,** but he only smokes out of doors or by an open window. The patient is not currently taking any medications.

PHYSICAL: The patient is alert and oriented, tachypneic, demonstrates mild air hunger, and has **audible expiratory wheezes.** Temp: 99.5°F; HR: 110; **RR: 35;** Ht and Wt 50th percentile. HEENT: (+) **nasal flaring;** tympanic membranes WNL; nose has clear exudate; mouth/throat have mucous membranes with **cyanosis,** nonerythematous, no postnasal drainage. Neck: supple, no lymphadenopathy. Lungs: **intercostal retractions, hyperresonant** to percussion, **prolonged expiratory phase,** no crackles or rhonchi; **wheezes** heard throughout chest. Extremities: no clubbing or edema; **cyanosis** is present and capillary refill is <2 sec. The patient is diaphoretic.

DIFFERENTIAL: Pneumonia (viral, bacterial, or mycoplasma); foreign body aspiration; asthma; cystic fibrosis; TB.

DIAGNOSTICS: Pulse ox 85% on room air; post albuterol nebulizer pulse ox is 96%. CXR: lung fields are **hyperinflated** bilaterally with flattening of diaphragm, with no atelectasis or infiltrate. Expiratory CXR: lung field and diaphragmatic levels are bilaterally symmetric. No opaque foreign body is visualized. CBC with diff: (+) lymphocytosis. PPD: negative. Sweat test (−).

DIAGNOSIS: Asthma (reactive airway disease—RAD).

(continued)

CASE 4   CC: "My son is wheezing and can't breathe." (Continued)

ASSESSMENT/PLAN: 5 y/o male infant with RAD. The condition is reversible with inhaled β₂-agonists or anticholinergics. Treat the patient with supplemental oxygen in hospital, inhaled **β₂-agonists, anticholinergics,** or **steroids** for acute exacerbations and **cromolyn** prophylactically.

Asthma: The history of multiple colds that "end in the chest," acute exacerbations of shortness of breath precipitated by exertion and cold weather, and attacks more commonly at night are typical of asthma. **Reversibility** of attacks is the key to diagnosing asthma. Spirometry in asthmatics shows a **decreased FEV₁/FVC ratio.** CXR in asthmatics can show hyperinflation due to air trapping in this **obstructive** condition (see Figure). Asthma can be familial with other people in the patient's family showing allergic conditions such as atopic dermatitis or eczema.

Tuberculosis: Primary tuberculosis generally is asymptomatic but can sometimes present with fever, malaise, and weight loss. CXR in TB shows **hilar lymphadenopathy** and a PPD would be positive.

Cystic fibrosis (CF): Although the patient is **white,** the history is negative for any **malabsorptive problems** (ht and wt are at the 50th percentile) that occur as a result of pancreatic insufficiency associated with CF. The result of the patient's **sweat test** for CF is negative.

Foreign body aspiration: Although aspiration of foreign bodies causes obstruction, air trapping and hyperinflation, it is usually **unilateral** (right > left because of the decreased angle of the right mainstem bronchus) instead of bilateral, as in this patient. The presentation of obstruction due to a foreign body generally is acute and severe and can present with a history of choking, gagging, or a paroxysmal cough. This patient has a history of wheezing, cough, and shortness of breath that started gradually.

Pneumonia (viral, bacterial or mycoplasma): The patient is afebrile. CXR shows no lung infiltration. In addition, the patient has a radiographic obstructive lung picture, which can be reversed with treatment.

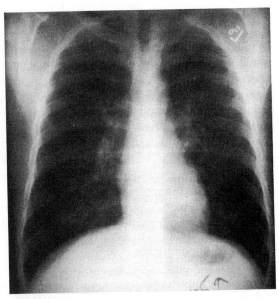

CASE 4 Asthma shown on a posteroanterior chest radiograph.

CASE 5   CC: "I'm having a lot of trouble breathing."

HISTORY: A 70 y/o man presents to the ED c/o **shortness of breath** and cough. The patient states that he has had an increase in SOB over the past **several months,** notable during exertion and at rest. The patient has an **intermittent cough** with scant sputum (no hemoptysis, no "rust" color) and the SOB preceded his cough. He denies asthma, TB exposure, previous history of DVT, orthopnea, or PND. He has an **88 pack-year history of smoking cigarettes** (2 packs/day for 44 years). The patient is a social drinker. He denies IVDU.

PHYSICAL: The patient is afebrile but appears in acute distress with RR of 27 breaths/min. No lymphadenopathy. The patient is thin; **he breathes through pursed lips** and uses **accessory respiratory mus-**

cles. **Increased A-P diameter** of chest. Lungs: **Prolonged expiration,** no wheezing, and no rales. Heart: RRR, no S3 or S4, no murmurs, and no JVD. Ext: nontender lower extremities with no edema.

DIFFERENTIAL: Acute exacerbation of COPD; acute asthmatic attack; pulmonary infection; pulmonary emboli; pulmonary neoplasm; CHF; carcinoid syndrome; pneumothorax; pleural effusion; anemia.

DIAGNOSTICS: ABG: slight **hypoxemia,** increased PCO_2, **O_2 sat 86%,** normal A-a gradient. CBC: normal. CXR: bilateral **hyperinflation;** flattened diaphragm; **narrowed cardiac silhouette.** Sputum cytology: no malignant cells; sputum culture: no growth. PFTs: **Decreased FEV_1, VC, peak expiratory flow rate;** increased TLC, RV. Electrolytes: WNL. ECG: WNL.

DIAGNOSIS: Acute exacerbation of COPD.

ASSESSMENT/PLAN: 70 y/o white man with a history of tobacco use who presents with SOB and cough. Administer oxygen at 2 to 4 L/min via a nasal cannula to achieve oxygen saturation >90%. Treat dyspnea with albuterol, terbutaline, anticholinergics, or aminophylline. The patient needs to be instructed on exercise, diet, and **smoking cessation.**

Acute asthmatic attack: This diagnosis is not likely, because the patient has **no history of asthma.** On physical exam, the patient has no wheezing or stridor, and he is not alkalotic. The patient's age is also late for presentation. Asthma would be the diagnosis if the patient's condition resolved with the administration of inhaled steroids or β-agonists.

Pulmonary infection: This diagnosis is not likely because the patient is **afebrile** with no purulent sputum and no tachycardia. Also, the result of the sputum Gram stain was negative, and the CXR showed no infiltrates.

Pulmonary emboli: This diagnosis is unlikely, because the patient has no **history of DVTs** or a hypercoaguable state. There is no **tachycardia** or pleuritic chest pain, and ABGs do not show **acute hypoxia.** Also, the patient's dyspnea has been gradual in onset (not **acute onset** as in pulmonary embolus).

Pulmonary neoplasm: This diagnosis is not likely even though the patient has a history of smoking, has gradual onset of dyspnea, and is thin. However, decreased breath sounds, decreased tactile fremitus, and increased A-P diameter are not signs of cancer. The CXR does not show any lesion that suggests a mass, nor does it show hilar lymphadenopathy.

Exacerbation of CHF: Although exacerbation of CHF can result in **increased dyspnea on exertion** and a **nonproductive cough,** the patient has no history of **PND** or orthopnea. On physical exam, there are no rales, no **S3,** no JVD, no hepatosplenomegaly, and no edema. PFTs would not be abnormal in a pt with an exacerbation of CHF.

Carcinoid: This diagnosis is not likely because the patient does not have **cutaneous flushing, diarrhea,** or **telangiectasias.** CXR does not demonstrate any pulmonary or mediastinal masses.

Pneumothorax: This diagnosis is unlikely even though a pneumothorax would cause dyspnea. The onset of a pneumothorax would be **acute,** rather than chronic. **Breath sounds** are not **absent,** and the **trachea** is not **shifted** (found in tension pneumothorax). CXR does not demonstrate a pneumothorax.

Pleural effusion: This diagnosis is not likely to be a pleural effusion, because there is no dullness to percussion, no rales, and no blunting of the costovertebral angle on CXR.

Anemia: The diagnosis is not likely to be anemia because the CBC is WNL and a peripheral blood smear does not show microcytic or macrocytic RBCs.

CASE 6 CC: "I have this incredible chest pain. I think I'm having a heart attack!"

HISTORY: A 55 y/o man presents to the ED with chest pain. The patient describes the pain as the **worst pain** that he has ever had. The pain started 2 hours ago while he was **exercising.** It is **crushing** and **substernal** and **radiates to his left jaw,** with an intensity of 10/10, and is not alleviated by rest or with change in body position. Inspiration does not intensify the pain [(−) pleurisy]. Sublingual nitroglycerin did not relieve the pain. He denies similar episodes in the past. The patient also c/o nausea, **profuse sweating,** and mild SOB. He denies syncope, palpitations, orthopnea, PND, ankle swelling, GERD, or pain after meals. PMH is significant for mild **HTN** and **hypercholesterolemia.** His father died at age 60 of a heart attack. The patient has a 40 pack-year history of **smoking,** drinks on the weekends and denies IVDU.

PHYSICAL: This individual is an overweight man who is diaphoretic, clutching his chest in pain, and in obvious distress. , Temp: 99°F, HR: 120, RR: 18, BP: 150/85. Tilt test: negative for orthostatic hypotension. Neck: carotid pulse shows decreased volume, (−) JVD, (−) HJR. Lungs: few B/L crackles at the lung bases, (−) wheezing or rhonchi. Heart: RRR, normal S1, S2; **(+) S3 and S4;** (−) murmurs, symmetric pulses B/L. Abd: (−) masses or ascites.

DIFFERENTIAL: Aortic dissection; unstable angina; MI; pulmonary embolism; pericarditis; perforated ulcer.

DIAGNOSTICS: ECG (see Figure): sinus tachycardia, normal axis, **ST segment elevation** >1 mm in anterior leads (e.g., V_2, V_4, V_6), (+) **Q waves.** Enzymes: total **CK—elevated, CKMB—elevated, cardiac troponin I—elevated.** 2-D echocardiography: hypokinesis in a segment of the anterior wall; (−) mural thrombi, (−) evidence of aortic aneurysm. ABG: normal O_2, CO_2, pH. CXR: (−) infiltrates, atelectasis, CVA blunting; (+) pulmonary edema (mild); (−) cardiomegaly or widened mediastinum. Cardiac panel: serum LDL is elevated, serum triglyceride is elevated, and serum HDL is low, serum glucose is normal.

DIAGNOSIS: Acute MI secondary to CAD.

ASSESSMENT/PLAN: A 55 y/o African-American man presents to the ED with substernal chest pain, nausea, diaphoresis, and mild SOB. Treatment includes **aspirin, supplemental O_2** via nasal cannula, IV morphine for pain, IV metoprolol to decrease HR and HTN, IV heparin for antithrombosis. Percutaneous transluminal coronary angioplasty (PTCA) is also a possibility, IV furosemide for pulmonary edema, bed rest, and **stool softeners to decrease strain** of defecation. Post MI complications include **arrhythmias,** cardiogenic shock, rupture of the left ventricular free wall, VSD, mitral regurgitation, pericarditis, and thromboembolism. The patient needs cardiac rehabilitation, cessation of smoking, and increased physical activity. Outpatient follow-up includes a thallium stress test and an echocardiogram to determine the

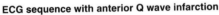

ECG sequence with anterior Q wave infarction

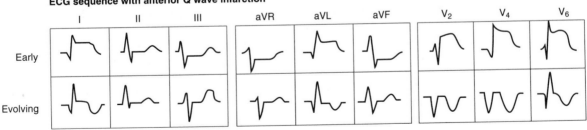

CASE 6 Sequence of depolarization and repolarization changes with acute anterior wall Q wave infarctions.

amount of remaining viable cardiac tissue. Aspirin, ACE inhibitors, and β-blockers should be used to decrease morbidity.

Aortic dissection: Patients present with **tearing substernal chest pain that radiates to the back** and lasts for hours. Aortic dissection results in **decreased distal pulses,** unlike this patient, who has equal pulses. CXR did not demonstrate **widening of the mediastinum.**

Unstable angina: Unstable angina is a potential diagnosis due to the new onset of severe chest pain that occurred during rest. However, nausea, diaphoresis, substernal chest pain, and ST segment elevations are characteristic of an MI, not unstable angina.

Pulmonary embolism (PE): PE produces **pleuritic chest pain, tachypnea,** tachycardia, and hypoxemia. This patient did not have pleuritic chest pain, nor did he have tachypnea. The ABG showed normal oxygen saturation, and the CXR showed neither atelectasis nor pleural effusion.

Pericarditis: Although pericarditis causes steady, substernal chest pain, nausea and diaphoresis are not symptoms of pericarditis. Cardiac auscultation revealed no **pericardial friction rub.**

Perforated ulcer: A perforated ulcer produces severe **epigastric/substernal chest pain,** hypotension, and some diaphoresis. However, this patient's history is not consistent with a perforated ulcer. He is not hypotensive from blood loss, and his Hct and Hgb are WNL.

CASE 7 | CC: "I feel terrible. I suddenly got this fever and this awful chest pain every time I cough."

HISTORY: A 47 y/o woman presents with a 24-hour history of sudden onset **fever,** shaking **chills,** stabbing pain in her left chest wall with deep inspiration, and a cough productive of **purulent rusty sputum** that is sometimes tinged with blood. She has also experienced nausea, vomiting, and myalgias. She has had no changes in stools, abdominal pain, changes in vision, or fainting but states that in the days prior to onset, she had an upper respiratory infection. She has no history of lung disease or breathing problems; she has had no recent hospitalizations; and she has not travelled recently. The patient has had a recent HIV test that was negative. Her past medical history and family history are noncontributory.

PHYSICAL: The patient is alert and mildly toxic; she has labored breathing with some **intercostal retractions** and use of **accessory muscles of respiration. T: 103.3°F; HR:120; RR: 33; Pulse ox: 90% on room air.** HEENT: conjunctivae noninjected; positive nasal discharge; no lesions in nasal or buccal mucosa. Neck supple with no lymphadenopathy. Heart: tachycardia, regular rhythm with no murmurs, rubs, or gallops. Lungs: **dullness to percussion over the right upper lobe;** increased **tactile fremitus,** bronchial breath sounds, **whispered pectoriloquy,** and **prominent crackles** in the right upper lobe. The left lung and lower right lung are clear to auscultation. Abdominal exam: WNL. Extremities: **(+) cyanosis,** but no clubbing or edema.

DIFFERENTIAL: Viral pneumonia, mycoplasma pneumonia, pneumococcal pneumonia, and tuberculosis.

DIAGNOSTICS: CBC: leukocytosis with a bandemia or **left shift.** Serum pH: 7.5 (alkalosis). Sputum sample-Gram stain: **Gram (+) lancet-shaped diplococci** in short chains; **(+) quelling reaction.** CXR: dense consolidation confined to the right upper lobe (see Figure A). PPD (−).

DIAGNOSIS: Pneumococcal pneumonia.

(continued)

CASE 7 CC: "I feel terrible. I suddenly got this fever and this awful chest pain every time I cough." (Continued)

ASSESSMENT/PLAN: 47 y/o woman with acute onset of right upper lobe pneumonia. Treat the patient with penicillin G or third-generation cephalosporin.

Pneumococcal pneumonia: Bacterial pneumonia very commonly presents with **lobar consolidation,** acute onset of cough, dyspnea, fever, and pleurisy. Sputum sample was positive for gram-positive, lancet-shaped diplococci that were quellung reaction positive. All of the clinical findings are consistent with pneumococcal (*Streptococcal pneumoniae*) pneumonia.

Mycoplasma, chlamydia, or virus: Mycoplasma and viral pneumonia are atypical in presentation. Generally, there is a 1- to 2-week period of low-grade fever, signs of upper respiratory illness, and **interstitial infiltrate** on CXR (see Figure B). Mycoplasma classically presents with a dry, hacking, nonproductive cough. Viral and mycoplasma pneumonia can be confirmed by serology. Mycoplasma can also be confirmed by **cold agglutinins.**

Tuberculosis: TB is generally asymptomatic in primary tuberculosis and presents with **hilar lymphadenopathy.** The PPD test result was negative.

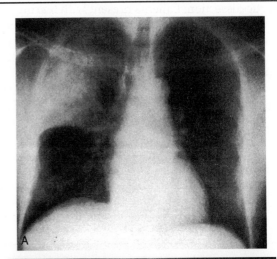

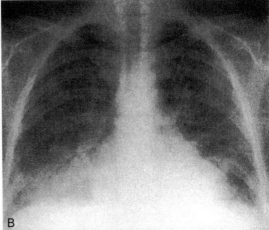

CASE 7 *A,* Lobar pneumonia from *Pneumococcus.* *B, Mycoplasma* pneumonia.

CASE 8 CC: "I've been bleeding every time I have a bowel movement and it's starting to scare me."

HISTORY: A 48 y/o man presents to the ED c/o **blood in his stools.** The patient states that the bloody stools began 1 month ago when he discovered red streaks on the toilet paper. He then noticed bright red blood on the surface of his stool and that the stools became thin ("**pencil-thin**"). The number of bloody stools has been increasing. There were episodes where he strained, but no defecation occurred [(+) **tenesmus**]. He also had intermittent **constipation** and **diarrhea.** During the past month, he has had diffuse, crampy abdominal pain of variable frequency with no relation to food intake or defecation. He has also had a 10-lb weight loss in the past month. The patient denies nausea, vomiting, steatorrhea, dehydration, fever, chills, night sweats, dyspnea, palpitations, orthopnea, or PND. He has a 28 pack-year history of **cig-**

arette smoking; he drinks socially; and he denies IVDU. The patient is in a monogamous relationship with his wife, with no history of STDs or anal intercourse. His diet consists of **high-fat, low-fiber food.** The patient's **uncle died of colon cancer.**

PHYSICAL: The patient appears anxious but in no acute distress. Temp: 98.6° F, HR: 95, RR: 15, BP: 150/95. Neck: no lymphadenopathy, (−) Virchow's node. Abd: soft, distended, **tender to palpation in LLQ,** no rebound, no guarding, no hepatomegaly, no splenomegaly, no palpable masses, hyperactive bowel sounds. Rectal: **Hemoccult test (+) for blood in stool,** no hemorrhoids, no anal fissures, prostate normal size. Ext: No rashes, no edema.

DIFFERENTIAL: Ulcerative colitis; Crohn's disease; infectious colitis; colonic polyps (adenoma); diverticulitis; adenocarcinoma of the colon.

DIAGNOSTICS: CBC: Hgb and Hct decreased, **microcytic anemia. CEA elevated.** Stool culture: ova and parasites negative. Serum lactate: normal. LFTs: WNL. CXR: no pulmonary masses, no mediastinal masses; no enlarged lymph nodes, no pleural effusions. NGT: no blood in stomach. Anoscopy: no hemorrhoids, no rectal ulcers, no anal fissures, no rectal fistulas. Double-contrast barium enema: annular constricting lesion ("**apple-core lesion**") in the descending colon (see Figure A), no cobblestone appearance, no "thumbprinting," no skip lesions, no "string sign," no continuous mucosal lesions, no shortening of the bowel. Colonoscopy: annular mass protruding into the lumen of the descending colon. The biopsy reveals **adenocarcinoma of the colon** (invasive tall columnar cells, moderately differentiated with some inflammation and fibrosis) (see Figure B) with extension into the muscular propria and no lymph node involvement.

DIAGNOSIS: Adenocarcinoma of the colon: stage B1 (T2 N0 M0).

ASSESSMENT/PLAN: 48 y/o white man c/o **hematochezia.** Therapy includes resection of the colon, the omentum, and regional lymph nodes. The patient has no evidence of lung metastases on the CXR; his LFTs were

(continued)

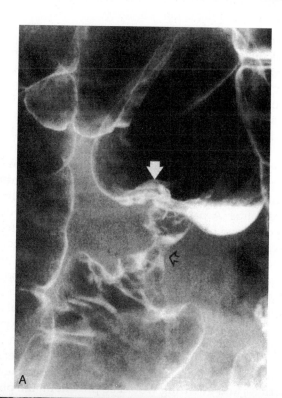

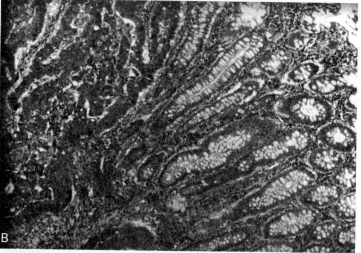

CASE 8 *A,* Adenocarcinoma of the jejunum. *B,* Adenocarcinoma of the colon.

CASE 8   CC: "I've been bleeding every time I have a bowel movement and it's starting to scare me." (Continued)

normal, indicating no metastases to the liver. The large intestine should be examined in its entirety by colonoscopy to determine if there are other polyps. The patient is a candidate for chemotherapy (5-FU and levamisole). Radiation therapy is not an effective treatment for left-sided colon cancer. **CEA levels should be measured** at 3-month intervals to assess increases in level, which would signify a recurrence of the cancer. An annual digital rectal examination (DRE) along with a Hemoccult test should be performed, and a colonoscopy should be done every 3 years to watch for recurrences. The 5-year survival rate of stage B1 adenocarcinoma of the colon is 85%.

Ulcerative colitis (UC): UC would have resulted in constipation, diarrhea, hematochezia, and LLQ pain; it would also have contributed to the anemia of chronic disease. However, this patient did not have any **extraintestinal manifestations** of UC, such as uveitis, sclerosing cholangitis, liver disease, arthritis, erythema nodosum, and aphthous stomatitis. CEA levels would not be elevated in UC. Barium enema in UC would have revealed **superficial, nontransmural ulcerations,** with **continuous involvement** of the colon and rectum.

Crohn's disease: Crohn's disease would have produced symptoms similar to UC and colonic adenocarcinoma. Also, **steatorrhea, malabsorption, enteric fistulas,** and **vitamin B$_{12}$ deficiency** are characteristic of Crohn's—signs that the patient did not have. CEA levels would not be elevated in Crohn's disease. Barium enema would have revealed "**cobblestoning**" (due to inflammation of the submucosa), "**thumbprinting,**" "**string sign,**" and **skip lesions** throughout the colon and small intestine.

Infectious colitis: A patient with infectious colitis would present with intermittent, diffuse abdominal pain, fever, and bloody diarrhea. This patient was afebrile, and his stool cultures were negative. Infectious colitis is self-resolving in 1 to 2 weeks and is not associated with elevated CEA levels, anemia of chronic disease, or "apple core lesions."

Adenomatous polyps: A patient with adenomatous polyps would have presented with hematochezia, "crampy" abdominal pain, and possibly an obstruction. The barium enema, however, would not have revealed an "apple core lesion." Colonoscopy would have demonstrated polyps, and the biopsy of these polyps would have revealed tubular, villous, or tubulovillous adenoma.

Diverticulitis: Diverticulitis would produce LLQ abdominal pain, fever, **leukocytosis,** and diarrhea. With diverticulitis, constipation and pain are relieved after a bowel movement. Double-contrast barium enema would have **demonstrated outpouchings of the mucosa and submucosa** (diverticula). **Rebound tenderness and guarding** would be present on the physical exam of the abdomen.

CASE 9   CC: "Why does my baby look like this? What happened?"

HISTORY: 1-day-old male patient is a product of a full-term (40 weeks) spontaneous vaginal delivery of a **37 y/o mother.** At 17 weeks of pregnancy, **maternal serum alpha-fetoprotein** was drawn and found to be low. Abnormalities were detected on fetal ultrasound and at birth. Pregnancy and birth were without complications.

PHYSICAL: Temp: 98.6 F, HR: 140 (normal: 120 to 160), RR: 35 (normal); ht, wt, and HC: 10–15%. General: alert 1-day-old male infant in no acute distress. HEENT: small and rounded head with a **flat occiput** (posterior part of skull); **low-set ears;** wide set eyes (**hypertelorism**) with upslanting palpebral fissures (eyelids) and white spots in the iris (**Brushfield spots**); **flat nasal bridge** with **epicanthal folds;** protuberant tongue; short neck. Lungs: clear to auscultation bilaterally. Heart: RRR with systolic ejection murmur.

Abd: normal. Genitourinary: normal male. Ext: upper extremities have transverse palmar crease (**simian crease**), short fourth and fifth fingers (**clinodactyly**); lower extremities have **wide space between first and second toe.** Musculoskeletal: **hypotonia** and hyperextensible large joints.

DIFFERENTIAL: Down's syndrome (trisomy 21 or 14:21 translocation); Patau's syndrome (trisomy 13); Edward's syndrome (trisomy 18).

DIAGNOSTICS: Karyotype: trisomy 21. Audiometry: level of **hearing abnormal.**

DIAGNOSIS: Down's syndrome (trisomy 21).

ASSESSMENT/PLAN: 1-day-old male infant with a constellation of findings that are typical of Down's syndrome with karyotypic trisomy 21 confirmation. Echocardiography is done to evaluate for a congenital heart lesion. Counsel the parents regarding the special needs of their child and future risks of having another child with this same syndrome.

Down's syndrome: The patient presented with most of the classic features of Down's syndrome. In addition to the findings above, Down's patients often have **duodenal atresia** ("**double-bubble**" on abdominal x-ray), increased risk for lymphoblastic leukemia, hypothyroidism, and Alzheimer's disease that presents at a younger age than is typical. Patients can also have atlantoaxial subluxation as a result of ligamentous laxity. **Congenital heart disease** is common, especially endocardial cushion defects as well as septal defects (e.g., ASD, VSD). Patients with Down's syndrome are generally mentally retarded with a mean IQ of 50. Mothers older than 35 years are at increased risk of having a child with trisomy 21. Mothers with a previous child with trisomy 21 have a **1% to 2% risk of recurrence** with future children. Mothers with a child with Down's syndrome as a result of a balanced translocation have approximately a 15% risk of recurrence. The prognosis of a child that survives the infant period is generally good, with survival to 60 years occurring in approximately 44% of patients with Down's syndrome.

Edward's syndrome (trisomy 18): This syndrome presents in the neonatal period with **micrognathia** (small jaw), **rocker-bottom feet, second and fifth fingers overlapping third and fourth**, respectively, congenital heart disease, hypertonia, and severe **mental retardation.** Patients with Edward's syndrome generally have a poor prognosis with life expectancy less than 1 year. Edward's syndrome also presents prenatally with **decreased α-fetoprotein levels.**

Patau's syndrome (trisomy 13): Presents with **microcephaly, cleft lip** with or without cleft palate, different degrees of **holoprosencephaly** (agenesis of midline structures), seizures, microphthalmia, **colobomas** of the iris, **polydactyly,** severe **mental retardation,** and congenital heart defects. Prognosis is generally even worse than Edward's syndrome, with life expectancy less than 1 year.

CASE 10 — CC: Follow-up visit for high-blood pressure.

HISTORY: 45 y/o white man sees his primary care physician for a follow-up appointment for hypertension that was first noted during his annual examination 6 months earlier. He has no new complaints and has no history of angina, orthopnea, changes in vision, cough, episodes of dizziness, urinary tract infections, headaches, weight loss, polyuria, polydipsia, muscle weakness, palpitations, diaphoresis, or mood changes. The patient is a salesman for a pharmaceutical company and spends most of his time on the road. The patient **does not exercise** and stated that he has not been in shape since he played college football.

(continued)

CASE 10   **CC: Follow-up visit for high-blood pressure.** (Continued)

The patient's diet consists mainly of **fried restaurant foods and pizza, with few fresh vegetables.** The patient does not smoke but does drink **alcohol** socially (1 to 2 beers about twice a week). The patient's **family history** is positive for a maternal grandfather who died at 60 years of age from an MI, and a paternal grandmother that died of an MI at 65 years of age. Parents: mother, 67 y/o, with well-controlled (by medication) hypertension; the father died at 35 y/o in a train wreck.

PHYSICAL: Well-appearing, well-proportioned, slightly obese 45 y/o man, appears stated age, alert, oriented, and in no acute distress. Temp: 98.5 F; HR: 75; Ht: 6′;Wt: 326 lb; BP: supine: 160/105 (upper extremity), 162/103 (lower extremity), 158/110 (standing). HEENT: Fundi normal, no **papilledema,** no carotid bruits heard bilaterally. Heart: RRR, normal S1, S2, no **m/r/g,** all pulses normal to palpation with no lag between radial and lower extremity pulses. Abd: no bruits heard over the kidneys bilaterally and no masses. Extremities: no c/c/e.

DIFFERENTIAL: Cushing's disease or syndrome, primary hyperaldosteronism, pheochromocytoma, coarctation of the aorta, essential hypertension.

DIAGNOSTICS: ECG: WNL. Blood electrolytes: potassium WNL, glucose WNL, BUN/creatinine WNL. Hct: WNL. UA: no cells or WBC, protein WNL, (−) glucose. 24-hour urine collection: (−) **cortisol** and (−) **catecholamines** (metanephrine, normetanephrine, and mandelic acid).

DIAGNOSIS: Essential hypertension.

ASSESSMENT/PLAN: 45 y/o white man with essential hypertension. No associated symptoms. Multiple risk factors for heart disease: obesity, high-cholesterol/high-fat diet, male, alcohol use, no exercise, and hypertension. The patient needs to be educated about the risk factors for cardiovascular disease and advised to follow a low-fat, low-salt, and low-cholesterol diet. Also, the patient should be encouraged to begin aerobic exercise three times per week. The patient should be started on captopril (an **ACE inhibitor**) therapy and should have a follow-up checkup in 4 weeks for a blood pressure check and adjustment of medication.

Essential hypertension: Essential hypertension is hypertension that is not secondary to a primary disease. More than **90%** of hypertensive patients have essential hypertension. Hypertension predisposes a patient to deadly cardiovascular accidents. Roughly, any diastolic blood pressure consistently above 85 or any systolic blood pressure above 135 is classified as hypertensive. This patient had no signs or symptoms of malignant hypertension (e.g., systolic blood pressure >200 and papilledema).

Secondary hypertension: Secondary hypertension is attributable to a specific organ defect that results in hypertension, which was not detected in this patient. The most common cause of secondary hypertension is **renal artery stenosis.**

Cushing's disease/syndrome: Although the patient is obese, there is no **central obesity** or **moon faces,** and extremity atrophy is not seen as would be the case in Cushing's disease/syndrome. Also, the **24-hour urine screen was negative for cortisol.**

Primary aldosteronism: This diagnosis is not likely because there is no history of muscle weakness secondary to **low serum potassium** level. The abdominal physical exam did not show a mass (adrenal tumor); however, this is not a very sensitive screen. If there were a higher level of suspicion for primary aldosteronism, a CT scan of the abdomen would be recommended to rule out this diagnosis.

Pheochromocytoma: This diagnosis is unlikely because there is no history of **episodic headaches, diaphoresis,** and **palpitations.** The 24-hour urine screen for metanephrine, normetanephrine, and mandelic acid (metabolites of norepinephrine and epinephrine) was WNL.

Coarctation of the aorta: This diagnosis is unlikely because there was no lag time between upper and lower extremity pulses. If this diagnosis was suspected, a chest x-ray would show **notching of the ribs** due to collateral blood flow.

CASE 11   CC: "Dude, what's going on? Where am I?"

HPI: A 25 y/o man is brought to the ED by EMS in a **confused** and **stuporous** state. The patient is inattentive, **not oriented to time or place,** cannot recall any of the three objects that he was asked to remember or complete the serial 7s test. The patient c/o nausea and constipation but cannot recall when these symptoms began. The patient denies abdominal pain, headache, or stiff neck. He is unsure of prior liver or renal disease or diabetes. He admits to **tobacco, alcohol,** and **IV drug use.**

PHYSICAL: The patient appears extremely stuporous and confused. Temp: 98.6°F; HR 40; RR 6/min; BP 120/80. The patient is thin and emaciated. Eyes: sclera are anicteric, conjunctiva are pink, pupils are **pinpoint** but reactive to light, (−) papilledema, (−) exudates, (−) hemorrhages on fundoscopy. Neck: (−) nuchal rigidity, (−) lymphadenopathy, (−) carotid bruits. Heart: RRR, normal S1, S2, (−) murmurs. Abd: distended abdomen. Neuro: **(+) asterixis,** decreased sensation in extremities, DTR normal, (−) Babinski. Ext: **needle tracks** in both arms, (−) petechiae.

DIFFERENTIAL: Drug overdose; alcohol intoxication; lead intoxication; myxedema coma; hepatic encephalopathy; uremia; meningitis; encephalitis; cerebral neoplasm; head trauma (subdural hematoma, cerebral contusion); CVA.

DIAGNOSTICS: Non-contrast CT: (−) evidence of mass lesions, herniation, hemorrhage, infarct. EEG: widespread **fast (beta) activity,** (−) evidence of seizure activity. LP: CSF pressure, protein, glucose, WBC are all WNL. CBC: WNL. Blood alcohol level—normal. Toxicology: (+) opioids, (−) cocaine. ABG: Respiratory acidosis (decreased PO_2, increased CO_2, increased pH). LFTs: WNL. Thyroid function tests: WNL.

DIAGNOSIS: Opioid intoxication due to IV drug use.

ASSESSMENT/PLAN: 25 y/o man with drug intoxication. If required, maintain a patent airway with tracheal intubation with mechanical ventilation. Maintain BP with IV fluids and pressor agents (dobutamine, dopamine); elevate the patient's head and torso to prevent aspiration of gastric contents into the lungs. IV **naloxone, thiamine, dextrose** should be given before the results of the electrolyte and toxicology screen. After recovery from acute opioid intoxication, the patient needs counseling. Consider methadone maintenance therapy to prevent opioid withdrawal.

Alcohol intoxication: Associated with confusion, respiratory depression, coma, and atelectasis. Pinpoint pupils are not seen. Blood alcohol level would be elevated.

Lead intoxication: No history of lead exposure could be elicited. Lead intoxication is characterized by **wrist drop** and **hypochromic microcytic anemia w/ basophilic stippling.**

Myxedema coma: Thyroid function tests are normal, and the patient is not hypo/hyperthermic. Also, there is no delay of DTRs.

Hepatic encephalopathy: **Stupor, confusion,** and **asterixis** are signs of this; but no evidence of jaundice, organomegaly, or cirrhosis (variceal bleeding, spider angioma, palmar erythema, gynecomastia) is seen with this patient. LFTs are abnormal, and serum ammonia is elevated in hepatic encephalopathy.

Uremia: No evidence of encephalopathy and atelectasis, pericarditis, or pleural effusion; no evidence of renal failure (BUN and Cr normal); and no peripheral edema.

Meningitis: The patient would be febrile with nuchal rigidity. CSF results are not consistent with meningitis (increased WBCs, decreased glucose, increased protein). Meningitis is not associated with pinpoint pupils but is associated with **photophobia.**

Encephalitis: Not associated with pinpoint pupils or acute respiratory acidosis. **Altered mentation** and a normal CSF are characteristic.

(continued)

CASE 11 CC: "Dude, what's going on? Where am I?" (Continued)

Head trauma: No history of head trauma and normal CT of head rules out this diagnosis.

CVA: The patient is very young to have a CVA; no risk factors (HTN, DM, hypercoagulable state). The patient has no focal deficits and reactive pupils rule out a brain stem infarct. A CT of the head shows no evidence of thrombosis, hemorrhage, or embolism.

CASE 12 CC: "I seem to be getting bigger and no one gives me a straight answer as to why and I don't know what to do."

HISTORY: A 40 y/o black woman presents to the ED with **an increasing abdominal girth.** The patient states that the increase in abdominal girth began a few weeks ago and has been gradually evolving. She denies abdominal pain, nausea, vomiting, diarrhea, constipation, or hemoptysis. There is no abdominal pain after fatty meals, no palpitations, no PND, and no wheezing. She also c/o **hemorrhoids** and noticed blood on some toilet paper a few days after the increase in abdominal girth. She has a **24-pack year history of cigarette smoking,** drinks alcohol socially, and admits to using **IV heroin** and cocaine. She also smokes crack.

PHYSICAL: The patient has an enlarged abdomen and appears uncomfortable. Temp: 98.6°F, HR: 75; RR: 16; BP: 120/85. Heart: no S3, no S4, no murmur, no JVD. Abd: soft, nontender, (+) **splenomegaly,** (+) shifting dullness [(+) **ascites**], no hepatomegaly, no caput medusae, (+) bowel sounds, **Hemoccult (+)** for blood in stool. Ext: no edema, no clubbing, no palmar erythema, (+) needle tracts. Neuro: cranial nerves II to XII intact and no asterixis.

DIFFERENTIAL: Portal hypertension (Budd-Chiari syndrome, cirrhosis, portal vein obstruction); nephrotic syndrome; CHF; Meigs' syndrome; metastatic cancer to the liver.

DIAGNOSTICS: Serology: anti-HAV Ab (−), HBsAg (−), anti-HBcAb (−), **anti-HBsAb (−), HCV Ab (+),** anti-HDV (−), Tb skin test (−). LFTs: elevated. BUN, Cr: WNL. UA: urine bilirubin elevated, urine dip WNL. AFP: WNL. Paracentesis of ascitic fluid: straw-colored fluid with **protein elevated,** cytology (−) for malignant cells. US of liver: (+) ascites, **patent hepatic vein, dilated portal vein,** liver nodules. CT-guided liver biopsy: diffuse **piecemeal** and **bridging necrosis,** diffuse fibrosis, liver cirrhosis, no Mallory bodies. Pelvic exam: WNL. Anoscopy: (+) internal hemorrhoids.

DIAGNOSIS: Portal hypertension secondary to hepatitis C–induced cirrhosis.

ASSESSMENT/PLAN: A 40 y/o black woman presents to the ER c/o increasing abdominal girth and hemorrhoids. Treat the portal HTN with decompression, either surgically (portal-systemic shunt) or by transjugular intrahepatic portosystemic shunt (**TIPS**). β-Blockers will also reduce the risk of variceal bleeding. Ascites and hemorrhoids will be alleviated after TIPS or surgery. Pt should be advised to **avoid alcohol, IVDU, and excessive protein intake** (may precipitate hepatic encephalopathy). Pt is at risk for variceal bleeding, SBP (spontaneous bacterial peritonitis), hepatorenal syndrome, and hepatic encephalopathy. Pt is most likely not a candidate for liver transplantation (the only cure for her portal HTN and liver cirrhosis) due to her IVDU.

Budd-Chiari syndrome: Postsinusoidal portal HTN is the result of Budd-Chiari syndrome, which mimics right-sided heart failure-induced liver congestion. However, this patient shows no evidence of a **hy-**

percoagulable state (a predisposition for getting Budd-Chiari), and her liver US showed **no obstruction of the hepatic vein.**

Portal vein obstruction: Obstruction of the portal vein (as a result of neoplasms, thrombosis, or schistosomiasis) results in presinusoidal portal HTN, which produces hemorrhoids, ascites, caput medusae, and esophageal varices. US of the liver did not show portal vein obstruction; dilatation of the portal vein is a sign of sinusoidal obstruction.

Nephrotic syndrome: One of the signs of nephrotic syndrome is **ascites.** The other signs are **edema, hyperlipidemia,** and **proteinuria,** none of which were present in this patient.

CHF: Right-sided heart failure produces hepatic congestion, splenomegaly, and edema. Chronic congestion results in cardiac cirrhosis, which may, in turn, lead to portal HTN. This patient had no signs of CHF (no S3 or S4 heart sounds, no peripheral edema).

Meigs' syndrome: Meigs' syndrome refers to the triad of **ascites, hydrothorax,** and **benign ovarian fibroma.** The patient's respiratory and pelvic exams were WNL and she had no gynecologic complaints.

Metastatic cancer to the liver: Metastases to the liver can produce ascites. This patient had no history of cancer, and the US of the liver revealed no masses indicative of cancer. The results of the ascitic fluid analysis were not consistent with metastases to the liver because the cytology did not contain malignant cells.

CASE 13 — CC: "My knee really hurts, and I feel achy all over."

HISTORY: 25 y/o white man presents with a 3-day history of pain in the right knee and a 5-day history of **general muscle aches and fatigue.** His knee has been aching and is now swollen and warm. The patient has no history of significant trauma to any joints during the past year. The patient denies having previous diagnosis of joint disease and has no other constitutional symptoms or history of a viral infection in the past month. The patient does have a history of a severe stiff neck and headaches 3 weeks ago after a **camping trip** along the Appalachian Trail, for which he was treated with nonsteroidal anti-inflammatory drugs. The patient denies being bitten by a tick or the presence of a rash around the time of his headache, but in the past week, he has noticed a couple of new red rashes on his left leg. Although the patient is sexually active, there is no history of sexually transmitted disease or pain on urination. There is no significant family history.

PHYSICAL: The patient is a well-appearing, well-developed 25 y/o man, alert, interactive, and in no acute distress. Temp: 98.6; HR: 63; RR: 14; BP: 122/85. HEENT: (−) lymphadenopathy. Lungs: CTA B/L. Heart: RRR. Abd: normal. Genitourinary: no rashes or discharges. Ext: right knee with slight decreased range of motion, warm to the touch, swollen, and painful when moved; two 3-cm **erythematous macules** on the left lower extremity on the flexor surface with some **central clearing,** (+) blanching.

DIFFERENTIAL: Lyme disease, septic arthritis, rheumatoid arthritis (RA), systemic lupus erythematosus (SLE), gouty arthritis.

DIAGNOSTICS: Joint aspirate of 70,000 WBC/ml (mainly PMNs). No uric acid crystals under polarizing microscope. The result of the Gram stain of the joint aspirate was negative, with 70,000 polymorphonuclear leukocytes. Serologic evaluation: (−) rheumatoid factors; (−) antinuclear antibodies; (−) double-stranded DNA antibodies; (+) ELISA antibody response to *Borrelia burgdorferi;* (+) Western blot for *B. burgdorferi* antibodies.

(continued)

CASE 13 — CC: "My knee really hurts, and I feel achy all over." (Continued)

DIAGNOSIS: Lyme disease.

ASSESSMENT /PLAN: 25 y/o man with Lyme disease. Treat with oral doxycycline for 30 days.

Lyme disease with late stage secondary Lyme arthritis: The history of joint and muscle pain with fatigue is consistent with untreated disseminated Lyme disease. The history of a camping trip with the subsequent onset of neck pain and headaches is also consistent with Lyme disease. The tick (*Ixodes dammini*) is common in the region from Maryland to Massachusetts and in some Midwestern states such as Wisconsin and Minnesota. In many cases, individuals do not recall being bitten by ticks or seeing the subsequent centrally clearing macular/papular non-painful erythematous rash (**erythema chronicum migrans**), because often the tick bite is on the flexor surfaces (behind the knees), in the hair, or in the groin or buttocks. A positive ELISA test for *B. burgdorferi* antibody followed by a confirmatory Western blot verifies the clinical suspicion.

Septic arthritis (bacterial): Usually *Staphylococcus aureus* or *Neisseria gonorrhoeae*. Although the patient has a **monarticular** arthritis, there is no history of joint trauma leading to bacterial joint seeding or systemic illness from bacteremia. Also, there is no history of STDs, penile discharge, or pain on urination.

Systemic lupus erythematosus: Even though he is experiencing muscle aches and fatigue, two symptoms of SLE, it is most often a disease found in **reproductive aged females.** Also, serum levels of **anti–double-stranded DNA,** which are 70% sensitive for SLE, and **antinuclear antibodies,** which are 95% sensitive for SLE, are both negative.

Rheumatoid arthritis (RA): Despite the presentation of arthritis, RA involves more than one joint **symmetrically** and typically affects the smaller joints (**PIP**) rather than the larger joints (hip and knee). RA usually spares the DIP joint. The serum **rheumatoid factor** is also negative lending to a diagnosis other than RA.

Gouty arthritis: Lack of **birefringent polarizing crystals** from the joint aspirate helps to rule out this diagnosis. Although gout could present as knee pain, it presents more commonly as **great toe pain** in an older male population.

CASE 14 — CC: "I have this terrible rash. And, I still feel achy, tired, and I haven't been able to beat this fever."

HISTORY: 37 y/o African-American **woman** presents with a 2-week history of **fever, muscle aches, fatigue, joint pain,** and stiffness. The woman saw her primary care physician 10 days ago with similar complaints, but without the **rash.** She was given the tentative diagnosis of a viral illness and sent home without therapy. The rash appeared 1 week after her initial visit, after she spent the day at her son's soccer tournament. The patient complains of no other changes in appetite or sleep and denies nausea/vomiting, diarrhea, dysphagia, and dysuria. She has general joint pain, stiffness, and fatigue but no muscle weakness or difficulty walking or climbing steps. She had been previously healthy up until 2 weeks ago. The patient denies any tick bites, recent camping or hiking trips, or exposure to wooded areas. She has never been hospitalized other than for giving birth to her two sons (7 y/o and 11 y/o). She is presently not taking medications, except for ibuprofen for muscle aches and pains. Her family history is noncontributory.

PHYSICAL: The patient is an alert and oriented, well-developed, non-obese female, appearing stated age, uncomfortable but in no acute distress. The patient is **febrile.** Temp: 101.3° F; HR: 85; RR: 18; BP: 125/85. HEENT: erythematous maculopapular rash on the nasal bridge and cheeks, sparing the nasolabial folds (**butterfly rash** or **malar rash**); two oral/pharyngeal ulcers, 0.5 cm in diameter, painless to touch. Ext: well perfused; no cyanosis, clubbing, or edema; minor joint stiffness; no nodules, telangiectasias, or rashes noted.

DIFFERENTIAL: Rheumatoid arthritis, Lyme disease, dermatomyositis, polymyositis, scleroderma, systemic lupus erythematosus (SLE), drug-induced lupus.

DIAGNOSTIC: Liver function test WNL. UA: **3+ protein, RBCs,** and **cellular casts.** Serum creatine kinase WNL. Serology: (+) antinuclear antibodies; (+) anti-ds DNA antibodies; (+) anti Smith (Sm) antigen antibodies; (−) anti-SCL-70 antibodies; (−) anticentromere antibodies; (−) antihistone antibody; (−) rheumatoid factor; (−) ELISA for *Borrelia burgdorferi* antibodies; decreased C3 and C4 complement levels.

DIAGNOSIS: Systemic lupus erythematosus.

ASSESSMENT/PLAN: 37 y/o African-American woman with a 2-week history of fever, muscle aches, fatigue, joint pain and stiffness, and a 3-day history of a photosensitive malar rash. Positive lab findings of serum antinuclear antibodies, anti-ds DNA antibodies, anti Sm antigen antibodies, decreased C3 and C4 levels, and a urinalysis positive for 3+ protein, RBCs and cellular casts are findings indicative of SLE. Daily doses of **hydroxychloroquine** (antimalarial) for SLE's skin and joint manifestations, oral **glucocorticoid** treatment for suppression of active SLE, and **nonsteroidal anti-inflammatory drugs** for muscle arthralgias are recommended. Renal biopsy is indicated for assessment of lupus nephritis. If the nephritis is of the **diffuse proliferative** type, consider monthly treatments of a cytotoxic agent such as **cyclophosphamide** to prevent progression to renal failure. The patient should also be advised to avoid exposure to sunlight and to use a **sunscreen**(SPF **D 15).**

  Systemic lupus erythematosus (SLE): SLE is the diagnosis because of the symptoms of generalized fatigue, arthralgias, fever, and photosensitive malar rash. Laboratory supportive findings include **positive ANA, ds-DNA, Sm antigen,** and **decreased C3** and **C4 complement levels.** The 3+ urine protein with RBCs and cell casts is suggestive of lupus nephritis.

Rheumatoid arthritis: This diagnosis is unlikely because of the lack of serum rheumatoid factor. Rheumatoid arthritis does not demonstrate a facial rash or involve the kidneys.

Scleroderma: This diagnosis is unlikely because there is no evidence of serum **anti SCL-70** or **anticentromere antibodies.** In addition, there is no history of subcutaneous calcifications (**calcinosis**), vasomotor instability (Raynaud's phenomenon), esophageal dysmotility, sclerodactyly, or telangiectasias. The constellation of these findings is consistent with a subset of scleroderma called CREST.

Lyme disease: The diagnosis is not likely to be Lyme disease, because there is no history of a **tick bite** or **erythema chronicum migrans** rash. Furthermore, the patient had a negative ELISA test result for *B. burgdorferi*.

Dermatomyositis or polymyositis: Although there is muscle pain and arthralgias, there was no history of any **proximal muscle weakness** or increased levels of serum creatine kinase.

Drug-induced lupus: This diagnosis is unlikely because the patient's serology is negative for antihistone antibodies and the patient is not on any medications that are known to cause lupus, such as **hydralazine, procainamide, isoniazid, chlorpromazine, methyldopa, quinidine, ethosuximide,** or D-**penicillamine.** Also, drug-induced lupus generally spares the kidneys.

CASE 15 CC: "I can't seem to beat this cold."

HISTORY: A 22 y/o **female** African-American law student presents with a 5-day history of fever, **night sweats,** cough, and **pruritus.** She stated that about 4 months ago she came in for a cold, because she had a cough, runny nose, and **swollen lymph nodes.** She was diagnosed with a viral illness and sent home. The runny nose resolved, but the cough and **lymphadenopathy** continued. She also thinks that she might have **lost some weight** because her clothes feel looser. She has noticed that in the past couple of days that her face appears to be a little "puffy." She is wondering if this is still the same cold or if something else is going on. She is currently on no medications except pseudoephedrine for a supposed URI. Her past medical and family history are noncontributory.

PHYSICAL: Temp: 100.4 F; HR: 77; RR: 20;Wt: 103 lb (last visit 115 lb). HEENT: Face demonstrates increased fullness; conjunctiva are noninjected; nose has no exudate; mouth/pharynx is nonerythematous and without lesions. Neck: supple, **(+) lymphadenopathy** with a right-sided supraclavicular lymph node, firm, mobile, approximately 2 cm in diameter; (+) jugular venous distention. Lungs: slight expiratory wheeze on the right. Heart: RRR. The rest of the physical exam is WNL.

DIFFERENTIAL: Toxoplasmosis, histoplasmosis, tuberculosis, non-Hodgkin's lymphoma, Hodgkin's lymphoma, sarcoidosis, infectious mononucleosis, bacterial/viral pharyngitis.

DIAGNOSTICS: CBC: **leukocytosis** with **increased PMNs** and lymphopenia; no atypical lymphocytes seen on the blood smear; heterophilic antibody test: negative; PPD: negative; HIV: negative; **increase in serum leukocyte alkaline phosphatase** and in erythrocyte sedimentation rate; indirect fluorescent serum antibody for toxoplasmosis: negative. CXR: 5 cm **mediastinal mass** with no other hilar lymphadenopathy. Biopsy of a cervical lymph node: lymphoid cells in nodules separated by bands of collagen; occasional binucleate cells with darkly staining nucleoli (**Reed-Sternberg cell**) (see Figure); no granuloma. No acid fast bacteria are seen. No fungi are seen on a silver stain. The lymph node fungal culture for histoplasmosis is negative.

DIAGNOSIS: Hodgkin's lymphoma (nodular sclerosing type).

ASSESSMENT/PLAN: 22 y/o African-American woman presenting with a 5-day history of fever, **night sweats,** increased facial fullness, pruritus, and a 4-month history of cough and lymphadenopathy. The CXR is positive for a mediastinal mass. The lymph node biopsy is positive for lymphoid nodules separated by collagen bands with Reed-Sternberg cells. Start the patient on a protocol for radiation therapy.

Hodgkin's lymphoma (nodular sclerosis type): The diagnosis is most likely Hodgkin's lymphoma due to the appearance of Reed-Sternberg cells on tissue biopsy and nodular sclerosing type due to the appearance of lymphoid nodules separated by collagen bands. Fever, night sweats, pruritus, and unexplained weight loss of at least 10% over a period of 6 months are symptoms associated with lymphoma. Facial fullness can be caused by the **superior vena cava syndrome,** where the mass compresses the SVC and obstructs the venous return from the upper extremities and the head. Wheezing can be caused by tracheal/bronchial obstruction by the mediastinal mass. Of the four types of Hodgkin's lymphoma (lymphocyte predominant, mixed cellu-

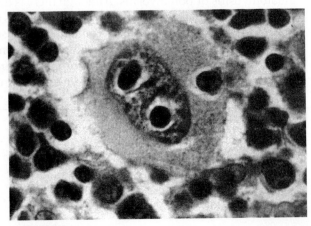

CASE 15 Classic Reed-Sternberg cell in Hodgkin's disease.

larity, nodular sclerosing, and lymphocyte depleted), the **nodular sclerosing type** is the most common type that occurs in women.

Toxoplasmosis: The patient has no evidence of being immunosuppressed because she is not taking steroids and her HIV test result is negative. Furthermore, the diagnosis is not likely to be toxoplasmosis, because of the negative result on the fluorescent antibody test.

Sarcoidosis: Although the clinical picture is similar to that of sarcoidosis, as the patient is a young, black woman with lymphadenopathy and an abnormal CXR, this diagnosis is unlikely because of the lack of **noncaseating epithelioid granulomas** in the tissue biopsy. Generally, with sarcoidosis, there is a leukopenia instead of leukocytosis.

Histoplasmosis: This diagnosis is generally associated with patients who are in an immunocompromised state. Although the patient did have respiratory complaints, there was only a single lesion seen on the CXR (vs. multiple lesions with calcifications found in histoplasmosis), there was no growth on the fungal culture, and no fungal forms were seen on the lymph node biopsy with the **silver stain.**

Tuberculosis (TB): Although the patient is experiencing night sweats, low-grade fever, weight loss, and cough, her cough is nonproductive and she has no hemoptysis. In addition, she reports no known exposure to TB or immunocompromised individuals. This diagnosis is ruled out by a negative PPD in a person without HIV.

Infectious mononucleosis: This disease is usually caused by the Epstein-Barr virus and is common in the college-aged population. It is characterized by symptoms of lymphadenopathy, fatigue, fever, and splenomegaly. Although this patient had lymphadenopathy, fatigue, and a low-grade fever, she did not have **splenomegaly.** This diagnosis is unlikely, because there were no **atypical lymphocytes** seen on the blood smear and the heterophilic antibody test result (Monospot test) was negative.

Viral or bacterial pharyngitis: This diagnosis is unlikely, because the patient did not complain of a sore throat during the course of her illness. In addition, on physical exam, there was no erythema, exudate, or lesions seen on the buccal or pharyngeal mucosa. Also, these diseases do not typically last for 4 months.

CASE 16 — CC: "My back keeps hurting."

HISTORY: 35 y/o white man comes in today complaining of left back/flank pain that radiates to his groin. The pain started 5 days ago and comes and goes. It started as point flank/ back tenderness that did not radiate but now **radiates to the groin area.** The pain starts slowly and continues to increase in intensity until he cannot stand it. He states that it is the worst pain that he has ever had, for which he has been taking ibuprofen. In the past day, the pt has had some nausea and chills but has not vomited. He reports no changes in his stools and denies abdominal pain or muscle aches. He states that in the last week his **urine has been getting darker** and now looks like there is **blood** in it. The patient has no urinary urgency, pain on urination, or trouble starting or stopping the stream. The patient denies any trauma or strain to his back or abdomen and has no occupational history of lifting heavy objects. The patient has no history of urinary tract infections. He has been healthy and has had no hospitalization or treatment for a medical illness. The patient has a 65 y/o mother with **recurrent kidney stones** and a father, 68 y/o, with hypertension and angina.

PHYSICAL: The patient is alert and oriented but distressed and clutching his left flank. Temp: 102.2 F; HR: 97; RR: 16; BP: 139/87. Patient has tenderness on his left flank/**costovertebral angle** but no abdominal masses or rebound tenderness. The genitourinary exam is normal. The rest of the examination is WNL.

DIFFERENTIAL: Appendicitis, cholecystitis, peptic ulcer, nephrolithiasis, pancreatitis, pyelonephritis, chronic pyelonephritis.

(continued)

AT THE BEDSIDE

CASE 16 | **CC: "My back keeps hurting."** (Continued)

DIAGNOSTICS: CBC: WNL, amylase: WNL, lipase: WNL, uric acid: WNL, **Ca: WNL, PTH: WNL.** Urinalysis: (+) RBCs, (+) WBCs, Gram stain shows no organisms, **increased urine calcium,** urine pH 6.0 (WNL). **AXR:** two **radiopaque objects** on the patient's left flank—one in the kidney parenchyma and one two thirds of the way down the ureter. Renal ultrasound: swollen left kidney.

DIAGNOSIS: Nephrolithiasis: Calcium phosphate stone from idiopathic hypercalciuria.

ASSESSMENT/PLAN: 35 y/o white man with a 5-day history of severe colicky left back and flank pain that radiates to the groin, hematuria, hypercalciuria, and positive findings of radiopaque kidney stones on abdominal radiographs, with no increase in serum PTH. The patient is beginning to pass stones. Treat as an inpatient with **morphine for pain** and observe the patient for passage of stones. If stones obstruct, consider treating with extracorporeal shock-wave lithotripsy. Treat idiopathic hypercalciuria nephrolithiasis with thiazide diuretics to lower urine calcium levels and decrease a recurrence.

Nephrolithiasis: The constellation of symptoms and signs, as well as radiopaque stones, hematuria, and increased urine calcium without an increased level of serum calcium or PTH and family history, all lead to a diagnosis of idiopathic hypercalciuria nephrolithiasis.

Appendicitis: The diagnosis is most likely not appendicitis because of the location and quality of the pain. Pain from appendicitis usually starts periumbilically and then moves to the lower right quadrant. One would also expect to see an increased level of WBCs in blood, and one would expect to find tenderness at **McBurney's point,** with rebound tenderness.

Cholecystitis: This diagnosis is not likely because the location of the colicky abdominal pain due to gallstones is usually in the upper right quadrant and is exacerbated by eating fatty foods.

Peptic ulcer disease (PUD): This diagnosis is unlikely because the location and quality of PUD pain are epigastric or low thoracic. Pain from an ulcer is generally a **gnawing,** burning pain that is relieved by food, milk, or antacid.

Pancreatitis: Pancreatitis is generally associated with severe **abdominal pain that radiates to the back.** The pain generally reaches maximal strength within minutes, instead of hours (as in this patient). **Serum amylase** would be elevated in a patient with pancreatitis early in the presentation of the disease.

Pyelonephritis/chronic pyelonephritis: This diagnosis is unlikely, because no organisms were seen on a urine Gram stain, and there was no previous history of UTIs. UTIs are infrequent in males beyond infancy. A male with a history of recurrent UTIs should be evaluated for anatomic abnormalities of the urinary tract.

CASE 17 | **CC: "My son has stopped walking."**

HISTORY: A mother brings her fussy and inconsolable 15 m/o **African-American** male infant to her primary care physician with a 1-day h/o of refusal to walk. One week earlier, the patient developed a URI that persisted until 3 days ago when he developed a fever and diarrhea. The diarrhea lasted for 2 days and has remitted since then. The patient has no recent history of trauma but has had a decrease in appetite. The mother denies that the infant has been vomiting or the appearance of any rashes or a change in the amount or smell of her child's urine. The patient is the product of a full-term, spontaneous vaginal delivery with no complications. The child has been healthy until this time. He has reached all of the appropriate landmarks (e.g., started to walk by 12 months). The family history is significant for a father with sickle cell disease and a mother with the sickle trait. He also has a healthy 8 y/o brother.

PHYSICAL: Temp: 101.3°; HR: 85; RR: 25; Ht: 60 percentile; Wt: 50 percentile. General: Alert, fussy, and **inconsolable** 15 m/o African-American male infant. HEENT: Conjunctiva are non-injected. Nares: no mucus or erythema. Mouth: tacky mucous membranes but no erythema or exudate. Neck: no lymphadenopathy. Lungs: CTA bilaterally, no wheezes, crackles, or rhonchi. Heart: RRR, no murmurs, rubs, or gallops. Abd: (+) bowel sounds, (+) **splenomegaly,** no hepatomegaly, non-tender, non-distended. Ext: feet and hands **tender,** bilateral swelling, no rash, no clubbing or cyanosis, no point tenderness could be elicited.

DIFFERENTIAL: Osteomyelitis; juvenile rheumatoid arthritis; sickle cell disease, trauma.

DIAGNOSTICS: CBC: **Hemoglobin and hematocrit low** with WBC **elevated.** Blood smear: **sickle cells** (see Figure), **poikilocytes,** and **target cells.** Hemoglobin electrophoresis: **hemoglobin S** (substituted valine for glutamine at position 6 on the beta chain). X-ray of extremities: no fractures. Blood culture: no growth. Radionucleotide scans with technetium phosphate: negative. Rheumatoid factor: negative. Antinuclear antibodies: negative.

DIAGNOSIS: Sickle cell disease—hand-foot syndrome.

ASSESSMENT/PLAN: 15 m/o African-American male infant in sickle cell **pain crisis** precipitated by URI with dehydration. Aggressively treat dehydration to prevent further sickling, and treat pain with narcotics. Immunization status should be confirmed, and polyvalent **pneumococcal vaccine** should be given. Consider prophylactic treatment daily doses of penicillin G to prevent pneumococcal infections. **Hydroxyurea,** a chemotherapeutic agent that increases **HbF,** should also be considered

Sickle cell disease: Dehydration can precipitate increased deoxygenation of blood, especially in the extremities. Initial pain crises, in children, frequently occur in the extremities, but later episodes can occur in other parts of the body. This pain in the extremities is called the hand-foot syndrome. The spleen is enlarged early in sickle cell disease but eventually becomes small due to multiple infarcts (**autosplenectomy**) by 2 to 5 years of age. Pain crisis can present in a number of forms. The **acute chest syndrome** (an emergency situation) is a pulmonary infarction causing decreased oxygenation of blood and promoting further sickling. Sickle cell patients can suffer cerebral vascular accidents, ischemic damage to the liver and kidneys, and **cholecystitis.** Children with sickle cell anemia are also at increased risk for encapsulated bacterial infections such as *S. pneumoniae* and *H. influenzae* because of splenic dysfunction. Sickle patients are also at risk **for aplastic anemia caused by parvovirus B-19** and **osteomyelitis due to salmonella.** Acute **splenic sequestration** occurs in infants with sickle cell anemia, in which large amounts of RBCs and platelets are pooled in the spleen, causing severe anemia and thrombocytopenia. Approximately 10% of African-Americans are heterozygous (positive) for the sickle trait.

Osteomyelitis: This diagnosis is unlikely as blood culture results were negative. *Staphylococcus aureus* is the most common cause of osteomyelitis. X-rays are usually not helpful or diagnostic until 7 to 10 days after symptoms. Bone scans are usually diagnostic within 24 hours of symptoms, but in this patient the results are negative. It would be unlikely that bone infections would simultaneously strike both hands and feet.

Juvenile rheumatoid arthritis: **Rheumatoid factor** is frequently negative in these patients and is diagnostically insignificant when negative. Antinuclear antibodies are frequently positive in systemic juvenile rheumatoid arthritis (JRA), but they are negative in this patient. There was also no salmon-colored morbilliform rash that preceded the pain, as in systemic JRA. JRA would present as a progressive disorder and not acutely, as in this patient.

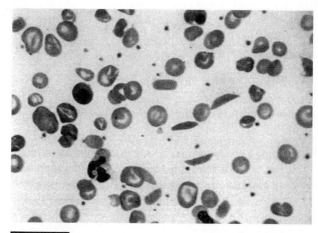

CASE 17 Sickle cell anemia shown on peripheral blood smear

CASE 18 **CC: "I can't feel my left arm and leg."**

HISTORY: A 55 y/o man states that he awoke from sleep early this morning and was unable to move his right arm and leg and has **lost "all feeling" on the right side.** The weakness has not progressed. He reports normal sensation and movement on the left. He also states that he has had some difficulty swallowing (dysphagia). He has had several episodes of weakness on his right side in the past month, but the episodes resolved after a few minutes. He denies difficulty speaking (dysarthria), weakness in his face, dizziness (vertigo), blurry vision, double vision (diplopia), spots in his eyes where he cannot see (scotomas), nausea, vomiting, urinary incontinence, tremors of the hands or feet, fever, chills, or cough. PMH is significant for **type II DM, HTN,** and **hypercholesterolemia.** He has a **35 pack year smoking history,** denies alcohol or IVDU. He takes glyburide and thiazide diuretics and has been **noncompliant** with his diet.

PHYSICAL: Overweight man who appears anxious. Temp: 98.6°F, HR: 90, RR: 14, BP: 160/100. HEENT: PERRLA, EOMI, (−) nystagmus, (−) lid droop, (−) horizontal/vertical conjugate gaze. Neck: supple, (−) Brudzinski's sign, (−) lymphadenopathy; (−) Lhermitte's sign. Lungs: CTA B/L. Heart: RRR, normal S1, S2 (−) m/r/g. Ext: (−)c/c/e, (−) Kernig's sign. Neuro: AA Ox3, CN II-XII intact. Muscle strength: left (arm: 5/5, leg: 5/5), right (arm: 1/5, leg: 1/5). Muscle tone: **spastic right arm and leg,** (−) muscle atrophy or fasiculations. Sensation: left arm and leg are normal to pinprick, vibration, and light touch; right arm and leg have decreased sensation to pinprick, vibration, and light touch. DTR: right side (**hyperreflexic 4+**), left side (normal 2+). Babinski's sign: **upgoing (+) on the right,** downgoing (−) on the left. Cerebellar signs: finger to nose test is slow but adequate, (−) cogwheel rigidity.

DIFFERENTIAL: Transient ischemic attack (TIA); thrombotic cerebrovascular accident CVA; embolic CVA; cerebral neoplasm; multiple sclerosis (MS); subdural hematoma; meningitis.

DIAGNOSTICS: Electrolytes: WNL. BUN/Cr: WNL. Serum glucose: mildly elevated. CBC: WNL. UA: WNL. PT/PTT: WNL. Lipid panel: TG elevated. ECG: (−) arrhythmia, (−) MI, (+) Left ventricular hypertropy (LVH). CXR: (+) mild cardiomegaly, (−) pulmonary edema, (−) aneurysms. CT of head: **hypodense area** in left cortex corresponding to cerebral infarction; (−) intracranial hemorrhage; (−) epidural/subdural hematomas; (−) masses; (−) aneurysms; (−) AV malformations. Carotid Doppler ultrasound: right common carotid is 40% stenosed, left common carotid is 50% stenosed. VDRL: nonreactive. Lumbar puncture: WNL.

DIAGNOSIS: Thrombotic CVA (stroke, brain attack).

ASSESSMENT/PLAN: 55 y/o man who presents with right hemiparesis and right hypesthesia. Thrombolytics are not helpful in this patient because they need to be administered within 3 to 4 hours of onset of the CVA. Give IV heparin, followed by warfarin after several days. Give aspirin or ticlopidine for antiplatelet effect. Treat cerebral edema, if it occurs, with mannitol and hyperventilation; do not attempt to lower the blood pressure at this point. Monitor electrolytes daily for a possible imbalance. Tube feeding may be needed if swallowing is not adequate. Prevent aspiration by elevating the head of the bed. Respiratory support may be needed. Initiate rehabilitation once the patient is stable.

Thrombotic cva (stroke, brain attack): The main symptom of this disease is the gradual onset of neurologic dysfunction, often with prior episodes of hemiplegia/hypesthesia. CT scan usually would **show only one hypodense infarcted area in the brain.**

Embolic CVA: In many cases, thrombotic CVA and embolic CVA present in a similar manner. However, the onset of symptoms with an embolic stroke is **rapid;** there are usually no previous episodes of hemiplegia. The patient is usually awake when an embolic stroke occurs. CT scan would demonstrate **multiple small hypodense areas** of infarction (see Figure 1).

TIA: This would produce the same symptoms as a CVA. However, the symptoms of a TIA **resolve within 24 hours.** The CT scan would not demonstrate infarcted areas. This patient demonstrated episodes of TIAs previously.

Cerebral neoplasm: A neoplasm impinging on the cortex could produce hemiplegia/hypesthesia, with gradually worsening symptoms. The CT scan showed no masses, and the lumbar puncture was normal (occasionally carcinomatous meningitis occurs with cerebral neoplasms).

MS: Patients with MS usually present initially with **optic neuritis.** This patient denied any visual symptoms, and the eye exam was normal. A positive Babinski and palmar grasp reflex do not usually occur in MS. **Lhermitte's sign** is not necessary to diagnose MS, but its presence is specific for it. A CT scan would show **plaques in the white matter.** This patient had a hypodense area in the left cortex, a finding that excludes MS.

Subdural hematoma: Typically, a patient with a subdural hematoma would lose consciousness immediately after trauma; then the patient would have an asymptomatic **period of lucency,** with gradual worsening of symptoms (e.g., hemiplegia/hypesthesia/dysphagia) hours later. This patient denies any trauma to the head. The symptoms would not occur several times in the past month if this patient had a subdural hematoma. A subdural hematoma would also cause alterations in consciousness or nausea/vomiting due to the increased ICP. The CT scan of the head demonstrated no evidence of subdural hematoma.

Meningitis: A patient with meningitis would have neck pain, a stiff neck, and a fever. This patient had a supple neck, a negative Brudzinski's sign, a negative Kernig's sign, and no cervical lymphadenopathy. The patient was afebrile, and the LP was normal.

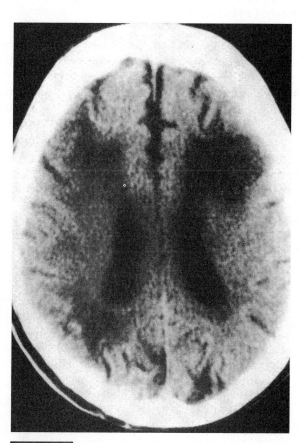

CASE 18 Magnetic resonance imaging findings in acute cerebral infarction.

CASE 19 — CC: "My son is not breathing right and turns blue."

HISTORY: A 15 m/o male infant of full-term spontaneous vaginal delivery presents with episodes of restlessness, **gasping for air, and blue lips.** The parents state that if the infant is playing hard or crying, he will subsequently get very restless, start gasping for air, assume a **squatting position,** and his lips will turn blue. After these episodes the patient will sleep for a couple of hours. The patient has previously been healthy with no recent history of rhinorrhea, nausea/vomiting, changes in appetite, stools, or urination. The infant's prenatal and neonatal history were without complication.

PHYSICAL: Temp: 99.5°F; HR: 110; RR: 35; Ht: 35th percentile; Wt: 32nd percentile. Gen: The patient is alert, breathing rapidly, and demonstrating air hunger. HEENT: Mucous membranes: moist and **cyanotic.** Neck: (−) without lymphadenopathy. Lungs: CTA bilaterally, without wheezes, rhonchi, or crackles.

(continued)

CASE 19 CC: "My son is not breathing right and turns blue." (Continued)

Heart: RRR, **systolic ejection murmur 4/6,** systolic **thrill** at the left sternal border. Ext: (+) **clubbing and cyanosis,** (−) edema or tenting.

DIFFERENTIAL: Cyanotic congenital heart disease (transposition of great vessels, truncus arteriosus, tricuspid atresia, total anomalous pulmonary return, tetralogy of Fallot).

DIAGNOSTICS: CBC: **increased hematocrit** (polycythemia). CXR: lungs clear; left heart border shows concavity in the area of the pulmonary artery, a narrow base, and rounded apical shadow above the diaphragm (boot-shaped heart, see Figure). ECG: right axis deviation and right ventricular hypertrophy. Echocardiography: **ventricular septal defect, pulmonary stenosis, right ventricular hypertrophy,** and an **overriding aorta** that is located above the right and left ventricles.

DIAGNOSIS: Tetralogy of Fallot.

ASSESSMENT/PLAN: 15 m/o male infant with a cyanotic congenital heart disease causing episodes of cyanosis and dyspnea. Prevention of dehydration to avoid hemoconcentration and subsequent thrombotic episodes; oral propranolol has been shown to decrease cyanotic episodes; iron supplements treat the relative iron deficiency; corrective surgery is necessary.

Tetralogy of Fallot: This is the most likely diagnosis because the patient demonstrated episodes of cyanosis due to increased cardiac demand from a heart that was already working at its maximum ability. Once the demand was greater than the supply, the child became cyanotic. It is typical for children to take a squatting stance to help relieve some of the demand on the overworked heart. The defects in tetralogy of Fallot cause cyanosis via a right to left shunt. In a neonate with severe pulmonary stenosis, cyanosis will be seen in the first hours or days of life when the ductus arteriosus begins to close. In these patients, immediate prostaglandin E_1 (alprostidil) treatment is necessary to maintain a patent ductus arteriosus.

Other congenital heart anomalies (VSD, ASD, and PDA): These defects do not cause cyanosis in an infant but rather result in a left to right shunt. The increased pressure and flow seen by the pulmonary system, due to the left to right shunt, lead to pulmonary hypertension. However, pulmonary hypertension usually does not develop until later in life. The increase in pulmonary resistance over time causes a reversal in the shunt. This reversal of flow is called **Eisenmenger's complex.** A PDA can be closed by use of indomethacin therapy.

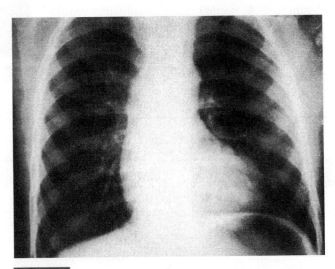

CASE 19 Tetralogy of Fallot.

CASE 20 CC: "My stomach hurts."

HISTORY: A 65 y/o man complains of stomach pains in the epigastric region that come and go throughout the day. He describes the pain as a **burning, gnawing** sensation. The pain started about 2 months ago as "discomfort" **after meals** that was relieved by **antacids.** The patient states that he thought it was indigestion and ignored it. In the past 4 days, the pain has worsened and is more constant. The pain is consistently in the same location; it does not radiate and is accompanied by no nausea, vomiting, or diarrhea. It is constant and accentuated by meals. The patient states that he is still using antacids, but lately they have not seemed to work as well. He has no other complaints. The patient has a history of rheumatoid arthritis and is currently being treated with **nonsteroidal anti-inflammatory drugs.** The past medical history and family history are noncontributory.

PHYSICAL: The patient is alert and oriented, appears the stated age, and is in no acute distress. Temp: 98.6°F; HR: 80; RR: 14; BP: 130/80. HEENT: WNL. Lungs: CTA, no wheezes, rhonchi, or crackles. Heart: RRR with no murmurs, rubs, or gallops. Abd: (+) bowel sounds, no hepatosplenomegaly, no masses, (+) **tenderness in the epigastric region** with **guarding.** Ext: WNL. Cranial nerves II to XII intact.

DIFFERENTIAL: Ménétrier's disease; gastrinoma (Zollinger-Ellison syndrome); gastric carcinoma; peptic ulcer (gastric or duodenal); Curling's or Cushing's ulcer.

DIAGNOSTICS: Endoscopy: reveals a **1-cm crater** with **sharply demarcated** margins; the crater base is covered by a gray-white exudate (see Figure); there is an area of hyperemia and edema directly around the ulcer; other gastric tissue appears normal. Cytology of crater tissue shows no signs of malignant transformation or that the ulcer has breached the muscularis mucosa. Culture from the crater area is (+) for urease positive gram-negative curved rods (i.e., *Helicobacter pylori*). X-ray studies with barium reveal gastric "**color button lesion**" in the lesser curvature of the gastric mucosa. Basal acid secretion rate: WNL. Serum gastrin: WNL.

DIAGNOSIS: Gastric ulcer.

ASSESSMENT/PLAN: A 65 y/o man with a gastric ulcer and no malignant transformation. Gastric mucosa is positive for *H. pylori.* Start the patient on a regimen of H_2 receptor blockers, misoprostol (PGE_1 analogue), and amoxicillin.

Gastric ulcers: Gastric ulcers occur most commonly along the lesser curvature of the stomach and often present with pain that increases with meals. On the other hand, duodenal ulcer pain is usually relieved by meals because of prandial bicarbonate secretion from the pancreas. *H. pylori* is associated with 70% of gastric ulcers and >90% of duodenal ulcers. The organism's production of **urease** damages the mucosa and predisposes it to injury.

Gastric cancer: Even though gastric cancers can present with epigastric pain, the ulcer borders would not be sharp and well demarcated. Cytology showed no signs of malignant change. Risk factors for gastric cancer include ethanol consumption, tobacco use, foods high in nitrates (e.g., smoked fish), and blood type A.

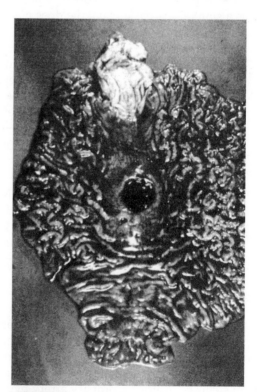

(continued) **CASE 20** Gastric ulcer.

CASE 20   CC: "My stomach hurts." (Continued)

Gastrinoma (Zollinger-Ellison syndrome): This is an unlikely diagnosis because patients with gastrinomas generally have **increased basal acid secretion,** large edematous gastric and duodenal folds, and increased levels of serum gastrin. Ulcers in patients with gastrinomas are generally duodenal (post bulbar) and not gastric.

Ménétrier's syndrome (hypertrophic gastritis): This disease is characterized by mucosal hypertrophy, excess mucus production, hypoproteinemia, and hypochlorhydria. Even though this syndrome can present with epigastric pain, on endoscopy the patient's rugae would be larger and increased in thickness.

Curling's or Cushing's ulcer: Curling's ulcers present in patients that are in severe shock, seriously **burned,** or following trauma. Cushing's ulcers present in patients that have **increased intracranial pressure** from surgery or trauma.

CASE 21   CC: "My chest really hurts."

HISTORY: A 52 y/o man presents to the ER c/o chest pain. The pt describes the chest pain as a **substernal tightness,** as if "a 300-lb weight was lying" on his chest. The pain **radiates to his left shoulder and arm;** its **intensity** is 9/10; and it lasts for less than **5 minutes.** The pain occurs **with exertion,** and it is **relieved by rest.** The patient has had this pain several times in the past; recently, it occurred with less exertion. He denies sweating, nausea, vomiting, pain with inspiration, pain while lying on his back, dysphagia, regurgitation of food, or dyspnea. He has no orthopnea or PND. The pain is not altered by changes in body position; it is not reduced when he leans forward. Also, the pain is not aggravated after meals. He is a **smoker** (54 pack-years); he does not drink or use IV drugs. The patient has a history of **type II DM** and **HTN.**

PHYSICAL: The patient is an **overweight** man in severe, acute pain. Temp: 98.6°F; HR: 80; RR: 12; BP: **150/90** (both arms). Neck: (−) JVD, (−) hepatojugular reflux. Lungs: CTA B/L, (−) crackles, wheezing, or rhonchi. Heart: RRR, normal S1 and S2, **(+) S4,** (−) murmurs. Abd: (+) BS, (−) hepatosplenomegaly. Ext: (−) cyanosis, clubbing, or edema; symmetric pulses B/L upper and lower.

DIFFERENTIAL: Angina pectoris; MI; aortic dissection; GERD; pneumonia; pulmonary embolus; pericarditis.

DIAGNOSTICS: Electrolytes normal. BUN/Cr normal. Total cholesterol elevated. Serum LDL elevated. ABG: normal O_2, normal CO_2, normal pH. ECG: sinus rhythm, normal axis, **ST segment depression, left ventricular hypertrophy.** Cardiac panel: CK-MB normal, cardiac troponin I normal. CXR: (−) infiltrates, pulmonary edema, or atelectasis; (−) blunting of costovertebral angle or widening of the mediastinum.

DIAGNOSIS: Stable angina pectoris.

ASSESSMENT/PLAN: 52 y/o white man with angina. Sublingual **nitroglycerine** should be given for the chest pain, and β-blockers or calcium channel blockers are also indicated. β-blockers are preferred (even though they may mask hypoglycemia) because they have been shown to increase life expectancy after an MI. Administer aspirin for its antithrombotic effect. A thallium stress test will help determine at what level of exercise ischemia occurs. Coronary **angiography** may be needed to determine the number and degree of stenosed arteries. Coronary artery bypass graft (CABG) is a possibility, as is percutaneous transluminal coronary angioplasty (PTCA) or stent placement. The patient should be advised to eliminate smoking, control HTN, begin exercise, control his diabetes, and reduce cholesterol level through either diet or medication (simvistatin, lovastatin). Long-term complications include stroke, MI, or CHF.

Pneumonia: Pleuritis due to pneumonia may result in chest pain. **Pleuritic pain** typically occurs **during inspiration.** This patient was afebrile, and there was no evidence of pleuritic pain. CXR showed no pulmonary infiltrates. The physical exam did not reveal **crackles or harsh breath sounds.**

Pulmonary embolus: Patients with pulmonary emboli present with **pleuritic chest pain, tachypnea, tachycardia,** and **hypoxemia.** This patient's pain was not pleuritic. He did not have tachycardia or tachypnea. ABGs showed normal blood O_2 levels. Also, the pain would have been acute, and it would not have been relieved by rest.

Pericarditis: Pain due to pericarditis can have both **pleuritic and steady components.** However, pericarditis is discovered by the **presence of a friction rub.** This patient had no friction rub. Also, pericarditis does not cause ST segment depression on an ECG.

MI: MI causes substernal tightness, which can radiate to the right shoulder. The pain is very intense, and it can be precipitated by exertion. However, the **pain lasts for more than 30 seconds and it is not relieved by rest.** The ECG changes for an MI are **ST segment elevation** and the **presence of Q waves.** Also, **cardiac troponin I, the CK-MB fraction,** and **the total CK** are **elevated** during an MI (see Figure). These lab tests were all normal in this patient.

Aortic dissection: The pain from an aortic dissection is a **sharp tearing pain** that lasts for hours and is **not relieved by rest.** This patient's pain was relieved by rest, and it lasted less than 5 minutes. Also, the pulses in the extremities were normal. In aortic dissection, the **pulses in the extremities would be decreased.** This patient's CXR did not show a **widened mediastinum,** which is characteristic of aortic dissection.

GERD: GERD causes an epigastric/substernal **burning sensation** that is worse in the morning and when the patient is **lying flat.** Also, the pain is relieved by antacids or food. This patient's pain was not relieved by these, nor was the pain altered by a change in body position.

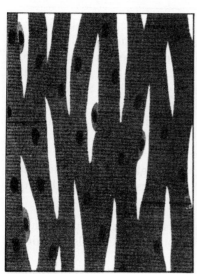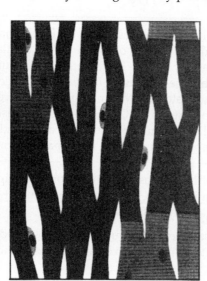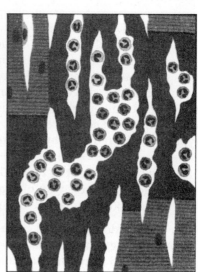

Normal   12–18 hours   1 day

CASE 21 Stages in the development of a myocardial infarction.

CASE 22 — CC: "I've felt nauseated, and I've thrown up four times since yesterday."

HISTORY: This 19 y/o female patient has been nauseated and vomited four times in the past 2 days. She also c/o of abdominal pain that is intermittent, diffuse, and dull. She denies fever, chills, diarrhea, constipation, or trauma to the abdomen. The **vomiting** is not associated with any particular time of day, nor does it occur with meals. The abdominal pain is not relieved by vomiting. The patient has not noticed early satiety; however, she does note a **10-lb weight loss** in the past month. Also, she has been **drinking a large quantity of water lately.** She had a **cold several weeks ago** and had some **stress** due to her final exams. Her last menstrual period was 3 weeks ago. She does not smoke; she drinks on weekends and denies IVDU. She is not taking any medication.

PHYSICAL: The patient appears in acute distress. Temp: 98.4°F; HR: 70; RR: 22; BP: 90/60. HEENT: Pink conjunctiva, anicteric sclera, dry oral mucosa, nonpalpable thyroid. Neck: (−) JVD. Lungs: CTA B/L, (−) c/w/r, (+) fast, deep breaths (**Kussmaul's respiration**). Heart: RRR, normal S1, S2, (−) S3 or S4, (−) m/r/g. Abd: soft, slight tenderness to palpation, (−) rebound, (+) bowel sounds. Neuro: (−) focal deficits, (−) asterixis. Ext: (−) c/c/e.

DIFFERENTIAL: Diabetic ketoacidosis (DKA); salicylate overdose; viral gastroenteritis; bacterial gastroenteritis; peptic ulcer disease (PUD); pregnancy; uremia; alcohol intoxication; hydrocephalus.

DIAGNOSTICS: Electrolytes: increased K^+, decreased bicarbonate, anion gap 24, **glucose 500 mg/dl.** ABG: pH 7.28, BUN/Cr WNL. CBC: leukocytosis, Hgb and Hct WNL, serum **acetoacetate** high. U/A: WNL. Urine dip: (+) **ketones**, (+) **glucose.** Blood alcohol level undetectable. β-hCG: neg.

DIAGNOSIS: DKA due to new onset of type I DM.

ASSESSMENT/PLAN: A 19 y/o white woman presents to the ER c/o nausea and vomiting. The ketoacidosis will not resolve without the administration of **insulin.** Give regular human insulin until the anion gap returns to normal (hypokalemia may result). Rehydrate with IV fluids; monitor electrolytes. Leukocytosis is most likely due to DKA because there is no indication of infection. When blood glucose drops to approx 250 mg/dl, IV dextrose and water (D5W) can be given to prevent hypoglycemia. Subcutaneous insulin can be given when the acidosis resolves. Counseling for the disease should follow including information about DM, its treatment, lifestyle modification, and acute and long-term complications (**DKA, hypoglycemia, retinopathy, nephropathy, peripheral neuropathy, stroke,** and **MI**).

DKA due to new onset of type I DM: Diagnosis due to abnormally high blood **glucose** level, high **acetoacetate** level, acidosis with high anion gap, (+) urine ketones, and (+) urine glucose. Signs and symptoms include polyphagia, polydipsia, polyuria, and weight loss.

Salicylate overdose: This will cause an increased anion gap acidosis and **Kussmaul's respirations.** However, serum glucose, acetoacetate, and urine glucose and ketones would not be elevated. Also, the drug screen would be positive for salicylates.

Pregnancy: **Nausea** and **vomiting** usually occur in the **morning** in pregnant women. Normal pregnancy would not cause a metabolic acidosis. Ketoacidosis can develop during the third trimester of pregnancy if the mother fasts. However, in starvation ketoacidosis, serum and urine glucose levels are rarely greater than 300 mg/dl. The serum β-**hCG** would reveal detectable levels if she were pregnant. Diabetes can occur as a result of pregnancy (gestational diabetes), which can lead to macrosomia. Gestational diabetes usually resolves after parturition, but it can rarely persist.

Uremia: This can cause an elevated anion gap metabolic acidosis; it can also cause nausea and vomiting, which occurs early in the morning. The patient does not have signs of renal insufficiency. There is also no edema or pericarditis (detected by a pericardial friction rub), no pleural effusions (detected by dullness to percussion of the lung fields), no asterixis, and no elevation of the BUN and Cr. UA does not show **proteinuria, RBCs, hyaline casts,** or **tubular casts.** The physical exam and lab tests exclude this diagnosis for this patient.

Peptic ulcer disease (PUD): Peptic ulcer disease frequently causes nausea and vomiting, which is usually relieved after vomiting. However, PUD does not lead to metabolic acidosis, increased ketones in blood or urine, or hyperglycemia.

Viral gastroenteritis: This can cause nausea, vomiting, and diffuse abdominal pain. Systemic symptoms are also characteristic; however, she denies fever, chills, nasal congestion, sore throat, or diarrhea. Viral gastroenteritis is not a cause of ketoacidosis or hyperglycemia.

Bacterial gastroenteritis: Nausea, vomiting, and abdominal pain are symptoms. The patient has leukocytosis, but there is no left shift (which would strongly suggest infection). She is afebrile and denies diarrhea. She would also not have ketoacidosis with bacterial gastroenteritis.

Alcohol intoxication: Ethanol use can result in nausea, vomiting, abdominal pain, gastritis, and ketoacidosis. Plasma free fatty acid levels approach those of DKA. The patient has lost weight recently and she has been under stress, which can point to alcohol ingestion. However, alcoholic ketoacidosis is usually associated with **hypoglycemia.** If hyperglycemia were present, levels in the blood would not exceed 300 mg/dl. Polydipsia and polyuria occurring with a weight loss are not characteristic of alcohol abuse. Blood alcohol level was 0.

Hydrocephalus: Increased intracranial pressure results in **projectile vomiting and nausea.** Central diabetes insipidus producing polyuria and polydipsia could occur as a result of increased intracranial pressure damaging the hypothalamus. However, the neurologic exam showed no focal deficits. Also, hydrocephalus would not result in ketoacidosis with hyperglycemia.

CASE 23 — CC: "I've been coughing up blood."

HISTORY: A 75 y/o man presented to the ER c/o of a productive cough for the past 2 days. His cough had been previously productive with yellow sputum. However, in the past 24 hours he has noticed an increasing amount of **bright red blood in his sputum.** The patient also c/o nausea and vomiting, and SOB, which **began several months ago** and has become **progressively worse.** He denies chills or night sweats. There is no pleurisy, PND, orthopnea, or ankle edema. He denies peptic ulcer disease, past medical history of lupus, or renal disease. The patient states that his **appetite has recently decreased,** and he has noted a **weight loss of 10 lb in the last month.** He has a **smoking history** of 112 pack-years (2 packs/day for 56 years).

PHYSICAL: The patient is frail and cachectic. Temp: 98.6°F; HR: 95; RR: 20; BP: 150/95. Skin: (−) telangiectasia. HEENT: anicteric sclera. Lungs: decreased breath sounds, hyperresonant to percussion, (+) **end expiratory wheezing,** (−) crackles. Heart: RRR, normal S1, S2, (−) S3 or S4, (−)m/r/g. Abd: soft, nontender, (−) masses or rebound, (−) hepatosplenomegaly. Ext: (−) cyanosis or edema, (+) **clubbing** of digits.

DIFFERENTIAL: Pulmonary neoplasm; pneumonia; brochiectasis; TB; pulmonary A-V fistula; Goodpasture's syndrome; Wegener's granulomatosis; pulmonary embolism; LV failure.

DIAGNOSTICS: Electrolytes: slightly increased Ca^{2+}, slightly decreased phosphate, normal BUN and Cr. U/A and dipstick: normal. ABG: slightly decreased P_{O_2}, slightly increased P_{CO_2}. Blood alcohol level: 0. Gastric lavage: no blood in stomach. Sputum stain: (−) acid-fast bacilli. Sputum culture:(−) growth Hemoccult test: (−) blood in stool. CXR: large **central mass near the hilum** of the right lung, **enlarged hilar lymph nodes** (see Figure), (−) atelectasis, pulmonary edema or blunting of costovertebral angle. Bronchoscopy: endotracheal mass in right lung. **Bx of mass reveals squamous cell carcinoma.**

(continued)

CASE 23   CC: "I've been coughing up blood." (Continued)

DIAGNOSIS: Hemopytsis due to squamous cell cancer (SCC) of the lung.

ASSESSMENT/PLAN: The patient is a 75 y/o black man w/ PMH of 112 pack-years of smoking who presented with hemoptysis and was diagnosed with SCC of lung. Start O_2 via a nasal cannula (2 to 4 L/min), maintain O_2 sat > 90%, suppress cough with dextromethorphan or hydrocodone. Hypercalcemia and hypophosphatemia are the result of elaboration of **PTH-like substance** from the tumor. If hypercalcemia is the result of an acute elevation, use IV normal saline followed by IV furosemide. If chronic, use pamidronate and oral phosphate. Staging of SCC should be done via a CT scan. Perform PFTs to evaluate the amount of pulmonary compromise. Treat the SCC with either surgery or radiation therapy. Smoking cessation is a necessity.

Hemoptysis due to SCC: This is the most likely diagnosis given the long history of smoking, weight loss, lack of fever, the CXR showing the hilar mass, and the confirmatory Bx.

Pneumonia: Hemoptysis and cough are symptoms of pneumonia. However, the progressive nature, lack of **fever, crackles, harsh breath sounds,** or **consolidation** on the CXR rule this out.

Bronchiectasis: This would result in massive hemoptysis. The patient's history of smoking can also contribute to this disease. However, the pulmonary exam usually demonstrates **dry crackles, no end-expiratory wheezing** or decreased breath sounds. CXR in bronchietasis would show **diffuse parenchymal changes without a hilar mass.**

Tuberculosis: Hemoptysis, weight loss, and a chronic cough are symptoms of TB. However, sputum Gram stain and culture were negative for acid-fast bacilli. Also TB does not usually present with an endotracheal mass.

Pulmonary arteriovenous fistula: Hemoptysis is the primary symptom; however, progressive dyspnea and a non-bloody productive cough that suddenly changes to a bloody cough are not characteristic features.

Goodpasture's syndrome: Patients with this disease have **lung disease and renal complications.** This patient denied hematuria, and his UA and dipstick were normal.

Wegener's granulomatosis: This disease presents with lung and renal complications. There is often a **rash** or evidence of vascular complications such as GI symptoms or arthritis.

Pulmonary embolism: The hemoptysis and dyspnea could indicate a massive PE, but the patient is not **severely hypoxic,** there is no pleurisy and no tachycardia. PE is characterized by acute rather than progressive dyspnea.

Left ventricular (LV) failure: Massive LV failure could produce hemoptysis; however, there is no **S3** sound, no crackles, no hepatomegaly, no edema, or JVD. The CXR does not show cardiomegaly.

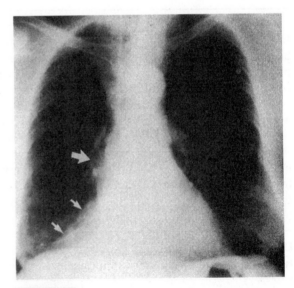

CASE 23 Tracheal carinal involvement in squamous cell carcinoma.

CASE 24 CC: "I can't fit into my shoes because my legs are so swollen."

HISTORY: This 65 y/o woman states that she has had **ankle swelling** for many months. Lately, the swelling has increased; it previously only involved her ankles, but now both of her legs are swollen. The swelling used to occur only at night, but more recently the swelling occurs during the day as well. There is no pain associated with the swelling. The patient states that she has had trouble breathing during the past week. This dyspnea especially occurs when she walks to the store (**dyspnea on exertion**) or when she lies down (**orthopnea**). She also wakes up in the middle of the night and has trouble catching her breath (**PND**). She has a history of **HTN** for which she takes propranolol. She states that she has been missing doses of her medication and **hasn't been compliant** with her low-salt diet. She denies fever, chills, nausea, vomiting, or urinary symptoms. She **smoked** 1 pack of cigarettes/day for 20 years but quit 25 years ago. She drinks alcohol occasionally and denies IVDU.

PHYSICAL: The patient appears her stated age and is in no apparent distress. Temp: 98.6°F; HR: 90; RR: 16; BP: 160/100. HEENT: anicteric sclera, pink conjunctiva, (−) periorbital edema. Neck: (+) **JVD**, (+) **HJR**, nonpalpable thyroid. Lungs: **bilateral crackles, dullness to percussion,** and **decreased breath sounds** at the bases, (−) rhonchi. Heart: tachycardia, normal S1, S2, (+) **S3, S4;** (−) murmurs or heaves, PMI displaced laterally to the 5th interspace at the anterior axillary line. Abd: soft, nontender, (+) BS, (−) rebound, (+) **hepatomegaly,** (+) **pulsatile liver** (right heart failure), (+) **bruit over liver** (right heart failure), (−) caput medusa, (−) spider angiomas. Ext: 3+ pitting edema, (−) cyanosis or clubbing, (−) calf tenderness or cords. Neuro: CN II-XII intact, no focal deficits, normal reflexes.

DIFFERENTIAL: Nephrotic syndrome; cirrhosis; congestive heart failure; myxedema; thrombophlebitis; acute glomerulonephritis.

DIAGNOSTICS: Electrolytes: WNL. BUN/Cr: WNL. Urine dip and U/A: (−) proteinuria, casts, RBCs, and WBCs. CBC: WNL. LFTs: normal serum bilirubin, normal albumin, normal alkaline phosphatase, normal AST and ALT. Thyroid function tests: normal TSH, T4, T3U. ABG: slightly decreased PO_2, slightly increased PCO_2, normal pH. CXR: cardiomegaly, cephalization of pulmonary blood flow, blunting of CVA B/L, pleural effusions B/L, B/L pulmonary edema. ECG: (+) sinus tachycardia, (−) ST segment changes, (−) T wave changes, (+) **LV hypertrophy,** (−) Q waves. Echocardiogram: **enlargement of all 4 chambers, no valvular abnormalities, ejection fraction (EF) 25%.**

DIAGNOSIS: Peripheral edema due to CHF.

ASSESSMENT/PLAN: A 65 y/o white woman presents to the office c/o peripheral edema, orthopnea, and DOE. Treat the pulmonary edema with oxygen via nasal cannula or mask to maintain the O_2 saturation over 90%. Give IV **furosemide** (loop diuretic) to cause an immediate diuresis that will clear the pulmonary edema. IV morphine can be given to reduce adrenergic vasoconstriction, IV sodium nitroprusside to reduce the after load, and IV digoxin to improve cardiac contractility. Once the patient has stabilized, an ACE inhibitor or β-blocker should be prescribed because they have been shown to decrease the morbidity and mortality of CHF. The patient's HTN should be diligently controlled to prevent further progression of the CHF.

Peripheral edema due to CHF: This is the most likely diagnosis because of the constellation of pitting edema in the extremities, along with pulmonary edema, JVD, HJR, S3 and S4 heart sounds, the displaced PMI, HTN, and the LV hypertrophy evident on the ECG.

Nephrotic syndrome: This can produce **peripheral edema, proteinuria, hypercholesterolemia,** and **hypoalbuminemia.** This patient had a normal UA and urine dipstick (which tends to rule out renal disease). Serum albumin levels were normal, and BUN and creatinine were not elevated as is consistent with renal disease.

(continued)

CASE 24   CC: "I can't fit into my shoes because my legs are so swollen." (Continued)

Acute glomerulonephritis (acute GN): This is characterized by **HTN, hematuria,** proteinuria, and edema. However, **cardiac output is normal** in acute GN. This patient has edema and HTN, but not the proteinuria and hematuria. Further, cardiac output was decreased as evidenced by the pulmonary edema, hepatomegaly, JVD, and S3 heart sound.

Cirrhosis: This disease can produce hepatomegaly, edema, and hypoalbuminemia. However, JVD, crackles, HJR, and the S3 heart sound are not present in this condition. LFTs were normal in this patient (they would be abnormal in cirrhosis). A patient with cirrhosis would not have a CXR, which showed cardiomegaly, cephalization of the pulmonary blood flow, and pulmonary edema.

Myxedema: **Severe hypothyroidism** can result in **pretibial edema, periorbital edema, and slow return phase of the DTRs.** This patient had leg and ankle edema, but there was no periorbital edema. Also, DTRs were normal. TFTs were completely normal; thus there was no evidence of hypothyroidism. The edema in hypothyroidism is non-pitting.

Thrombophlebitis: This produces localized edema. It is possible that this patient had bilateral thrombophlebitis, but there was no evidence of **inflammation,** which is normally associated with thrombophlebitis. There was no evidence of erythema, masses in the legs, or calf tenderness. Thrombophlebitis would not cause JVD, HJR, crackles, hepatomegaly, or the S3 heart sound.

CASE 25   CC: "My son doesn't seem to be growing right and he can't walk straight."

HISTORY: A 20-month-old African-American male infant was brought in by his mother after she noticed **bowing of her son's legs,** as well as his toes turned in during walking. The child was the product of a full-term, spontaneous vaginal delivery, and the infant appeared normal upon delivery. Immunizations are current, and the past medical history is significant for otitis media, mild constipation, and **3 ED visits due to fractures.** The mother is concerned that her child hasn't been growing as much as other babies and that he has been irritable. No significant family history exists.

PHYSICAL: Vital signs: WNL. Ht: 15th percentile, Wt: 20th percentile. HEENT: **craniotabes** of skull with widening of sutures. Lungs: CTA B/L. Heart: RRR. Abd: soft, nontender, nondistended, (+) bowel sounds, (−) masses. Ext: **bowing of legs on walking.** Musculoskeletal: **rachitic rosary, Harrison's groove.**

DIFFERENTIAL: Vitamin D–dependent rickets; vitamin D–resistant rickets; rickets due to nutritional vitamin D deficiency; absorption syndromes; renal osteodystrophy; achondroplasia; DiGeorge syndrome; osteoporosis due to glucocorticoid administration; primary chondrodystrophy; anticonvulsant therapy.

DIAGNOSTICS: Electrolytes: **decreased serum calcium and phosphorus.** BUN/creatinine: WNL. Decreased **serum 25(OH)D** levels with subsequent decrease in $1,25(OH)_2D$; increased serum alkaline phosphatase and PTH; serum glucocorticoid level normal; serum phenytoin level 0. UA: increased urinary cAMP. X-ray shows **bowing of shafts of the tibia, thickening of the epiphyseal growth plate,** and decreased bone density. Genetic analysis: normal karyotype.

DIAGNOSIS: Rickets due to nutritional vitamin D deficiency.

ASSESSMENT/PLAN: 20-month-old African-American male infant presenting with bowed legs, craniotabes, decreased vitamin D level, and rickets. No family history of similar disorder and x-rays show decreased bone density. Treat with vitamin D_2 or D_3 given orally for 6 to 12 weeks followed by daily supplements.

Rickets due to nutritional deficiency: This is the most likely diagnosis because the physical findings and lab values correlate. Underprivileged, dark-skinned infants living in crowded northern cities are most susceptible in the U.S.

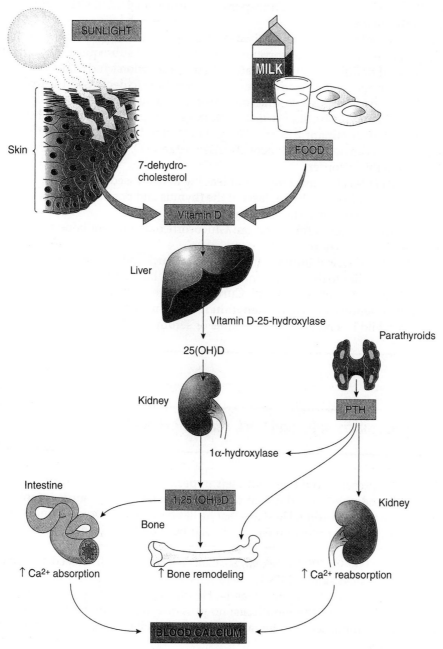

CASE 25 Metabolism of vitamin D and the regulation of blood calcium.

(continued)

CASE 25 CC: "My son doesn't seem to be growing right and he can't walk straight." (Continued)

Vitamin D–dependent rickets: Autosomal recessive deficiency of 1-α-hydroxylase where calcium, phosphorus, and 1,25(OH)$_2$D are low, but **normal 25(OH)D.** The infant's 25(OH)D levels do not correlate because they are decreased (see Figure).

Vitamin D–resistant rickets: This disease is also called familial hypophosphatemia, an X-linked disease in which there is a defective Na$^+$/phosphate transporter in the proximal tubule. The patient does not have a family history of this disease.

Absorption syndromes: Cystic fibrosis, celiac disease, steatorrhea, pancreatitis, and chronic biliary obstruction lead to impaired vitamin D absorption from the gut and subsequent hyperparathyroidism. Lab values and physical findings do not correlate with malabsorption syndrome.

Renal osteodystrophy: Chronic renal failure can result in rickets due to decreased 1-α-hydroxylase; however, BUN/creatinine are normal, which rules out chronic renal failure.

Achondroplasia: **Short bowing limbs, short trunk with large cranium,** and **flat nasal bridge** are characteristic of this **autosomal dominant** disease. The patient's family history is negative, although the achondroplasia mutation can occur spontaneously. Also, vitamin D, calcium, phosphate, and PTH levels would be normal in this disorder.

Di George's syndrome: **PTH levels would be absent** leading to decreased calcium deposition in bone. A pt with this disease would also have hypoplasia of the thymus and possible hypoplasia of the external auditory canal, interruption of the aortic arch, and cardiac anomalies.

Osteoporosis due to glucocorticoid administration: Glucocorticoids prevent bone formation; however, serum glucocorticoid level was normal.

Primary chondrodystrophy: Physical findings in this disease, such as bowing of the legs, short stature, and waddling gait, are similar to dietary vitamin D deficiency, but serum calcium, phosphate, alkaline phosphatase, and vitamin D levels are normal. Currently, there is no effective treatment.

Anticonvulsant therapy: **Phenobarbital** and **phenytoin** increase metabolism of calcidiol and lead to low vitamin D levels. The child has no history of seizures or serum levels of anticonvulsants.

CASE 26 CC: "My stomach, side, and back really hurt, and I've been throwing up a lot."

HISTORY: A 50 y/o man presents to the ED with left upper quadrant pain. The man states that he has had **constant pain** in his **abdomen** for 1 day that **radiates to his back** and is **more intense when he lies down.** He also has nausea and **vomiting.** He states that he has been hospitalized six times before for **fainting in a public place** and twice for pneumonia, and he has been told that he has cirrhosis.

PHYSICAL: Temp: 100.3°F; HR: 95; RR: 22; BP: 90/60. Gen: The patient is distressed and anxious and appears thin and frail with flushed skin. HEENT: sclera **icteric,** conjunctiva pale. Lungs: decreased breath sounds in the left lower lung field, (+) **gynecomastia.** Heart: RRR, no m/r/g, (−) S3 or S4. Abd: noticeable **series of veins appear around the umbilicus;** no pulsatile masses are palpable in the midline abdomen; bowel sounds are diminished; (+) **hepatomegaly;** (+) **ascites.** Back: green-brown discoloration of the lower back (**Turner's sign**).

DIFFERENTIAL: Acute pancreatitis due to chronic alcohol ingestion; biliary tract disease; trauma to abdomen; drug hypersensitivity induced pancreatitis; acute pyelonephritis; perforated peptic ulcer; diabetic ketoacidosis.

DIAGNOSTICS: BUN/Cr: WNL. Urine dip and U/A: WNL. Increased serum pancreatic **amylase,** increased serum pancreatic **lipase.** WBC: **leukocytosis.** Electrolytes: hyperglycemia, **hypocalcemia.** LFTs: ALT and AST elevated with AST/ALT ratio > 2. Creatine kinase: WNL. Cardiac troponin I: WNL. Blood alcohol level elevated. CT scan of the abdomen: pancreatic necrosis.

DIAGNOSIS: Acute pancreatitis due to chronic alcohol ingestion.

ASSESSMENT/PLAN: A 50 y/o white man with a history of ethanol consumption presents with acute abdominal pain. Treat the acute pancreatitis with analgesics for pain, IV fluids to maintain volume, NPO (nothing by mouth), and nasogastric suction to reduce the gastric contents from entering the duodenum and stimulating the pancreas. The acute pancreatitis will usually resolve within 3 to 7 days. Provide counseling for alcoholism.

Acute pancreatitis due to chronic alcohol ingestion: The patient's complaints of abdominal pain with radiation to the back and nausea and vomiting are all consistent with acute pancreatitis. The patient's history of chronic alcohol consumption as well as the elevated amylase and lipase confirm the physical findings (see Figure). Alcohol and gallstones are the most common causes of acute pancreatitis in the United States.

Biliary tract disease: The symptoms of fever, nausea, and vomiting as well as leukocytosis are all consistent with acute cholecystitis. However, the pain is typically **right sided** and **crampy** with this condition. If a gallstone is passed through the common bile duct and lodges in the distal pancreatic duct, acute pancreatitis may occur in conjunction with biliary tract obstruction.

Trauma to the abdomen: The patient has no history of trauma and no abrasions or lacerations are visible, although this diagnosis cannot be ruled out given the patient's history of alcoholism.

Drug hypersensitivity-induced pancreatitis: The patient has no history of **azathioprine, 6-mercaptopurine, sulfonamide, diuretics, estrogen, tetracycline, valproic acid, pentamidine,** or **ddI** intake, all of which may induce acute pancreatitis.

Acute pyelonephritis: Whereas acute pyelonephritis would cause flank pain, fever, nausea, vomiting, and leukocytosis, the patient's urine dip and U/A are normal. In addition, pyelonephritis typically follows urinary tract infections, which the patient has no history of having.

Perforated peptic ulcer: This disease may result in epigastric pain, nausea, vomiting, leukocytosis, and hematemesis. No evidence of **free air** in the abdomen was seen on a CT scan. However, this patient has a history of chronic alcohol consumption, which places him at a higher risk for peptic ulcer disease.

Diabetic ketoacidosis (DKA): The abdominal pain of DKA can often mimic acute pancreatitis. In addition, DKA can produce an increased serum amylase, but **serum lipase is not elevated.** Absence of an elevated anion gap, high blood glucose level, or high urine ketone level can help rule out DKA.

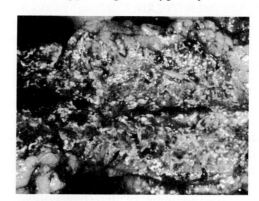

CASE 26 Acute hemorrhagic pancreatitis.

CASE 27 CC: "My child is not breathing right and has a fever."

HISTORY: A 10 y/o **white** girl presents to the ER with her mother, complaining of difficulty breathing and feeling feverish. The girl's mother states that the child has **cystic fibrosis** (CF) and has had difficulty breathing for 2 days, along with a fever. She is coughing up thick **green/yellow mucus** with small amounts of blood. She has only eaten one meal over the past 2 days but has no nausea, vomiting, or diarrhea. She has been treated successfully for five pulmonary infections before with tobramycin and a cephalosporin (e.g., ceftazidime). She was hospitalized at birth for meconium ileus. She uses inhaled β-agonists when she has difficulty breathing and takes **pancreatic enzymes** with each meal. She receives injections of **vitamins A, D, E, and K** and is a regular visitor to the physical therapy center for her CF. She does not have exposure to second-hand smoke and has no known allergies.

PHYSICAL: Temp: 104°F; HR: 110; **RR: 28;** BP: 110/70; Ht: 10th percentile; Wt: 5th percentile. Gen: **cyanotic** in mild respiratory distress. HEENT: (−) lymphadenopathy. Lungs: using **accessory muscles** to breathe; **increased A/P chest diameter;** intercostal and substernal retractions; increased breath sounds, **dullness to percussion,** and **increased tactile fremitus** found in the left lower lung. Heart: tachycardic, regular rhythm. Abd: soft, nontender, no masses, no guarding. Ext: distal pulses 2/4 (normal), (+) **clubbing** of distal phalanges.

DIFFERENTIAL: Pneumonia due to exacerbation of CF; upper respiratory infection; bronchitis; chemical irritant inhalant; asthma.

DIAGNOSTICS: CBC: leukocytosis. ABG: hypoxia and hypercapnia. Blood culture: no bacterial growth. CXR: lung opacities in the left lower lobe and overinflated lung fields bilaterally. Sputum sample: grows *Pseudomonas aeruginosa*. PFTs: **decreased FEV_1, increased FVC, increased RV/TLC ratio.** Stool sample: **increased fat content.**

DIAGNOSIS: Pneumonia due to exacerbation of CF.

ASSESSMENT/PLAN: 15 y/o white girl has a fever and trouble breathing with a history of CF. Treat the patient's pneumonia with IV tobramycin (macrolide antibiotic) and ceftazidime as treated before; maintain hydration with IV fluids; use acetaminophen to control the fever; and maintain replacement of the pancreatic enzymes as before. CF is an **autosomal recessive disease,** which is prominent in **whites.** It caused by a defect in the **CFTR gene** (cystic fibrosis transmembrane receptor), which disrupts normal chloride ion transport across cell membranes (see Figure). CF can affect the lungs (predisposing to pneumonia), exocrine pancreas (causing poor excretion of digestive enzymes into the duodenum), and vas deferens (leading to sterility in males) and causes abnormal ion concentration in sweat. It is diagnosed by the **chloride sweat test.**

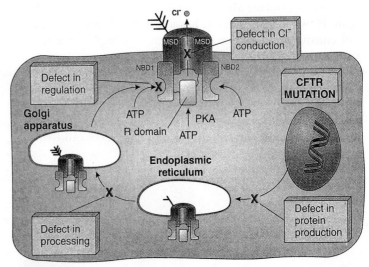

CASE 27 Cellular sites of the disruptions in the synthesis and function of CFTR in cystic fibrosis.

Pneumonia due to CF: Characteristic **lobar infiltration on x-ray.** Thick greenish mucus is characteristic of CF patients colonized with *Pseudomonas* *aeruginosa* and is consistent with the sputum culture growing *Pseudomonas aeruginosa*. Decrease in FEV$_1$ is due to long-standing CF.

Upper respiratory tract infection (URI): Most often viral thus should reveal no growth. A URI can present with various symptoms but often produces **low-grade fever, dry and unproductive cough,** with nasal erythema, congestion, and clear exudate.

Bronchitis: Similar to upper respiratory tract infection with nonproductive cough and low-grade fever.

Chemical irritant inhalant: This diagnosis is unlikely because there is no history of exposure, no associated neurologic findings, no rashes, no eye or mucosal irritation, no nausea, vomiting, or diarrhea.

Asthma: This disease can be diagnosed by observing a **15% or more increase in FEV$_1$ after two puffs of a β-agonist** or by observing airway constriction after administration of methacholine (methacholine challenge test).

CASE 28 — CC: "My roommate is trying to kill me."

HISTORY: A **19-year-old** college sophomore is brought to student mental health services by her roommates because she claims that **voices** have been telling her that her roommate is trying to kill her. She has been **socially withdrawn** for 6 months and will not return phone calls from her family. She has not washed or groomed for 7 days. Her friends report that her grades have dropped from As to Cs since the last semester. The patient is agitated and distracted, making a history difficult to elicit. She denies any drug use. She does reveal that her mother had been hospitalized when the patient was a young girl because she is "crazy."

PHYSICAL: The patient is a well-developed, well-nourished 19-year-old in no apparent distress. She is **alert and oriented** to person, place, and time. She demonstrates a **flattened affect,** and she responds to questions inappropriately (e.g., laughs when she is asked serious questions). Her thoughts are disconnected and have **loose association.** She refuses to cooperate with a physical exam.

DIFFERENTIAL: Schizophrenia; personality disorders; mood disorder; brief reactive psychosis; schizoaffective disorder; schizophreniform disorder; organic mental disorders; malingering.

DIAGNOSTICS: CBC, Chem 7, vitamin B$_{12}$, folate, thyroid function tests, and LFTs are all normal. Urine drug screen was negative for opioids, cocaine, or THC. A CT scan shows **cortical atrophy** and enlarged lateral ventricles.

DIAGNOSIS: Schizophrenia; most likely the paranoid type.

ASSESSMENT/PLAN: A 19-year-old white woman presenting with schizophrenia. Treat with antipsychotic drugs (e.g., thorazine or clozapine) and intense individual and family psychotherapy.

Schizophrenia: Most commonly presents in **young adults** (age 15 to 35), and **lifetime prevalence is 1%** of the general population. The disorder affects men and women equally; it is cross-cultural and is more prevalent in lower socioeconomic groups, blacks, and Hispanics. However, some think that the illness itself causes a decline in social status and may account for such statistics (**drift vs. breeder hypothesis**). Look for the "four As": **blunted affect, loose associations, autism,** and **ambivalence.** These characteristic symptoms must be present for at least 6 months for the diagnosis of schizophrenia to be made. Schizophrenia includes psychotic symptoms, which impair behavior and cognition, and may also include delu-

(continued)

CASE 28 CC: "My roommate is trying to kill me." (Continued)

sions and **hallucinations (mainly auditory).** Symptoms are divided into **positive** and **negative** categories, the predominance of which can determine the subtype of schizophrenia. (Subtypes include: **catatonic, paranoid, residual, disorganized,** and **undifferentiated.**) Positive symptoms are delusions, hallucinations, behavior changes, and loose associations. Negative symptoms are withdrawal, blunted affect, and lack of motivation. Diagnosis is made by observation and history. A CT scan may show cortical atrophy and lateral ventricle enlargement. Patients are alert and oriented, but illogical thought and loose associations are prevalent. Family history is a key part of the diagnosis, and evidence of a **genetic link** is strong (as evidenced by concordance, consanguinity, and adoption studies). The disease is chronic and may include flare-ups (often with increased stress) and remissions. Half of schizophrenic patients will attempt **suicide,** and one tenth will succeed. The etiology is multifactorial, but an increase in dopamine activity is thought to play a major role. The "**dopamine hypothesis**" is supported by the fact that antipsychotic drugs block dopamine (D_2 receptor), whereas dopaminergic drugs (amphetamines, cocaine) can cause schizophrenic-type behavior.

Personality disorders: In general, symptoms are present for a longer time and interfere with many different aspects of life. A person who displays some schizophrenic characteristics may have one of the following personality disorders: schizotypal, schizoid, paranoid, or borderline.

Mood disorders: Mania and depression can have a similar initial presentation to schizophrenia, but hallucinations and delusions do not persist after the mood disorder resolves.

Brief reactive psychosis: Usually precipitated by an identifiable, highly **stressful event** and lasts **less than 1 month.** If this patient had been evaluated within 1 month of the onset of symptoms, this would be the most likely diagnosis.

Schizophreniform disorder: This diagnosis is given for patients with schizophrenic symptoms that last for **less than 6 months.** If this patient had been seen between 1 month and 6 months after the onset of symptoms, this would be the most likely diagnosis.

Schizoaffective disorder: **Both mood changes and schizophrenic symptoms** are present, but hallucinations and delusions may remain for up to 2 weeks after the schizophrenic symptoms end.

Organic mental disorders: May be caused by substance abuse (i.e., **PCP, cocaine**), infections, or **complex partial seizures.** This disorder is usually associated with memory loss, diminished orientation, and signs of CNS damage. This patient's history and urinary drug screen are inconsistent with this diagnosis.

Malingering: Patients may mimic schizophrenic symptoms to receive attention or to obtain some other **secondary gain.** Because there are no definitive diagnostic tests for schizophrenia, malingering must be a consideration in evaluating a patient with the aforementioned history. Malingering is unlikely in this case, because the patient was brought in by others.

CASE 29 CC: "I found a lump in my left breast while I was in the shower last week."

HISTORY: A 58-year-old white woman presents with a hard, bumpy mass in her lower left breast. She is 2 years **post-menopause** and does not take hormone replacement therapy (HRT). Menses began at age 11. She denies breast or nipple discharge but has noticed some puckering of the nipple since early last month. Her **mother died of breast cancer** at the age of 48; she has no sisters or aunts. She has **never been pregnant** and has no history of fibrocystic changes or reproductive cancers.

PHYSICAL: The patient's vital signs are normal. The patient appears her stated age and is in no apparent distress. Her skin is normal with the exception of some puckering in the lower right quadrant of her left areola. A **hard, nodular mass** is palpable in the lower right quadrant of her left breast. The exam is otherwise unremarkable.

DIFFERENTIAL: Malignant mass; benign mass; fibrocystic change; fibroadenoma; acute mastitis; intraductal papilloma.

DIAGNOSTICS: Mammogram demonstrates a radiopaque mass with surrounding **calcifications** in the right lower quadrant of her left breast. The right breast shows no lesions. A biopsy of the left breast reveals large cells in nests, cords, and sheets (a histologic pattern consistent with invasive ductal carcinoma).

DIAGNOSIS: Invasive ductal carcinoma of the breast.

ASSESSMENT/PLAN: A 58-year-old white woman appearing in generally good health with an invasive ductal carcinoma of her left breast. Refer to surgery for **left segmental mastectomy** and **axillary node dissection.** The mass should be sent for estrogen receptor and progesterone receptor analysis. If the mass is receptor-positive, it has a better prognosis, because it will be more likely to respond to **hormone therapy (tamoxifen).** If the mass is receptor-negative, the patient should receive adjuvant chemotherapy (CMF: cyclophosphamide, methotrexate, and 5-fluorouracil).

Invasive ductal carcinoma: 65% to 80% of all breast cancers. This tumor is a very hard, circumscribed mass averaging 1 to 2 cm in size. The tumor may infiltrate the chest wall causing **skin dimpling and nipple retraction.** Malignant cells appear as **nests, cords, tubules, and glands** and are highly atypical (see Figure). Invasive ductal carcinoma can invade the underlying connective tissue, nerves, and vasculature.

Other malignant breast diseases:

Intraductal carcinoma in situ: Does not invade through basement membrane; thus it is non-metastatic but may spread to adjacent cells in the affected breast. When the nipple is involved, it may appear like Paget's disease.

Medullary carcinoma: This tumor is described as a flesh mass 5 cm or greater and is typically **softer to palpation** than other carcinomas. Histology demonstrates solid sheets of large, plump, pleiomorphic cells with intervening lymphocytic invasion. It has a **better prognosis** than do other carcinomas. The 10-year survival rate is 70%.

Mucinous carcinoma: Slow-growing tumor that tends to be seen in **older women.** The carcinoma consists of gelatinous material, which appears blue-gray on gross inspection. "Mixed" forms occur with other types of infiltrating duct neoplasms.

Paget's disease of the breast: Tumor spreads via growth in the excretory ducts, which **invade (via the epithelium) the nipple and areola.** This carcinoma is always associated with ductal carcinoma in-situ or invasive ductal carcinoma of the breast. The **nipple is usually bloody and ulcerated.**

Benign masses:

Duct ectasia: Dilatation of the ducts with **granulomatous inflammation** around the ducts and in the interstitium. Usually occurs in multiparous women in their 40s and 50s and may be associated with pituitary adenoma.

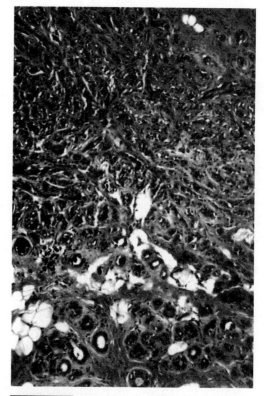

(continued)   **CASE 29** Breast cancer

CASE 29   CC: "I found a lump in my left breast while I was in the shower last week."
(Continued)

Fat necrosis: **Trauma** to breast, as a result of surgery or radiation, may cause necrosis followed by inflammation and fibrosis. It usually occurs in a localized area.

Fibrocystic change: This benign disease may appear like a carcinoma on physical examination. It does not
usually predispose women to future carcinoma, but cancer risk is increased by the amount of atypical
hyperplasia seen at biopsy. This condition is very common and is seen in 29% of women at autopsy.

Fibroadenoma: This condition is more common in women **younger than 30 years of age.** It is described
as a round, clearly demarcated nodule that is **freely moveable.** The mass contains fibrous and glandular tissue. It may be affected by hormonal changes and grow at the end stages of the menstrual cycle or during pregnancy.

Acute mastitis: This disease presents as **purulent discharge** from the nipple, which is most often a complication of **lactation after pregnancy.** *Staphylococcus aureus* is the most common cause. Patients present with local inflammation, soreness, and redness. Temperature may be elevated. This presentation
is not consistent with the patient's history.

Intraductal papilloma: Pathologically seen as solitary masses in principal lactiferous ducts. It most commonly presents with **bloody nipple discharge** and a small tumor below the areola. Infrequently, nipple retraction is seen.

General discussion: Breast cancer is the **most common cancer in women** (1 in 9 will be diagnosed at some
point in their lives), but the second leading cause of cancer death after lung cancer. Regular mammog-
raphy has been shown to reduce mortality but has a 15% false-negative rate. Therefore, **all masses must
be biopsied** regardless of appearance on mammogram. Sites of metastatic breast cancer, in order of decreasing frequency, are lungs, bones, liver, adrenal glands, and brain. Sites of nodal spread, in order of
decreasing frequency, include axillary, internal mammary, and supraclavicular. Risk factors are family history, genetic (BRCA1, BRCA2), early menarche, late menopause, nulliparous or first pregnancy
after age 30, fibrocystic changes, increased age, estrogen replacement therapy, and oral contraceptives
use prior to the first pregnancy.

CASE 30   CC: "The pain in my toe is unbearable."

HISTORY: A 60-year-old African-American woman presents to the emergency department with a
swollen, tender, erythematous **great toe.** She has a mild fever but denies any trauma, joint pain, swelling,
or fatigue. She has no history of degenerative joint disease, gonorrhea, or syphilis. She is hypertensive and
takes verapamil prescribed by her previous physician. She began taking a **thiazide** diuretic yesterday. She
does not recall any trauma to her foot. She denies any alcohol use or cigarette smoking and has not
changed her diet recently or had an **unusually heavy meal.**

PHYSICAL: A 60-year-old African-American woman appearing her stated age. Temp: 100.3° F; HR: 80; RR:
16; BP 140/80. HEENT: unremarkable. Lungs: CTA. Heart: RRR. Ext: No clubbing, edema or cyanosis;
warm, erythematous right **metatarsophalangeal (MTP) joint** appearing twice its normal size (**podagra**);
all other joints WNL. Skin: WNL. Neurologic exam: intact.

DIFFERENTIAL: Primary gout; pseudogout; septic arthritis; trauma; sarcoid.

DIAGNOSTICS: Fine-needle aspirate of synovial fluid from the affected joint is cloudy, xanthochromic,
and contains **needle-like, strongly negative birefringent monosodium urate crystals;** an increased
number of PMNs are also evident. Synovial fluid analysis: Gram stain is negative for organisms, glu-

cose is decreased, and WBCs are elevated with 85% PMNs (usually 60%). Serum uric acid is 9 mg/dl (3.5 to 7.2).

DIAGNOSIS: Primary gout.

ASSESSMENT/PLAN: A 60-year-old African-American woman with podagra secondary to thiazide-induced gout. Acute treatment consists of **indomethacin** and **colchicine. Allopurinol, probenecid,** and **sulfinpyrazone** can be used prophylactically. Allopurinol is used for overproducers of uric acid (see Figure).

Primary gout: This is the most likely diagnosis. Hyperuricemia causes uric acid to accumulate in joints, which incites a **phagocytic response** and subsequent inflammation. Acute attacks may be brought on by alcohol ingestion, high-protein meals, salicylates, and, as in this case, diuretics. Gout has three phases: (1) acute attack; (2) interval asymptomatic period; and (3) chronic 10 to 20 years after onset. The chronic phase involves the deposit of **tophi** in the synovium of the olecranon, bursa, and pinna (ear). Destruction of the articular cartilage can deform the joint. Most hyperuricemia is idiopathic (most patients **undersecrete uric acid** into the urine at the renal tubule). Elevated uric acid levels may also be caused by hypoxanthine-guanine phosphoribosyl transferase (**HGPRT**) **deficiency in Lesch-Nyhan syndrome, lead intoxication,** or **psoriasis.** Finally, **myeloproliferation** may cause increased cell turnover leading to hyperuricemia.

Pseudogout: **Calcium pyrophosphate** deposition may occur with hyperparathyroidism, hypothyroidism, and hemochromatosis. X-ray may show **linear calcification in larger joints,** especially the knee. Weakly positive birefringent crystals are present in the joint aspirate.

Septic arthritis: This disease is primarily caused by **gonorrhea** in sexually active young adults. *Staphylococcus aureus* is most common in other groups. Alcoholics, diabetics, IV-DUs, and immunosuppressed individuals are at increased risk. Opaque synovial fluid demonstrates considerable **leukocytosis** and infectious organisms. The joint aspirate results in this patient are inconsistent with septic arthritis.

Trauma: This diagnosis is inconsistent with the patient's history. However, trauma to a joint, especially a large joint such as the knee, can lead to seeding of the joint with bacterial organisms and precipitate septic arthritis.

Sarcoid: The joint manifestations of sarcoid usually involve the **proximal interphalangeal (PIP) joints** and the **knee joints.** Sarcoidosis also has other systemic manifestations, including respiratory complications, lymphadenopathy, ocular lesions, splenomegaly, and **erythema nodosum.**

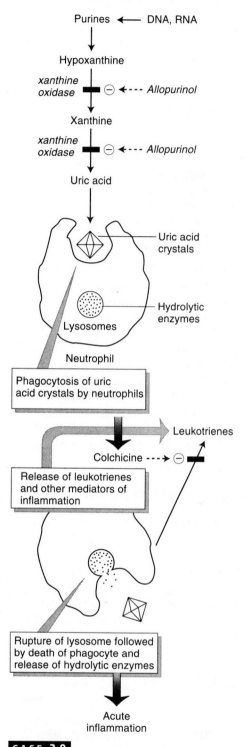

CASE 30 Role of uric acid in the inflammation of gout.

CASE 31 CC: "My bones ache so much that I can't sleep."

HISTORY: A 70-year-old Japanese man presents with a complaint of excruciating **bone pain** in his back and legs for the past month. He reports that he has been weak and tired lately and has had pain in his wrists that is worse at night. He has also noticed that his ankles are swollen and he feels bloated. He denies a history of smoking, cough, cancer, urinary infection, or STD.

PHYSICAL: Vital signs normal. Gen: 70-year-old man appearing his stated age, thin and anxious. Lungs: CTA. Heart: 2/6 systolic flow murmur is heard over the left sternal border. Abd: (+) CVA tenderness. Ext: 2+ pitting edema is evident in the lower extremities.

DIFFERENTIAL: Multiple myeloma; metastatic bone lesions; osteoarthritis; spondylolysis; nephrotic syndrome.

DIAGNOSTICS: CBC: anemia. Electrolytes: **serum calcium is elevated.** Serum alkaline phosphatase normal. LFTs: WNL. UA: demonstrates mild **Bence-Jones proteinuria** and pyuria, but no casts or RBCs are present. XR: diffuse **lytic lesions** of **skull** and **pathologic fractures** on the left tibia and fibula. CXR: negative for lung mass. Serum protein and urinary electrophoresis: hyperlipidemia, hypoalbuminemia and a monoclonal "spike." Bone marrow biopsy: **hypercellular** with >10% immature **plasma cells** in the marrow.

DIAGNOSIS: Multiple myeloma.

ASSESSMENT/PLAN: A 70-year-old man with multiple myeloma. Secondary effects include lytic lesions in his skull, back, and bones of lower extremity, **carpal tunnel syndrome** from **amyloid deposits** in the median nerves, and fatigue from **anemia.** Increase in light chain proteins causes peripheral **edema.** Give the patient large quantities of fluid to preserve renal function. Radiation therapy and chemotherapy are given to treat painful bone lysis, including melphalan (or another alkylating agent), steroids, and vincristine.

Multiple myeloma: This disease is a cancer of plasma cells, which prolifer-

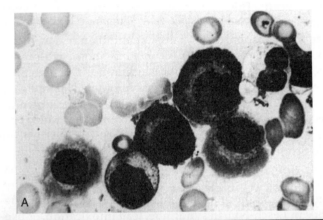

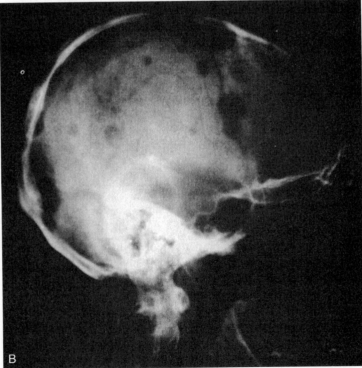

CASE 31 *A,* Multiple myeloma—a smear of bone marrow aspirate. *B,* Multiple myeloma—a radiograph of the skull. *(continued)*

ates in bone marrow and causes **pancytopenia.** Clinical presentation may include bone pain caused by osteolysis and pathologic fractures, weakness from anemia, and nephrotic syndrome from increased light chain production. Myeloma nephrosis causes classic nephrotic symptoms and Bence-Jones (light chain) proteins are often evident on UA. Consequent IgG and IgA immunoglobulinemia leads to neurologic problems (e.g., carpal tunnel syndrome) and manifests as an **M spike** on plasma electrophoresis. Chronic **infections,** including pneumonia and pyelonephritis, are due to abnormal immunoglobulin production and often cause death (see Figure).

Metastatic cancer: Most common metastases to the bone are from cancers of the breast, lung, testes, thyroid, kidney, and prostate. However, none of these cancers would result in an M spike or Bence-Jones proteinuria.

Nephrotic syndrome: This disease would account for the proteinuria, edema, and hyperlipidemia but would not cause bone pain, lytic lesions, or fractures. Neurologic symptoms and M spike would not be evident in nephrotic syndrome.

Osteoarthritis (OA): This disease most often presents in the hands, hips, and knees but may also affect the lumbar and cervical spine, resulting in spinal stenosis. OA is not associated with kidney disease, carpal tunnel syndrome, or osteolytic lesions.

Alkylosing spondylitis (AS): Inflammation and ossification of spinal ligaments and joints lead to fusion of the spine (**bamboo spine**), which prevents rotational motion causing postural problems and restrictive lung disease. AS tends to cluster in families and is associated with **HLA-B27.** This disease presents with pain and stiffness in patients younger than 40. XR does not show lytic lesions.

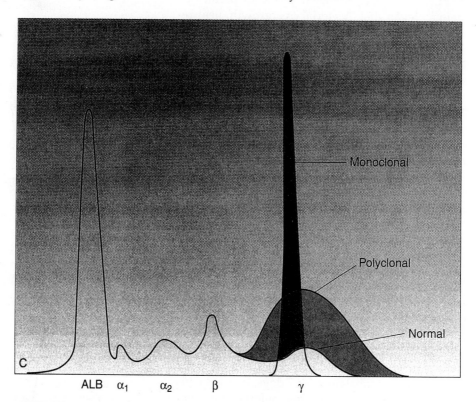

CASE 31 *(continued) C,* Serum protein electrophoretic patterns in multiple myeloma.

CASE 32

CC: "I haven't been myself lately—forgetting things and confused. And I have these marks all over me."

HISTORY: A 57-year-old white woman presents with confusion and forgetfulness over the past 2 months. She has bruises over all extremities. The patient states that she has been "out of it" lately and has been forgetting names and addresses. She has been bumping into furniture and often misses her footing while walking to the market. She does not feel any soreness or tenderness but has experienced increasing fatigue over the past few months. She denies weight loss, vomiting, diarrhea, or fever. She reports a balanced diet, which includes meat and vegetables, but she does not eat fish. She does not smoke, and she drinks alcohol about three times a year. She has been postmenopausal for 6 years.

PHYSICAL: Temp: 98.7° F; HR: 75; RR: 16; BP: 130/60. Gen: The patient is thin and pale but is in no apparent distress. HEENT: Head is normocephalic; conjunctiva are pale; the disk is sharp; jugular and cervical lymph nodes are enlarged; the tongue is swollen and red. Lungs: CTA. Heart: remarkable for a 2/6 systolic flow murmur heard along the left sternal border. Abd: nontender and bowel sounds are audible; no abdominal scars are present. Ext: old and new bruises are on both legs and the lateral aspects of the patient's arms and shoulders. Neurologic exam: **decreased vibration and position sense** bilaterally in both arms and legs.

DIFFERENTIAL: B_{12} deficiency due to pernicious anemia; vegan diet; bacterial overgrowth; ileal resection/malabsorption; D. latum (fish tapeworm); folate deficiency due to alcoholism; altered metabolism due to antimetabolic drugs (methotrexate, trimethoprim, pyrimethamine, sulfasalazine).

DIAGNOSTICS: CBC with manual diff: MCV is increased; peripheral blood smear shows macro-ovalocytes, **hyperlobular PMNs** (>5 segments), and a low reticulocyte count (see Figure A). WBC: WNL. LDH: elevated. Methylmalonic acid (MMA) and homocysteine levels: elevated. Indirect bilirubin: elevated. Serum B_{12}: decreased. Serum folate level: decreased. **Anti-IF and antiparietal antibodies** are present in the serum. Bone marrow biopsy: erythroid hypercellularity and cells have enlarged nuclei with dispersed chromatin. **A positive Schilling test** confirms the diagnosis.

DIAGNOSIS: Pernicious anemia.

ASSESSMENT/PLAN: A 57-year-old white woman with pernicious anemia. Treatment is with intramuscular cyanocobalamin for 7 days, then once per week for 4 to 8 weeks until hemoglobin is normal. Do not treat with folic acid alone, because anemia will correct but neuropathy will persist.

Autoimmune pernicious anemia: This disease is the **most common cause of B_{12} deficiency** and results from anti-IF and antiparietal cell antibodies (see Figure B and C). It is more common in Scandi-

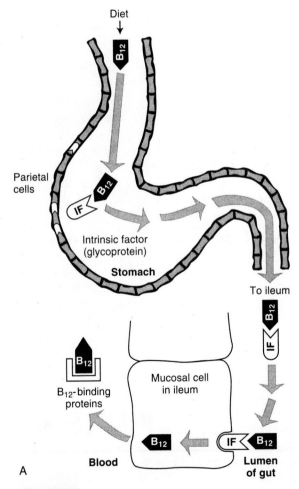

CASE 32 *A*, Absorption of vitamin B_{12}—pernicious anemia. *(continued)*

navian descendants in their fifth through eighth decades. **Atrophic gastritis** stops intrinsic factor (IF) production by the parietal cells in the gastric fundus and leads to **achlorhydria.** HCl and IF are required to form the IF-B$_{12}$ complex, which is required for transport and absorption in the ileum. Lymphocytic infiltrate is demonstrated on biopsy.

Vegan diet: Vitamin B$_{12}$ is only available from animal protein. However, the deficiency takes years to develop because body stores of the vitamin are vast. This patient's diet includes meat.

Folic acid deficiency: This deficiency is most commonly caused by **malnutrition** (dietary deficiency in fruits and vegetables) associated with **alcoholism.** Unlike vitamin B$_{12}$ deficiency, no neurologic symptoms are seen in folic acid deficiency. Only homocysteine levels would be elevated in a deficiency of folic acid, but both homocysteine and MMA are elevated in this patient.

Antimetabolites: Methotrexate, trimethoprim, pyrimethamine, and sulfasalazine interfere with DNA synthesis and may cause macrocytic anemia. However, the patient denies taking any medication other than vitamins.

Ileal resection/malabsorption: The patient denies surgery and has no abdominal scars. Malabsorption may be caused by inflammatory bowel disease (i.e., Crohn's and ulcerative colitis) and celiac sprue. Other vitamin deficiencies (A, E, D, and K) would be evident before vitamin B$_{12}$ deficiency, because vitamin B$_{12}$ stores are so vast.

Bacterial overgrowth/ D. latum: The patient does not have an increased WBC count, has not been taking antibiotics, and does not eat fish. In these disorders, vitamin B$_{12}$ deficiency would result from interference of absorption along the gut lining.

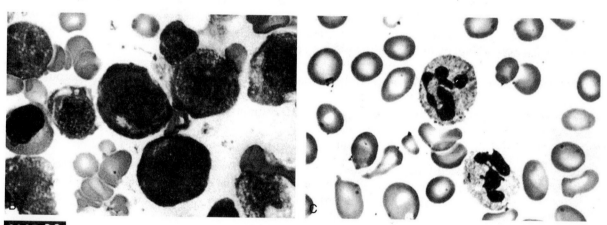

CASE 32 (continued) B, Megaloblastic bone marrow aspirate. C, Megaloblastic anemia–smear of peripheral blood cells.

CASE 33 CC: "I've stopped getting my period."

HISTORY: A 25-year-old white woman presents with a 6-month history of amenorrhea and a 1-year history of infertility (the patient is attempting to get pregnant). She reports that she is **training for the Boston Marathon** and has been running over 35 miles each week. She has also **cut down on fats and carbohydrates** and has dropped two clothing sizes in the past 7 months. She reports that she is not dieting intentionally but has always wanted to lose a few pounds. She denies any previous pregnancy, STDs, or radiation therapy. She denies vaginal dryness, hot flashes, or nipple discharge. Onset of menarche occurred at age 14, and her periods were of moderate flow and on average lasted for 5 days. She has no family his-

(continued)

CASE 33 **CC: "I've stopped getting my period."** (Continued)

tory of diabetes, heart disease, or cancer. She occasionally takes multivitamins and denies any history of contraceptive use.

PHYSICAL: Vital signs are normal. Gen: The patient presents with wasting and pale skin. She weighs 94 lb and is 5'7" tall. She appears malnourished and nervous. HEENT: **Cephalic hair is thinned** but present. Neck: supple, (−) lymphadenopathy. Lungs: CTA B/L. Heart: RRR. Genitourinary: pubic and axillary hair is consistent with a normal female pattern. Ext: (−) c/c/e, distal pulses are present. Neurologic exam: intact.

DIFFERENTIAL: Secondary amenorrhea due to: pregnancy, anorexia/exercise, hypothalamic dysfunction, pituitary neoplasm, ovarian dysfunction.

DIAGNOSTICS: CBC, Chem 7, and UA: WNL. β-hCG negative. Progesterone administration does not yield uterine bleeding after 2 weeks. **GnRH levels are decreased. LH, FSH, and estrogen are all slightly below normal.** Prolactin levels normal. No antibodies against ovarian antigens or TSH antigen found; TSH, ACTH, ADH, and GH all normal. MRI is negative for pituitary enlargement.

DIAGNOSIS: Amenorrhea secondary to anorexia and strenuous exercise.

ASSESSMENT/PLAN: A 25-year-old white woman presenting with secondary amenorrhea. Pt began menarche at age 14, which excludes primary amenorrhea as the diagnosis. The symptoms of her amenorrhea have lasted for 6 months and are due to exercise and diet-induced anorexia. The patient requires psychological counseling, including dietary therapy and a decrease in rigorous exercise.

Anorexia and exercise: This is the most plausible diagnosis due to her recent weight loss, rigorous physical training, and endocrine profile. Anorexia **causes a hypothalamic decrease in GnRH release,** leading to an overall depression of sex hormone levels. Secondary amenorrhea is common in long-distance runners (e.g., this patient), gymnasts, and ballerinas.

Pregnancy: β-hCG is negative.

Pituitary neoplasm/prolactinoma: Secondary amenorrhea may be due to a prolactin-producing adenoma. The adenoma may be associated with galactorrhea. This diagnosis is unlikely in this case because FSH would be normal or increased and prolactin would be increased. In a pituitary adenoma, the MRI would show a mass lesion in the pituitary gland.

Ovarian neoplasm/ dysfunction: This disorder leads to an increase in testosterone production and precipitates hirsutism and virilization. These symptoms are not present in this patient. In addition, an ovarian neoplasm would not alter FSH and LH levels.

Polycystic ovarian syndrome (Stein-Leventhal syndrome): Symptoms of this disease include obesity, infertility, hirsutism, and androgen excess. An increased LH:FSH ratio would be expected.

General discussion: Causes of primary amenorrhea

In primary amenorrhea, menarche never takes place.

Turner's syndrome: This is the **number one cause of primary amenorrhea.** Karyotype is 45 XO with gonadal dysgenesis affecting 1/3000 women. Clinical features include short stature, webbed neck, and coarctation of the aorta.

17-hydroxylase deficiency (congenital adrenal hyperplasia): This deficiency results from an inability to make corticosteroids or estrogen, with consequent increase in mineralocorticoids. Primary amenorrhea, lack of secondary sex characteristics, and hypertension are characteristics of this disease.

Testicular feminization: Individuals with this disease are genotypically males, but phenotypically females. They have primary amenorrhea and scant pubic and axillary hair, but they develop normal breasts and secondary female sexual characteristics. The lack of male development of these individuals is due to a receptor defect, which causes **androgen insensitivity.**

CASE 34 CC: "I have a huge lump on my throat."

HISTORY: A 36-year-old Hispanic **woman** presents with a large mass in the midline of her neck. She reports that she has been having panic attacks for the past few weeks, with **diaphoresis** and **palpitations.** She has been **unable to sleep** and has experienced intermittent diarrhea and loss of appetite for the past 3 weeks. She insists on keeping the windows open even though it is December. She reports a recent onset of **diplopia (double vision)** that she assumes is related to her anxiety. She has three children and has taken oral contraceptives since 1985. She has not had her period for 2 months. She denies any cardiac problems or additional medications. She has **lost weight** even though she has not been dieting or taking weight loss aids.

PHYSICAL: Temp: 100.6°F; **HR: 112;** RR 17; BP: 135/80. Gen: This is a well-developed, well-nourished Hispanic woman who appears nervous and jittery. HEENT: **Exophthalmos** is present. The fundoscopic exam is normal, and visual acuity and visual fields are intact bilaterally. Neck: (−) lymphadenopathy or JVD, (+) smooth and enlarged thyroid gland is found in the midline, a bruit is heard over the thyroid. Lungs: CTA. Heart: tachycardia with a loud S1 and S2. S3 is barely audible, a 2 / 6 systolic ejection murmur can be heard on the left sternal border. Ext: nails are brittle, but no splinters or hemorrhages are noted, (+) **clubbing** of fingers and thickening of the 3rd and 4th digits on the right hand, distal pulses are normal. Skin: feels "velvety," is hyperpigmented, warm, and moist and has raised lesions on the anterior leg. Neuro: (+) **brisk proximal reflexes** and **resting tremor.**

DIFFERENTIAL: Graves' disease; toxic adenoma; toxic multinodular goiter; subacute (de Quervain's) thyroiditis; chronic (Hashimoto's) thyroiditis; factitious hyperthyroidism; ectopic thyroid hormone production (struma ovarii).

DIAGNOSTICS: Thyroid function tests: total T4 is elevated, free T4 is elevated, total T3 is elevated, **TSH is greatly decreased,** radioactive iodine uptake is increased, **TSI** (thyroid stimulating immunoglobulin) is present. β-hCG is negative.

DIAGNOSIS: Graves' disease.

ASSESSMENT/PLAN: This is a 36-year-old Hispanic woman with a goiter from Graves' disease. Treat the patient with propylthiouracil or methimazole for 12 to18 months. Give propranolol for symptomatic relief of cardiac manifestations. Radioactive iodine for 3 to 24 weeks will destroy part of the gland and reduce thyroid hormone. Consider a subtotal thyroidectomy if the patient's condition is refractive to medical treatment.

Graves' disease: This is the **most common cause of hyperthyroidism.** It is a prototypical autoimmune disorder and is caused by IgG antibody binding to TSH receptors, which leads to gland enlargement and hyperactivity (see Figure). Increased thyroid hormone production causes an elevated basal metabolic rate with increased appetite and weight loss. Patients become **heat intolerant.** Hair becomes silky and fine and vasodilatation causes skin to become moist. Sinus tachycardia may lead to A-fib and PVCs. Typically, patients are **anxious** and exhibit restlessness and irritability. Fatigue and weakness may be present. Ophthalmopathy is present in most cases and may include stare and lid lag. Exophthalmos is unique to Graves' disease and is secondary to the inflammation of the orbital tissues, conjunctival swelling, and ocular muscle weakness.

Toxic adenoma: This usually presents as a **benign** solitary nodule in older patients. **"Hot" lobe (metabolically active lobe)** is seen on thyroid scan. A very elevated T3 and moderately elevated T4 are characteristic.

Toxic multinodular goiter: This condition usually occurs in older patients with long-standing goiter and with advanced signs such as arrhythmias and heart failure. Labs are similar to those used for Graves'

(continued)

CASE 34 CC: "I have a huge lump on my throat." (Continued)

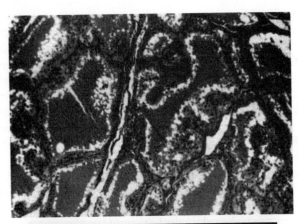

disease, but a thyroid scan shows multiple nodules with discrete areas of hyperactive tissue that suppress the activity of normal tissue.

Subacute (de Quervain's) thyroiditis: This disease presents as acute thyroid gland inflammation, which may be secondary to viral infection. The hallmark of subacute thyroiditis is a **very tender thyroid gland** with anterior neck pain and fever. Lab results change with the course of the disease. The patient is initially hyperthyroid but will progress to euthyroid and eventually to hypothyroid before it reverts to euthyroid.

Chronic (Hashimoto's) thyroiditis: Lymphocytic invasion destroys normal thyroid tissue causing hypothyroidism. Initially, this disease may present as hyperthyroidism due to active release of T3 and T4, secondary to follicle destruction. **TgAb (thyroglobin antibody)** is high, and T3 and T4 are normal or low.

Factitious hyperthyroidism: This is typically due to ingestion of thyroid hormone by patients **trying to lose weight** or taking amiodarone therapy or patients who have Münchausen's syndrome.

Ectopic thyroid hormone production: **Struma ovarii** (ovarian teratomas containing thyroid tissue) or hydatidiform moles may produce ectopic thyroid hormone; however, β-hCG would be positive in these patients.

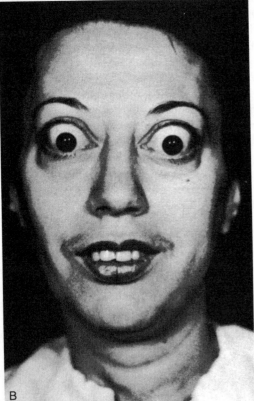

B

CASE 34 *A*, Graves' disease—follicles with hyperplastic, tall columnar cells. *B*, Graves' disease—a patient with hyperthyroidism and exophthalmos.

CASE 35 CC: "It hurts when I pee."

HISTORY: A 21-year-old Hispanic man presents to the university student health service with a 3-day history of **burning on urination** and a **thick yellow discharge from his urethra.** He is sexually active and began having intercourse with his new girlfriend last weekend. He did not use a condom, because they agreed to a monogamous relationship. He denies any fever, suprapubic or flank pain, weight loss, cough, diarrhea, or other constitutional symptoms. He states that he has been in good health and has never had an STD.

PHYSICAL: Vital signs normal. Gen: A well-developed 21-year-old man in no apparent distress. HEENT: oropharynx and conjunctiva are clear of discharge or exudate, vision and hearing are normal. Neck: supple, no nodes or JVD are present. Lungs: CTA. Heart: RRR. Abd: non-tender, (+) bowel sounds, no CVA tenderness or suprapubic pain. Genitourinary: notable for purulent urethral discharge; no masses or nodules are found on rectal exam. Neuro: intact. Skin: normal.

DIFFERENTIAL: Gonococcal urethritis; nongonococcal urethritis (*Chlamydia trachomatis, Ureaplasma urealyticum, Trichomonas vaginalis*); interstitial cystitis.

DIAGNOSTICS: CBC and chem 7 are normal. UA: (+) WBCs with no RBCs or casts. A Gram stain of urethral discharge demonstrates **gram-negative diplococci,** and the sample grows on **Thayer-Martin chocolate agar.** The HIV test is pending. RPR / VDRL tests for syphilis are negative.

DIAGNOSIS: Gonococcal urethritis.

ASSESSMENT/PLAN: A 21-year-old man with gonococcal urethritis. Culture the urethra and oral cavity for chlamydia because patients are often coinfected. Give one dose of 250-mg intramuscular ceftriaxone and 100 mg doxycycline orally for 7 days.

Gonorrhea: The risk for contracting this STD in men is 20% after a single unprotected encounter with an infected female. Symptoms usually develop 2 to 7 days after infection and **coinfection with chlamydia is very common.** *N. gonorrhoeae* virulence factors include **pili** and **IgA protease.** Infected women present with painful cervicitis ("**chandelier sign**"), which may lead to pelvic inflammatory disease (PID) and eventually to infertility. Extragenital infection can manifest as arthritis, polysynovitis, and dermatitis.

Nongonococcal urethritis (NGU): Nonspontaneous mucoid discharge would be present in patients infected with NGU, rather than the purulent discharge as is the case with this patient. Generally, nongonococcal urethritis has a longer incubation period (7 to 14 days) than gonococcus. This patient presented less than 1 week after exposure. The most common organism that causes NGU is chlamydia. In addition, chlamydial infection is the most common STD because it is often untreated.

Cystitis: Suprapubic pain and flank pain would be present with this condition. Pyuria and elevated WBCs in the urine would be indicative of cystitis. Even though this patient had some WBCs in the urine, his other symptoms did not point toward this diagnosis. Furthermore, the diagnosis of cystitis (usually secondary to a urinary tract infection) is uncommon in a male.

CASE 36 CC: "I can't breathe right."

HISTORY: A 76-year-old Asian-American woman hospitalized for 1 week after a left cerebrovascular accident (CVA) is discovered to be **short of breath** and **cyanotic** on morning work rounds. She complains that her right leg is bigger than her left leg. She has been bedridden for the last week, and her heparin therapy (given for her CVA) was briefly discontinued before she received a CT scan with contrast 3 days ago. She denies chills or cough but feels slightly warm.

PHYSICAL: Temp: 100°F; **HR: 130; RR: 30;** BP: 120/70. Gen: The patient is a thin ill-appearing woman in respiratory distress. Lungs: **tachypneic** with shallow breaths, breath sounds diminished B/L, chest pain with inspiration [(+) pleurisy]. Heart: **tachycardia** with a loud S2. Ext: cyanosis present in the hands and feet, 3+ pitting edema in her right leg, no clubbing, right leg tender to palpation. Neuro: she has a total right hemiparesis unchanged since her CVA.

DIFFERENTIAL: Pulmonary embolism; pneumonia; acute respiratory distress syndrome.

DIAGNOSTICS: CBC and chem 7 normal. ABG: pH WNL, PCO_2 decreased, PO_2 WNL. **A-a gradient** (calculated A-a = $[(713 \times FIO_2) - (PaCO_2/0.8)] - PaO_2$) is **elevated.** ECG demonstrates sinus tachycardia and signs of pulmonary embolism. CXR shows **consolidation** in the left lower lobe (LLL), atelectasis, and pleural effusions. Doppler ultrasound demonstrates a **deep vein thrombosis** in the right upper thigh. V/Q scan shows a mismatch in the left lower lobe. Pulmonary angiography is deferred because clinical data are conclusive, although it is the gold standard.

DIAGNOSIS: Pulmonary embolus in the LLL secondary to DVT (see Figure).

ASSESSMENT/PLAN: A 76-year-old Asian-American woman with a pulmonary embolus in her left lower lobe secondary to a DVT. Supportive care includes supplemental O_2 and IV saline to correct volume depletion. Prophylaxis includes an IV bolus of heparin followed by continuous infusion. PTT should be maintained at 1.5 to 2.5 times greater than normal for 5 to 10 days. PT should remain between 2 and 3 times normal. Surgical insertion of an IVC filter may be considered if another embolus occurs.

Pulmonary embolism (PE): This condition is most often secondary to mobilization of a deep vein thrombosis in the lower extremities. Risk factors include **immobility, postoperative stage, hip fracture, hypercoagulable states, birth control pills, pregnancy,** and **visceral cancers.** Hemoptysis and syncope, which are not present in this patient, would indicate a pulmonary infarct as a result of the PE. The CXR is usually normal, and a V/Q scan mismatch is diagnostic. **Pulmonary angiography** is the gold standard diagnostic test but is done only when other results are equivocal, because it is associated with increased morbidity and mortality.

Pneumonia: This patient is at risk for bacterial pneumonia secondary to aspiration or nosocomial infec-

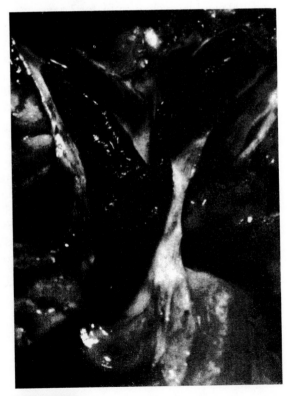

CASE 36 Pulmonary embolism.

tion because she is a hospitalized stroke patient. However, she does not have a cough or purulent sputum, which would be expected. The most common pathogens in hospitalized patients include *S. aureus* and gram-negative agents, including *H. influenzae* and *Klebsiella*.

Acute respiratory distress syndrome (ARDS): Conditions including trauma, aspiration, and sepsis can injure the alveolar-capillary membrane leading to the deposition of neutrophils, blood products, and protein-rich fluid in the alveolar space. Patients with this condition present with severe hypoxemia refractive to oxygen administration and a normal pulmonary artery wedge pressure. The CXR shows **"white out"** in advanced stages.

CASE 37 CC: "I want to kill myself."

HISTORY: A 40-year-old white woman presents to the ED threatening to shoot herself with a gun. She has a history of recurrent major depression. This depressive episode has lasted 8 months and began when her mother died. During the exam the patient **looks only at the floor.** She complains of intense guilt and feeling of **worthlessness.** She has lost touch with her friends and family because she does not want to trouble them with her problems. She has not seen her children in 3 months because she thinks they must hate her. She was fired from her job because she stopped showing up to work. She is currently taking amitriptyline (tricyclic antidepressant), and attending psychotherapy four times a week. She tried to commit suicide 3 years ago but has not had other suicidal ideations until recently. She has been tired lately but feels better as the day progresses. She says that she no longer enjoys her hobbies and hasn't laughed in months. She now eats only one meal a day and has lost 10 lb in 1 month. She has been having difficulty sleeping and has no interest in sex with her boyfriend. She denies any recent pregnancy, headaches, health problems, or substance abuse.

PHYSICAL: VS: normal. Gen: A lethargic 40-year-old white woman looking gaunt and wearing loose-fitting clothes. Neuro (mini-mental status): AAO ×3, immediate memory: intact; recent memory: The patient can recall two of three words that she is asked to remember after 5 minutes. Her distant memory is intact. Her affect is blunted but appropriate. She shows evidence of psychomotor retardation. The physical exam is unremarkable.

DIFFERENTIAL: Major depression; organic mood disorder; substance abuse; pseudodementia; dysthymia; grief; schizophrenia.

DIAGNOSTICS: CBC and chem-7: normal; thyroid function tests: WNL; vitamin B_{12} level: WNL. 24-hour urine analysis: **lower than normal levels of catecholamine metabolites (HVA, MHPG, and 5-HIAA).** A CT scan is unremarkable. The result of a **dexamethasone suppression test is positive.**

DIAGNOSIS: Depression.

ASSESSMENT/PLAN: This is a 40-year-old white woman who presents with signs and symptoms consistent with major depression. Patients with this condition must have five or more of the following nine symptoms over the same 2-week period for this diagnosis to be made. **Depressed mood or anhedonia must be present.**

1. Depressed mood
2. Anhedonia (inability to experience joy)
3. Sleep difficulties (insomnia, early morning awakening)

(continued)

CASE 37   CC: "I want to kill myself." (Continued)

4. Change in appetite or weight
5. Psychomotor agitation or retardation
6. Lack of motivation, fatigability
7. Feelings of worthlessness or guilt
8. Inability to make a decision or concentrate
9. Thoughts of suicide

Major depression: This condition usually lasts from 5 to 12 months and may be intermittent or chronic. If accompanied by episodes of mania, it is considered bipolar disorder. If delusions and hallucinations are present, it is called depression with psychotic features. Monoamine and neuroendocrine disorders are common. In depressed patients, 60% have suicidal ideation, and 15% successfully commit suicide. Women tend to have more suicidal ideation, but men more successfully complete suicide because they tend to use more lethal methods. Of those who commit suicide, **80% seek medical care shortly before they take their life.** Major depression presents differently at different ages. Children have somatic complaints; adolescents express their depression through drug abuse; and depression in the elderly often appears as cognitive deficits. 20% of women and 10% of men can expect a major depressive episode in their lifetime. All races are affected equally, but risk is increased with a **family history of depression or alcohol abuse** and lower socioeconomic status.

Organic mood disorder (OMD): In this disorder depression or mania occurs along with cognitive deficits. It is usually secondary to **drugs (e.g., cocaine and amphetamines), illness,** metabolic abnormalities, brain tumor, steroids, and propranolol.

Pseudodementia: This cognitive impairment is unique to elderly patients with depression. It may be confused with Alzheimer's dementia, but pseudodementia resolves with antidepressant medication.

Dysthymia: This disorder is similar to major depression, but less severe, and is more often associated with losses or stressors. It occurs most commonly in **women** in their **third and fourth decades.** Symptoms tend to be **worse later in the day,** and it is not associated with hallucinations or delusions.

Grief: Grief may present like major depression but usually resolves within 1 year. Normal grief reactions include **shock, denial, anger, and somatic symptoms.** Normal grieving is not associated with suicidal thoughts or hopelessness.

Schizophrenia: This disease can easily be mistaken for depression with psychotic features. Prior health history, family history, and response to medications such as Haldol can be used to differentiate schizophrenia from depression. Schizophrenia typically presents in young adulthood usually before 35 years of age and is more common in people born in the winter.

CASE 38   CC: "My daughter has a rash."

HISTORY: The mother of an inner-city 4 y/o African-American infant states that her daughter has been **itching** for 3 days. The mother first noticed the child scratching her neck, but now she is scratching all over. She also noticed that the child had several areas of rash on her neck, shoulders, and abdomen. The child denies headache, fever, malaise, anorexia, abdominal pain, pain or swelling in her joints, or sore throat. She does not have asthma or allergies and has had all her immunizations including chickenpox. She has not been ill recently and does not take any medication.

PHYSICAL: Vital signs: WNL. Gen: Uncomfortable and irritable 4-year-old girl who is scratching her neck and abdomen. Lungs: CTA. Heart: RRR. Abd: Soft, nontender, nondistended, (+) bowel sounds. Ext: (−) c/c/e, no rashes on lower extremities. Skin: several **well-defined circular areas with raised bor-**

ders and flat, **erythematous centers** located on neck, back, shoulders, and abdomen; some lesions are scabbed over.

DIFFERENTIAL: Dermatophytosis (e.g., tinea, ringworm), scabies, atopic dermatitis (eczema), allergic urticaria, Henoch-Schönlein purpura (HSP), erythema infectiosum (fifth disease), roseola infantum (exanthem subitum)

DIAGNOSTICS: Electrolytes: WNL. CBC: WNL. U/A: WNL. PT/PTT: WNL. Potassium hydroxide (KOH) prep: (+) hyphae. Wood's lamp: (−) fluorescence. Throat culture: no growth.

DIAGNOSIS: Dermatophytosis (e.g., tinea, ringworm)

ASSESSMENT/PLAN: This is a 4-year-old African-American girl with a typical case of a tinea fungal infection. It is caused by fungi such as Microsporum, Trichophyton, or Epidermophyton species. Tinea corporis (ringworm) develops on the trunk, extremities, or face and is characterized by circular lesions with raised borders and flat, erythematous centers. These lesions are **pruritic** and can become scabbed over if they are regularly scratched. Tinea can also develop on the scalp and hair (*Tinea capitis*), the groin and thigh (*Tinea cruris*), and on the foot (*Tinea pedis* or athlete's foot). Diagnosis can be made using a **Wood lamp,** which will cause a *Microsporum* infection to fluoresce. A **KOH prep** of a lesion, viewed under a microscope, will reveal hyphae. A fungal culture can confirm the diagnosis. For minor infections, treatment can be topical with an antifungal such as **ketoconazole.** For infections requiring systemic treatment, the drug of choice is griseofulvin.

Atopic dermatitis (eczema): This disease is characterized by a **chronic and relapsing course.** In infants and children, **erythematous, papulovesicular, and exudative lesions** appear on the face and extensor surfaces. In older children, the lesions tend to be more dry and lichenified and appear on the flexural surfaces. Over 80% of cases show elevated **IgE** levels to a specific environmental antigen. More than 90% of cases begin at 5 years of age and follow a fluctuating course with seasonal variation in severity. Typical patients also have allergies and asthma. Treatment is oral antihistamines to reduce itching, liberal skin lubrication and moisturization, and topical corticosteroids in severe cases.

Allergic urticaria: **Hives (urticaria)** are the characteristic lesion in this disease. Typically, urticaria is a **type I (IgE-mediated) hypersensitivity reaction** to a variety of stimuli including viral infections, bee stings, and foods such as nuts, eggs, dairy, or shellfish. Other causes include immune complex diseases, drugs that release histamine such as morphine, codeine, or curare, complement activation by agents such as radiocontrast dyes and blood transfusions. Prolonged pressure to the skin and exposure to cold can also result in hives. This patient was not on any medication, nor did she have any allergies. In addition, IgE-mediated urticaria does not last for 3 days. It typically becomes evident 5 to 30 minutes after the inciting event and lasts up to 60 minutes.

Scabies: This disease is caused by a 0.4-mm round **mite.** The mite burrows into the skin and causes a very pruritic, erythematous rash. The rash can be focal or generalized and is found especially in the **folds between the fingers and toes.** Scrapings of the burrows with mineral oil and observation under a microscope can reveal the mites, but this test often produces negative results. The diagnosis is usually made by the history and the characteristic rash. Treatment involves the use of permethrin (applied to the body).

Henoch-Schönlein purpura (HSP): The characteristic features of this disease are a **maculopapular rash** that typically occurs over the **lower half of the body,** abdominal pain, one or more painful/swollen joints, and gross or microscopic hematuria. The maculopapular rash is caused by **deposition of immune complexes.** The diagnosis can usually be accomplished by identifying the characteristic rash. However, normal platelet and coagulation studies can differentiate this disease from other hemorrhagic disorders. The disease is self-limited; it lasts for 4 to 6 weeks but may recur.

Erythema infectiosum (fifth disease): This childhood illness is caused by **parvovirus B-19.** It is typically not associated with a prodrome or fever, but arthralgias may be present in adults. It is characterized by

(continued)

CASE 38 CC: "My daughter has a rash." (Continued)

a three-stage process. First, an erythematous rash appears on the cheek, giving the so-called "slapped cheeks" appearance. Second, the rash becomes maculopapular with a reticular pattern and extends to the arms, body, and lower extremities. Finally, the rash will fluctuate in severity usually over 2 to 3 weeks. This stage may persist for months and can include a low-grade fever. Supportive care is the treatment for this disease.

Roseola infantum (exanthem subitum): This disease of young children is caused by **human herpesvirus 6.** It is characterized by a 1- to 5-day fever ranging from 103°F to 106°F and no other systemic symptoms. Following a return to normal body temperature, a **rash** appears on the trunk and then spreads to the periphery. This rash often resolves 1 day after its appearance. A leukocyte count on the first or second day of the illness may reach 20,000/mm^3, but after the second day there is usually leukopenia and neutropenia. Treatment is supportive.

Figure Acknowledgments

Case 1. From Rubin E and Farber JL: *Pathology,* 3rd ed. Philadelphia, Lippincott-Raven, 1999, p 317. Used by permission of Lippincott Williams & Wilkins.

Case 3. From Brant WE and Helms CA: *Fundamentals of Diagnostic Radiology,* 2nd ed. Philadelphia, Lippincott Williams & Wilkins, 1999, p 839.

Case 4. From Brant WE and Helms CA: *Fundamentals of Diagnostic Radiology,* 2nd ed. Philadelphia, Lippincott Williams & Wilkins, 1999, p 446.

Case 7A & B. From Brant WE and Helms CA: *Fundamentals of Diagnostic Radiology,* 2nd ed. Philadelphia, Lippincott Williams & Wilkins, 1999, pp 402, 404.

Case 8A. From Brant WE and Helms CA: *Fundamentals of Diagnostic Radiology,* 2nd ed. Philadelphia, Lippincott Williams & Wilkins, 1999, p 753.

Case 8B. From Rubin E and Farber JL: *Pathology,* 3rd ed. Philadelphia, Lippincott-Raven, 1999, p 745. Used by permission of Lippincott Williams & Wilkins.

Case 15. From Rubin E and Farber JL: *Pathology,* 3rd ed. Philadelphia, Lippincott-Raven, 1999, p 1144. Used by permission of Lippincott Williams & Wilkins.

Case 17. From Rubin E and Farber JL: *Pathology,* 3rd ed. Philadelphia, Lippincott-Raven, 1999, p 1081. Used by permission of Lippincott Williams & Wilkins.

Case 18. From Brant WE and Helms CA: *Fundamentals of Diagnostic Radiology,* 2nd ed. Philadelphia, Lippincott Williams & Wilkins, 1999, p 97.

Case 19. From Brant WE and Helms CA: *Fundamentals of Diagnostic Radiology,* 2nd ed. Philadelphia, Lippincott Williams & Wilkins, 1999, p 1150.

Case 20. From Rubin E and Farber JL: *Pathology,* 3rd ed. Philadelphia, Lippincott-Raven, 1999, p 693. Used by permission of Lippincott Williams & Wilkins.

Case 21. From Rubin E and Farber JL: *Pathology,* 3rd ed. Philadelphia, Lippincott-Raven, 1999, p 559. Used by permission of Lippincott Williams & Wilkins.

Case 23. From Brant WE and Helms CA: *Fundamentals of Diagnostic Radiology,* 2nd ed. Philadelphia, Lippincott Williams & Wilkins, 1999, p 392.

Case 25. From Rubin E & Farber JL: *Pathology,* 3rd ed. Philadelphia, Lippincott-Raven, 1999, p 1370. Used by permission of Lippincott Williams & Wilkins.

Case 26. From Rubin E and Farber JL: *Pathology,* 3rd ed. Philadelphia, Lippincott-Raven, 1999, pp 846–847. Used by permission of Lippincott Williams & Wilkins.

Case 27. From Rubin E and Farber JL: *Pathology,* 3rd ed. Philadelphia, Lippincott-Raven, 1999, pp 846–847. Used by permission of Lippincott Williams & Wilkins.

Case 29. From Damjanov I: *Histopathology, A Color Atlas and Textbook.* Baltimore, Williams & Wilkins, 1996. Fig 14.13A, p 364. Used by permission of Lippincott Williams & Wilkins.

Case 30. Adapted from Mycek MJ, Harvey RA, and Champe PC: *Lippincott's Illustrated Reviews: Pharmacology, 2nd edition.* Philadelphia, Lippincott-Raven Publishers. 1997. p. 415. Used by permission of Lippincott Williams & Wilkins.

Case 31A, B & C. From Rubin E and Farber JL: *Pathology,* 3rd ed. Philadelphia, Lippincott-Raven, 1999, pp 1148–1149. Used by permission of Lippincott Williams & Wilkins.

Case 32A & B. From Rubin E and Farber JL: *Pathology,* 3rd ed. Philadelphia, Lippincott-Raven, 1999, p 1076. Used by permission of Lippincott Williams & Wilkins.

Case 34A. From Rubin E and Farber JL: *Pathology,* 3rd ed. Philadelphia, Lippincott-Raven, 1999, p 1169. Used by permission of Lippincott Williams & Wilkins.

Case 34B. From Cotran RS, Kumar V, Robbins SL, Schoen FJ (eds.): *Robbins Pathologic Basis of Disease, 5th edition.* Philadelphia, W. B. Saunders Company, 1994, p. 1124.

Case 36. From Rubin E and Farber JL: *Pathology,* 3rd ed. Philadelphia, Lippincott-Raven, 1999, p 289. Used by permission of Lippincott Williams & Wilkins.

Glossary

ABG • Arterial blood gas

Accuracy • Degree to which a measurement represents the actual value

Acne vulgaris • Simple acne, usually occurs during puberty

AD • Right ear

Addison's disease • Insufficient production of cortisol by the adrenal gland

AFOF • Anterior fontanelle open and flat

AFP • α-Fetoprotein

AKA • Above-knee amputation

Albuminocytologic dissociation • Increased protein in cerebrospinal fluid without an increased cell count, found in Guillain-Barré syndrome

Allotype • Antigenic differences of immunoglobulins that differ among individuals (e.g., variations in H chains are allotypes)

Amenorrhea • Absence or abnormal cessation of menses

Argyll Robertson pupil • Loss of pupillary light reflex, but accommodation retained; found in syphilis

Arthus reaction • A localized allergic inflammatory reaction

AS • Left ear

Asherman's syndrome • Amenorrhea and infertility secondary to scarring of the uterus (usually caused by excessive curettage)

ASO • Antibody to streptolysin O; streptolysin O made by group A β-hemolytic streptococcus

Auer rods • Rod-shaped structures in myeloblasts, found in acute myelogenous leukemia

BE • Barium enema

Bence Jones protein • Immunoglobulin light chains found in the urine of patients with multiple myeloma

BKA • Below-knee amputation

BPD • Biparietal distance; also bronchopulmonary dysplasia

Brushfield spots • Speckled spots of the iris; found in Down's syndrome

Bullous pemphigoid • Tense skin vesicles with antibodies to the epidermal basement membrane

C & S • Culture and smear

Café au lait spots • Hyperpigmented cutaneous lesions associated with neurofibromatosis type 1 (von Recklinghausen's disease)

Cauda equina syndrome • Sacral pain, pelvic analgesia, and bowel and bladder dysfunction

Chancre • Painless lesion of primary syphilis

Chancroid • Painful genital ulcer caused by *Haemophilus ducreyi*

Chandelier sign • Found in pelvic inflammatory disease; severe pain on pelvic exam causing a woman to "jump up and hit the chandelier"

Charcot triad • (1) Found in multiple sclerosis: nystagmus, tremor, and scanning speech; (2) found in cholangitis: fever, upper abdominal pain, and jaundice

Charcot-Leyden crystals • Found in asthma; elongated double pyramid-shaped crystals

Chem 7 (Screen 7) • Serum electrolyte tests for sodium, potassium, chloride, bicarbonate, blood urea nitrogen, creatinine, and glucose

Chocolate cysts • Ovarian cyst containing an old hematoma often found in endometriosis

Chvostek's sign • Tapping the facial nerve causes a unilateral spasm of the facial muscles; found in hypocalcemic tetany

Clue cells • Cells with a "rough" border and intracellular "dots"; found in bacterial vaginosis

CMT • Cervical motion tenderness

Condyloma lata • Flat-topped papules often in the anal region; found in secondary syphilis

Corrigan's pulse • Also called a "water-hammer pulse"; quickly rising and falling pulse; found in aortic valve regurgitation

Craniotabes • Thinning and softening of the skull; found in syphilis and rickets

CREST • Calcinosis, Reynaud's phenomenon, esophageal disorders, sclerodactyly, telangiectasia

CRI • Chronic renal insufficiency

CTX • Contractions

Cullen's sign • Periumbilical ecchymoses; sign of retroperitoneal hemorrhage

CVAT • Costovertebral tenderness

CXR • Chest x-ray

DKA • Diabetic ketoacidosis

Donovan bodies • Clusters of blue or black-staining chromatin condensations seen in mononuclear cells infected with *Calymmatobacterium granulomatis* (granuloma inguinale)

DVT • Deep vein thrombosis

Dysmenorrhea • Painful menses

Dyspnea • Shortness of breath

ECC • Endocervical curettage

Eclampsia • Preeclampsia (hypertension, proteinuria, and edema) and seizures; occurs during pregnancy

Eczema • Acute or chronic inflammation of the skin described as edematous, papular, vesicular, and crusting; often very itchy

Epitope • Simplest antigenic determinant

Erythema chronicum migrans • A spreading circular red rash with a clear center at the bite site; found in Lyme disease

Erythema marginatum • Distinctive rash, often involving the trunk and extremities; rheumatic fever

Erythema multiforme • Macules, papules, or subdermal vesicles often on the hands and arms; can be an allergic or drug-induced reaction; called Stevens-Johnson syndrome if severe

Ewing's sarcoma • Malignant neoplasm of bone usually found in young men; associated with 11:22 translocation

Exstrophy • A congenital defect resulting in a hollow organ with inside grossly visible, as in exstrophy of the bladder

Ferruginous bodies • Foreign body in the lungs coated with hemosiderin; found in asbestosis/mesothelioma

FEV • Forced expiratory volume

FEV$_1$ • Forced expiratory volume in the first second of expiration

FLP • Fasting lipid panel

Foam cell • Histiocytes that have ingested lipid; found characteristically in hypercholesterolemia

Gardner's syndrome • Autosomal dominant-inherited disease characterized by multiple tumors of the colon, osteomas of the skull, epidermoid cysts, and fibromas that occur before 10 years of age

Genomic imprinting • Differences in the expression of a gene that depend on whether it has been inherited from the mother or the father

Goiter • Enlarged thyroid gland

Gower's maneuver • Using the arms to stand from a prone position, due to muscle weakness in the legs; found in muscular dystrophy

Gravid • Pregnancy

Grey Turner's sign • Flank ecchymosis in a butterfly pattern in the retroperitoneum; found in acute hemorrhage of the pancreas

Hapten • Antigen that must be combined with a carrier protein to induce antibody production

Harrison's groove • Rib deformity; found in rickets

Heinz bodies • Intracellular inclusions of denatured hemoglobin in red blood cells; found in thalassemia, enzyme defects, and hemoglobinopathies, especially glucose-6-phosphate dehydrogenase deficiency

HELLP • Hemolysis, elevated liver enzymes, low platelets; found in pregnancy

Hematochezia • Bloody stool

Hemoptysis • Coughing up blood

Henoch-Schönlein purpura • Purpuric lesions, joint pain and swelling, colic, and bloody stools; usually found in children

Heterophil antibodies • Antibodies found in mononucleosis, caused by Epstein-Barr virus

Hirsutism • Excessive male pattern body and facial hair found in women

Homer-Wright pseudorosettes • Characteristic arrangement of tumor cells often seen in medulloblastomas

Idiotype • Antigenic determinant in their hypervariable regions, unique to a clonal cell line of antibody-producing cells (e.g., IgG antibodies to measles and mumps viruses are idiotypes)

Impetigo • Superficial infection of the skin caused by *Staphylococcus* or *Streptococcus*; begins as a vesicle that ruptures and becomes yellow and crusty; often occurs on the face

Involucrum • Sheath of new bone that forms around necrotic bone (sequestrum)

Isotype • Antigenic differences of immunoglobulins in their constant regions, but they are found in all members of a given species (e.g., IgM and IgG are isotypes)

IVDU • Intravenous drug use

Jarisch-Herxheimer reaction • Inflammatory reaction induced by antibiotic treatment of syphilis

JVD • Jugular venous distention

Kartagener's syndrome • Situs inversus, bronchiectasis, chronic sinusitis, impaired cilia; causes reduced fertility in women and sterility in men; autosomal recessive disease of the dynein arms

Kawasaki's disease • Fever, conjunctivitis, pharyngitis, cervical lymphadenopathy, acute necrotizing vasculitis; can lead to coronary artery aneurysms; found in children especially younger than 2 years of age

Kayser-Fleischer rings • Green pigment encircling the cornea; found in Wilson's disease

Keratin pearls • Characteristic microscopic findings in squamous cell carcinoma

Kimmelsteil-Wilson nodules • Characteristic glomerular nodules found in diabetic nephropathy

Koilocytes • Cells with a clear perinuclear halo, characteristic of hepatitis B virus infection

Koplik spots • Red lesions with a blue-white center on the buccal mucosa; characteristic of early measles

Kussmaul breathing • Deep, rapid breathing with an increase in both tidal volume and respiratory rate; often seen in diabetic ketoacidosis or other types of acidosis

Kussmaul's sign • Increase in jugulovenous pressure with inspiration; cardiac tamponade

Lhermitte's sign • Flexing of the head causes electric-like shocks to be felt down the spine

Libman-Sacks endocarditis • Aseptic endocarditis with warty lesions of the cardiac valves, found in systemic lupus erythematosus

Lichen planus • Flat, shiny papules on buccal mucosa, male genitalia, and flexor surfaces; unknown cause

Lichen sclerosis • White atrophic patches (leukoplakia) of vulva

LLQ • Left lower quadrant

Lou Gehrig's syndrome • Also called amyotrophic lateral sclerosis; disease of the motor tracts of the lateral columns of the spinal cord that causes muscular atrophy

LUQ • Left upper quadrant

Macrosomia • Abnormally large body size

Malar • Cheek or cheek bones

Mallory-Weiss syndrome • Tear of the lower esophagus associated with bloody vomitus, usually found in alcoholics

McBurney's point • Located two thirds of the way down on a line connecting the umbilicus with the anterior superior iliac spine; a point of pain in appendicitis

Meigs' syndrome • Ovarian fibroma, ascites, and hydrothorax

Menorrhagia • Profuse bleeding during menses

Menorrhalgia • Painful menses

Metrorrhagia • Irregular bleeding from the uterus between menstrual cycles

MMPI • Minnesota Multiphasic Personality Test

Molluscum contagiosum • Disease of the skin caused by a virus characterized by pearl-colored papular lesions

MRSA • Methicillin-resistant *Staphylococcus aureus*

Mycosis fungoides • Progressive lymphoma and inflammatory process of the skin

Myotome • Mesoderm that gives rise to skeletal muscle; innervated by a common nerve

NEC • Necrotizing enterocolitis

Negri bodies • Inclusion bodies found in nerve cells in rabies; eosinophilic and sharply demarcated

Neurofibrillary tangles • Found in Alzheimer's disease

NIFS • Noninvasive flow study

NPO • Latin for "nothing by mouth"

NSS • Normal saline solution

Obturator sign • Right lower quadrant pain on external rotation of the hip; usually associated with appendicitis

OCP • Oral contraceptive pills

OOBTC • Out of bed to a chair

Opsonization • Process by which bacteria are made easier to phagocytize

Orthopnea • Shortness of breath on lying down

Pancoast's tumor • Tumor of the apex of the lung resulting in Horner's syndrome and brachial plexus compression

Pannus • Grayish membrane that covers the upper portion of the cornea; found in trachoma

Parity • Having given birth to a child

Pemphigus vulgaris • Serious illness marked by flaccid vesicles over the entire body

PFOF • Posterior fontanelle open and flat

PFT • Pulmonary function tests

PICC • Peripherally inserted central catheter

Pleurisy • Inflammation of lung pleura

Plummer-Vinson syndrome • Dysphagia with esophageal webs and hypochromic microcytic anemia

PND • Paroxysmal nocturnal dyspnea; often a symptom of heart failure

PO • Latin for "by mouth"

Polymenorrhea • Increased frequency of menstrual cycles

Pott's disease • Tuberculosis of the spine

Precision • Degree to which a measurement is reproducible, but not necessarily correct (e.g., a thermometer that always shows a temperature that is 5 degrees higher than the actual temperature is precise but not accurate)

Psammoma bodies • Microscopic hyalinized concretions surrounded by cells; found in ovarian serous papillary cystadenocarcinoma, thyroid papillary adenocarcinoma, meningioma, and mesothelioma

Pseudocyesis • False pregnancy

Psoas sign • Right lower quadrant pain on hip flexion; often associated with appendicitis

Psoriasis • Reddish maculopapules with silvery scaling; occurs on the flexor surfaces, scalp, and trunk

PVD • Peripheral vascular disease

Rachitic rosary • Junction of the ribs with cartilage looks like beads on a string; found in children with rickets

Raynaud's phenomenon • Spasm of arteries of the hand causing blanching, numbness, and pain in the fingers; found in CREST syndrome

Reed-Sternberg cells • Binucleate cells, "owl eyes"; found in Hodgkin's lymphoma

Reinke crystals • Rod-shaped crystals with pointed or rounded ends present in Leydig cell tumors

Reye's syndrome • Loss of consciousness, cerebral edema, and fatty change in the liver; often fatal; associated with aspirin ingestion in children with influenza

RLQ • Right lower quadrant

Romaña's sign • Painless edema of the tissue surrounding the orbit; occurs from the bite of the Reduvid bug, which transmits Chagas' disease

Rorschach test • Inkblot test; a psychological test used as a subjective personality assessment

Rouleaux formation • Red blood cells stacked like poker chips; found in multiple myeloma

Rovsing's sign • Pain is felt in the lower right quadrant upon palpation of the lower left quadrant; often seen in appendicitis

RUQ • Right upper quadrant

RV • Residual volume

S/P • Status post

Sensitivity • Number of people who test positive for a disease divided by the total number of people who actually have the disease

Sequestrum • Necrotic tissue, often bone, which has separated from the surrounding tissue

Serum sickness • Immune complex disease appears days after an injection of foreign serum; characterized by urticaria, fever, lymphadenopathy, edema, and joint pain

Sézary syndrome • Variant of *Mycosis fungoides*; characterized by pruritus and exfoliative dermatitis

Sheehan's syndrome • Pituitary necrosis and resultant hypopituitarism following parturition

Simmond's disease • Anterior pituitary insufficiency, often following parturition, characterized by

hypotension, asthenia, loss of weight and hair, and endocrine dysfunction

Sipple's syndrome • Multiple endocrine neoplasia (MEN) type 2: pheochromocytoma, medullary thyroid carcinoma, and neural tumors

SLE • Systemic lupus erythematosus

Smith antigen • Highly characteristic antigen found in systemic lupus erythematosus

SOB • Shortness of breath

Somite • Paired embryonic cell masses originating from mesoderm; differentiate into cartilage, bone, muscle, and dermis of the skin

Specificity • Number of people who test negative for a disease divided by the total number of people who do not have the disease

Standard deviation • Measure of variation from the central tendency

Standard error • The amount that the mean of a population sample deviates from the true mean of a population

Stein-Leventhal syndrome • Polycystic ovary syndrome

String sign • Narrowed region of small bowel as seen on an abdominal x-ray with contrast

Subcutaneous nodules • Small painless swellings over bony prominences; found in rheumatic fever

Sydenham's chorea • Dance-like movements of the extremities appearing weeks to months after rheumatic fever

Tabes dorsalis • Neurosyphilis; posterior roots of the spinal cord are usually infected, resulting in ataxia, impotence, hypotonic bladder, Romberg's sign, Argyll Robinson pupils, and Charcot joints

Target cells • Erythrocyte with a dark center and a surrounding clearing encircled by a dark border (looks like a target); most commonly found in thalassemias and sickle cell disease

Tinkles • High-pitched bowel sounds; often heard in obstruction of the bowels

Tophi • Uric acid deposition in fibrous tissues such as cartilage; found in gout

TORCHES • Toxoplasmosis, *o*ther infections, *r*ubella, *c*ytomegalovirus, *h*erpes, *s*yphilis; cause birth defects if the mother is infected during pregnancy

Trousseau's sign • Carpal pedal spasm, evident when the upper arm is compressed as with a blood pressure cuff; found in hypocalcemic tetany

Turcot's syndrome • Rare disease characterized by multiple intestinal polyps and brain tumors

U/A • Urinalysis

UGI • Upper gastrointestinal

Urticaria • Hives

Vaginismus • Vaginal contraction caused by attempted penile penetration

VC • Vital capacity

Virchow's node • Enlarged, palpable, supraclavicular lymph node, usually on the left; highly suggestive of a thoracic or abdominal malignancy

von Hippel-Lindau disease • Autosomal dominant disease consisting primarily of hemangiomas of the central nervous system and hamartomas of the internal organs

VRE • Vancomycin-resistant enterococcus

Water-hammer pulse • See Corrigan's pulse

Waterhouse-Friderichsen syndrome • Infection, usually meningeal; found mainly in children younger than 10 years of age; characterized by purpura, diarrhea, vomiting, cyanosis, convulsions, circulatory collapse, and hemorrhage into the adrenal glands

WD/WN • Well developed/ well nourished

Wegener's granulomatosis • Disease of necrotizing granulomas of the lungs and glomerulonephritis; the underlying cause of disease is due to a vasculitis

Wermer's syndrome • Multiple endocrine neoplasia (MEN) type 1; characterized by tumors of the parathyroid, pancreatic islets, and pituitary or other endocrine organ

Wernicke's aphasia • Inability to comprehend the spoken word, even though normal hearing is intact

Whipple's disease • A disease characterized by steatorrhea, lymphadenopathy, arthritis, fever, and cough; foamy macrophages are found in the jejunum

Winterbottom's sign • Lymphadenopathy of the posterior cervical chain found in African trypanosomiasis (African sleeping sickness)

Wire-loop glomeruli • Thickened basement membrane of glomeruli; characteristic lesion found in patients with systemic lupus erythematosus

WNL • Within normal limits

y/o • Years old

Zollinger-Ellison syndrome • Gastric hypersecretion and a tumor of the non-insulin-producing cells of the pancreatic islets

Index

Page numbers in *italics* designate figures; page numbers followed by "t" designate tables; (*see also*) cross-references designate related topics or more detailed topic breakdowns.